LIFE UNIVERSITY
1269 BARCLAY CIRCLE
MARIETTA, GA 30060
(770) 426-2688

LIFE UNIVERSITY
1269 BARCLAY CIRCLE
MARIETTA, GA 30060
(770) 426-2688

Springer

Tokyo
Berlin
Heidelberg
New York
Barcelona
Hong Kong
London
Milan
Paris
Singapore

H.E. Takahashi (Ed.)

Mechanical Loading of Bones and Joints

With 154 Figures Including 7 in Color

LIFE UNIVERSITY
1269 BARCLAY CIRCLE
MARIETTA, GA 30060
(770) 426-2688

WITHDRAWN
LIFE UNIVERSITY LIBRARY

RC
931
.O73
M43
1999

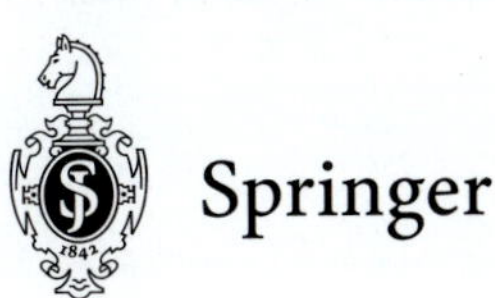 Springer

Hideaki E. Takahashi, M.D., Ph.D.
Professor and Chair, Department of Orthopedic Surgery
Niigata University School of Medicine
1-757 Asahimachi-dori, Niigata, 951-8510, Japan

ISBN 4-431-70242-3 Springer-Verlag Tokyo Berlin Heidelberg New York

Library of Congress Cataloging-in-Publication Data

Mechanical loading of bones and joints / H.E. Takahashi (ed.).
    p. cm.
    Includes bibliographical references and index.
    ISBN 4-431-70242-3 (hard cover : alk. paper)
    1. Osteoporosis—Pathophysiology Congresses. 2. Bones—Mechanical
properties Congresses. 3. Joints—Mechanical properties Congresses.
I. Takahashi, Hideaki, 1933– .
    [DNLM: 1. Osteoporosis—physiopathology Congresses. 2. Stress,
Mechanical Congresses. 3. Bone Density—physiology Congresses.
4. Joint Instability—physiopathology Congresses. 5. Spinal Cord—
physiology Congresses. 6. Cauda Equina—physiology Congresses.
WE 250 M486 1999]
RC931.O73M43   1999
616.7′16—DC21
DNLM/DLC
for Library of Congress   99-19475

Printed on acid-free paper

© Springer-Verlag Tokyo 1999
Printed in Japan
This work is subject to copyright. All rights are reserved, whether the whole or part of the material is concerned, specifically the rights of translation, reprinting, reuse of illustrations, recitation, broadcasting, reproduction on microfilms or in other ways, and storage in data banks.
The use of registered names, trademarks, etc. in this publication does not imply, even in the absence of a specific statement, that such names are exempt from the relevant protective laws and regulations and therefore free for general use.
Product liability: The publisher can give no guarantee for information about drug dosage and application thereof contained in this book. In every individual case the respective user must check its accuracy by consulting other pharmaceutical literature.

Typesetting: Best-set Typesetter Ltd., Hong Kong
Printing and binding: Obun, Japan
SPIN: 10688818

Preface

Bones and joints of both the appendicular and axial skeleton are always under mechanical loading, a key concept for understanding bone metabolism. Each bone of the skeleton has its peculiar shape because of functional adaptation. Osteoporosis and osteoarthritis are the most important and common diseases of bones and joints in the elderly. Because of the unique shape of the spine, dynamic changes in mechanical loading to the spinal column give rise to local problems of content and container—that is, the spinal cord, cauda equina, and vertebrae—resulting in stenosis of the spinal column at the cervical, thoracic, and lumbar levels. Inflammation such as chronic rheumatoid arthritis also results in joint destruction, accelerated by mechanical loading.

This volume contains basic and clinical information about bones and joints, including the spinal column, related to mechanical loading at the tissue, cellular, and molecular levels. The clinical relevance of mechanical loading on bones and joints is provided for clinicians, basic scientists, and engineers. Most of the papers were presented at the 12th annual meeting of the Orthopaedic Research Meeting of the Japanese Orthopaedic Association (Japanese Orthopaedic Research Society) held October 17–18, 1997, in Niigata, Japan. This volume includes the symposia, the instructional course lectures, and other events in this annual meeting. The symposia were titled "Mechanical Loading and Its Regulation on Bone," moderated by Drs. Toshiaki Hara and Toshitaka Nakamura; "Joint Destruction and Its Regulation in Rheumatoid Arthritis," moderated by Drs. Toru Abo and Takahiro Ochi; "Response of the Spinal Cord and Cauda Equina to Dynamic Stress," moderated by Drs. Tetsuya Tamaki and Megumu Yoshimura; and "Advances in Basic Research to Analyze the Pathophysiology of Osteoporosis, Focused on Bone-Forming Cells," moderated by Drs. Hiromichi Norimatsu and Akira Yamaguchi. The special lectures were "From Wolff's Law to the Mechanostat: A New 'Face' of Physiology," by Dr. Harold M. Frost, and "Mechanotransduction and Fuctional Response of the Skeleton to Physical Loads," by Dr. Charles H. Turner.

I am particularly grateful to the staff members of the Department of Orthopedic Surgery and to the alumni of the Orthopedic Department of the Niigata University School of Medicine, especially the former president Dr. Mizuo Nyui and the current president Dr. Naoshi Hayashi. I also thank Ms. Yukino Ikegami and Ms. Tomoko Yuasa, who provided excellent secretarial work and support. Finally, I would like to thank the staff of Springer-Verlag Tokyo for their patience and continuous efforts in the publication of this book.

HIDEAKI E. TAKAHASHI
Editor

Contents

Part 2 Mechanical Loading and Its Regulation in Bone

Part 3 Joint Destruction and Its Regulation in Rheumatoid Arthritis

Part 4 Response of Spinal Cord and Cauda Equina to Dynamic Stress

Part 5 Human Iliac CFU-F Properties and Potential Uses

Contributors

Color Plates

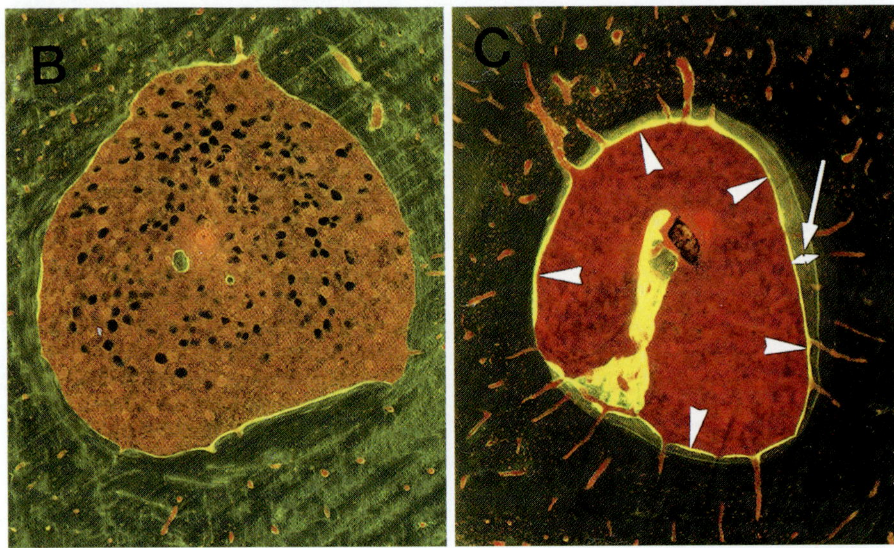

F_IG. 2B,C. Fluorescent micrographs of representative endocortical regions of the cross sections of tibial shafts. **B** OVX control animals with vehicle treatment (Group 4). **C** OVX rats with PTH treatment (Group 5). A well-mineralized layer of subendocortical bone (*arrowheads*) can be observed in the PTH-treated tibiae. Virtually 100% of the endocortical surface was labeled with calcein and tetracycline in the PTH-treated OVX rats. In PTH-treated rats, almost visible is the formation draft in the endocortical surface (*arrowheads*). The new endocortical bone (*arrow*) appeared to be well-mineralized bone which is lining the cortex ×40. (*See* page 64)

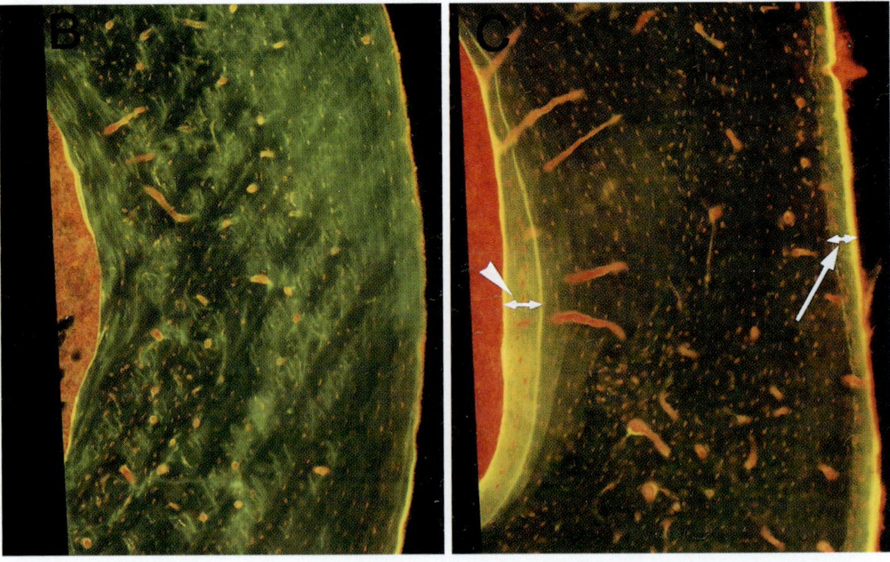

No flow (f-actin/c-fos)   Flow 1 h (f-actin/c-fos)

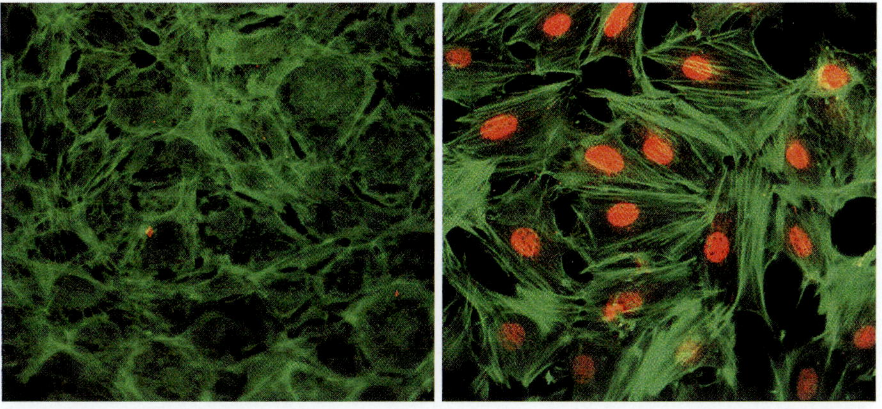

FIG. 7. MC3T3-E1 osteoblasts subjected to fluid shear (12 dynes/cm^2) for 60 min undergo dramatic reorganization of the actin cytoskeleton and express the early response gene c-fos. *Left panel*: Control cells not subjected to flow have poorly organized stress fibers labeled with Texas red-phalloidin (*green*), and expression of c-fos is not present. *Right panel*: Cells subjected to fluid flow for 60 min develop prominent stress fibers labeled with Texas red-phalloidin and demonstrate clear nuclear staining of c-fos protein (*red*). Copyright 1998 by Neil X. Chen, used with permission. (*See* page 88)

FIG. 3B,C. Fluorescent micrographs of periosteal and endocortical surfaces in the tibial shafts: **B**, Group 4; **C**, Group 5. The newly added subperiosteal (*arrow*) and subendocortical bone (*arrowhead*) were added circumferentially, and the new bone was well-mineralized layer bone and thickened the cortex. The faint yellow tetracycline label administered before the initiation of therapy helped to identify the newly formed bone and the previous location of the subendocortical and subperiosteal surfaces (**C**). ×60. (*See* page 64)

Part 1
Osteoporosis
Basic and Clinical Research

The Biomechanical "Face" of Osteoporosis: Emerging Views with Insights from the Utah Paradigm

Harold M. Frost

Summary. Bone strains help to control the adaptations of a bone's strength and "mass" to its mechanical loads, and muscles cause the largest strains. Chiefly bone modeling and remodeling provide those adaptations. Normally that arrangement keeps voluntary muscle forces from breaking bones or causing bone pain. Declining muscle strength with aging or in disease makes normal bone-adaptive mechanisms cause an osteopenia in which spontaneous fractures and/or bone pain do not occur. But, adaptive mechanism disorders can reduce bone strength and "mass" so much that spontaneous fractures and/or bone pain do occur. Such biomechanical grounds could define at least four kinds of "osteoporosis" or osteopenias that were long known under other names. They reveal the need for some new directions in osteoporosis research, diagnosis and treatment, and for skeletal research in general, and the text discusses some of them.

Key words. Osteoporosis, Biomechanics, Research, Absorptiometry

Introduction

In the 1990s we began to recognize some general rules that govern the adaptations of all skeletal tissues and organs to their mechanical loads. This chapter suggests how those insights could apply to "osteoporosis". Most past efforts to understand it depended on a 1960 paradigm of bone physiology [1] that could not account for things that were understood later. The Utah paradigm that supplemented it [2,3] injects new ideas about the nature of osteoporoses, how to manage these ideas, and what needs more research.

Since loss of bone strength is the main problem in osteoporosis, this text will review its determinants as they are currently understood, describe four osteopenias that depend on those determinants, and suggest some implications of that physiology.

Department of Orthopaedic Surgery, Southern Colorado Clinic, 41 Montebello, Pueblo, CO 81001, USA

Determinants of Bone Strength

Physical Determinants of Bone Strength

A bone's strength depends on four things [4]:

1. The strength of bone as a material
2. The amount of bone in its cross section (the mass contribution to its strength)
3. Its cross-sectional size and shape, and its length (the architectural contribution)
4. The amount of microdamage (microscopic fatigue damage).

Normally bone strength and mass (the amount of bone) increase during growth, plateau in young adults, and then decline slowly until death [5].

Microdamage makes a bone weaker without affecting its architecture or mass. Some microdamage occurs in all of us. Repeated strains cause it, and the remodeling described below usually repairs it [2,6]. Normally bone can repair any microdamage caused by strains below a particular size, but larger strains can incite too much to repair and cause fatigue fractures of trabeculae or whole bones [7,8]. This "microdamage threshold" strain range centers near 3000 microstrain (bone's ultimate strength $\approx$ 25 000 microstrain [9]).

Biologic Determinants of Bone Strength and Mass [10–12]

Modeling by formation drifts and resorption drifts can move bone surfaces in tissue space to increase bone strength and mass (Fig. 1). Where longitudinal bone strains exceed a "modeling threshold" range centered near 1000 microstrain in young adults, this modeling is turned on to strengthen the bone and lower its strains toward the bottom of that threshold [2,13]. Where strains stay below that threshold, mechanically controlled modeling stays *off* or inactive. By making bones strong enough to keep strains below the microdamage threshold, modeling minimizes fatigue fractures [11]. Failure to do that can cause those fractures. The bone made by formation drifts lies on smooth or "arrest" cement lines [10].

Remodeling by Multicellular Mechanisms Called Basic Multicellular Units (BMUs). This remodeling can turn bone over in small packets (Fig. 2) [10,11]. Where longitudinal strains stay below a remodeling threshold range, disuse-mode remodeling removes bone next to marrow, and only there, by causing completed BMUs to make less bone than they resorb. Where strains exceed this threshold, conservation-mode remodeling can conserve bone strength and mass, by making completed BMUs equalize their formation and resorption. BMUs also repair microdamage to keep it from accumulating [6–8]. Impaired repair can cause fatigue fractures ("spontaneous" fractures, which are not really spontaneous). The bone made by BMUs lies on scalloped or reversal cement lines [10].

On the Role of Muscle. The above arrangements adapt a bone's strength to its largest strains (and loads), which come from muscles, not body weight [9]. To move us around, muscles must overcome the resistances of body weight multiplied by the bad lever arms most muscles work against. For such reasons it takes more than 2 kg of muscle force on bones to move each kilogram of body weight around, and muscle strength strongly affects bone strength and *mass* [2,16,17]. Usually muscle strength

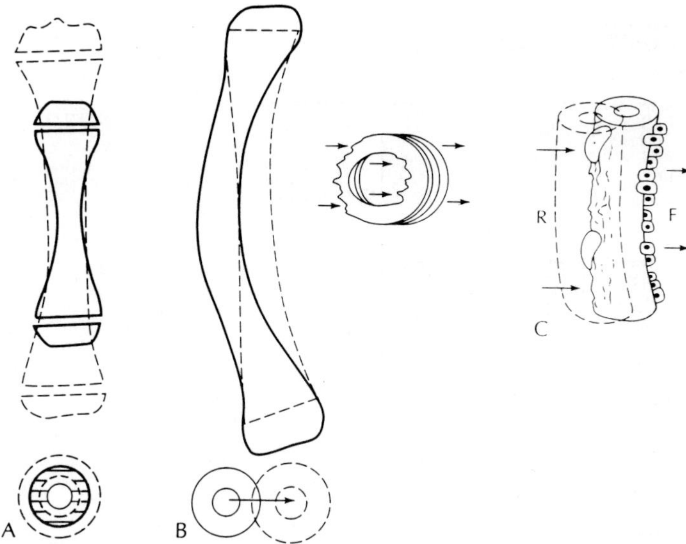

FIG. 1. Bone modeling by drifts. *A* An infant's long bone with its original size and shape in *solid line*. To keep this shape as it grows in length and diameter, its surfaces move in tissue space as the *dashed lines* suggest. Formation drifts make and control new osteoblasts to build up some surfaces. Separate resorption drifts make and control new osteoclasts to remove material from other surfaces. *B* A different drift pattern can correct the fracture malunion in a child, shown in *solid line*. The cross-sectional view on the *right* shows the cortical-endosteal as well as the periosteal drifts that do that. *C* Schematic drawing of how the drifts in *B* would move the whole segment to the right. Drifts can also thicken and strengthen trabeculae. They are created when and where needed. They include capillaries, precursor and supporting cells and some wandering cells. They are multicellular entities in the same sense as renal nephrons. Modified from [12]

increases during growth, it plateaus in young adults, and then it declines slowly until death [14,15].

The Mechanostat. This putative mechanism helps to control the effects of modeling and remodeling on bone strength and mass [18]. It would include modeling, remodeling, and their thresholds, plus still unidentified cells and mechanisms. One could view it as the *master control* of bone strength and *mass*, and modeling and remodeling as its *hands*. Normally it makes bones strong enough to keep their largest voluntary loads from breaking them or causing pain, and for life. Similar mechanisms do the same for joints, tendons, and ligaments [2,12].

In Summary. (a) Bone adapts to hypervigorous mechanical usage by making modeling increase bone strength and *mass* and making remodeling keep both. (b) Bone adapts to disuse by turning modeling off and making disuse-mode remodeling remove bone next to marrow to cause an osteopenia. (c) Modeling can increase but does not decrease bone strength and mass, while remodeling can conserve or reduce them but does not increase them. (d) Normal mechanical usage of osteopenic bones increases their strains and microdamage, which increases the fragility due to the osteopenia alone. (e) Strains can "inform" a bone's biologic mechanisms about the fit of its strength for its mechanical usage. Where strains exceed the modeling threshold,

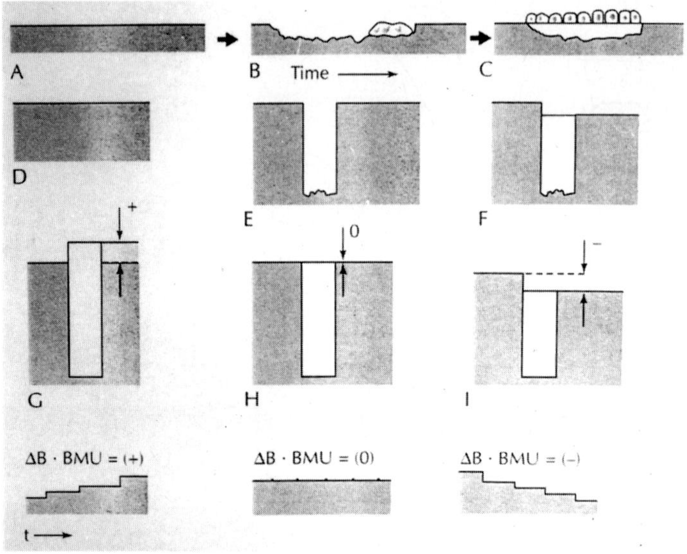

FIG. 2. Bone remodeling basic multicellular units (BMUs). *Top row*: An activation event on a bone surface at **A** causes a packet of bone resorption at **B**, and then replacement of that bone by osteoblasts at **C**. The BMU makes and controls the new osteoclasts and osteoblasts that do this. *Second row*: This emphasizes the amounts of bone resorbed **E** and formed **F** by completed BMUs. *Third row*: In these "BMU graphs" (after Frost [2]), **G** on the left shows a small excess of formation over resorption. **H** shows "conservation mode" remodeling where resorption and formation are nearly equal, as on haversian surfaces. **I** on the right shows "disuse mode" remodeling, where less formation than resorption occurs, as on endocortical and trabecular surfaces. *Bottom row*: These "stair graphs" (after PJ Meunier [2]) show the effects on the local bone "mass" of the BMUs immediately above. BMUs are created when and where they are needed. They include a capillary, precursor and "supporting" cells and some wandering cells. They are multicellular entities in the same sense as renal nephrons. Modified from [12]

more strength is needed and modeling adds it. Where strains stay below the remodeling threshold, bone is not needed and disuse-mode remodeling removes it.

Four Kinds of Osteoporosis

The following definitions depend on the biomechanical causes of osteopenias (less bone than normal) [19,20], not on the accompanying medical problems [5] or the osteopenia's severity [21]. These conditions were known for decades under other names [5].

Physiologic Osteopenia

Chronically weak muscles and/or chronic physical inactivity usually cause corresponding losses of bone strength and *mass* in which voluntary activities do not cause spontaneous fractures and/or bone pain. Most aging adults develop this osteopenia, and so do people with chronic debilitating problems like those in Table 1. Fractures

TABLE 1. Some conditions that cause muscle weakness and disuse in humans (and related osteopenias[a])

Asthma	Emphysema	Pulmonary fibrosis
Renal failure	Hepatic failure	Cardiac failure
Malnutrition	Anemia	Polyarthritis
Metastatic cancer	Depression	Stroke
Muscular dystrophy	Multiple sclerosis	Alzheimer's disease
Organic brain syndrome	Huntington's chorea	Myelomeningocele
Lou Gehrig disease	Paralyses	Leukemia
Cystic fibrosis	Still's disease	Alcoholism
Drug addiction	Nursing home residence	Myasthenia gravis

[a] In causing an osteopenia, the relative importance of the mechanical disuse, muscle weakness, and the biochemical-endocrinologic abnormalities accompanying some of these entries is uncertain, since past studies of the matter did not really evaluate the mechanical usage effects and tended to assume that the nonmechanical factors were dominant. In the new paradigm's view, the mechanical usage and muscle strength effects would dominate most (not all) biochemical-endocrinologic ones (modified from [2]).

occur only from injuries and usually affect extremity bones. These common osteopenias can affect men, women, and children. An intrinsic bone disorder does not cause them.

True Osteoporosis

Disordered modeling and/or remodeling can reduce bone strength and *mass* so much that voluntary activities *do* cause spontaneous fractures and/or bone pain. Those less common conditions affect the spine and women more than extremity bones and men. Of course, falls can fracture extremity bones too. An intrinsic bone disorder must cause this affection. Presumably it involves the mechanostat and increased microdamage.

Combined States

In some people, features of those two conditions can combine in different ways (Frost, personal observations).

Transient Osteopenias

As a severe injury like a burn, fracture, or spinal fusion heals, a regional loss of bone usually occurs. After the injury heals and normal physical activities resume, most of the lost bone returns without treatment intended to achieve it [20]. Presumably the attendant disuse and a regional acceleratory phenomenon [2] combine to cause this temporary osteopenia. It probably should not be viewed as a disease.

Quo Vadis?

The above physiology has many implications for osteoporosis research as well as for skeletal research in general, and some of them are mentioned below. But first another matter deserves comment.

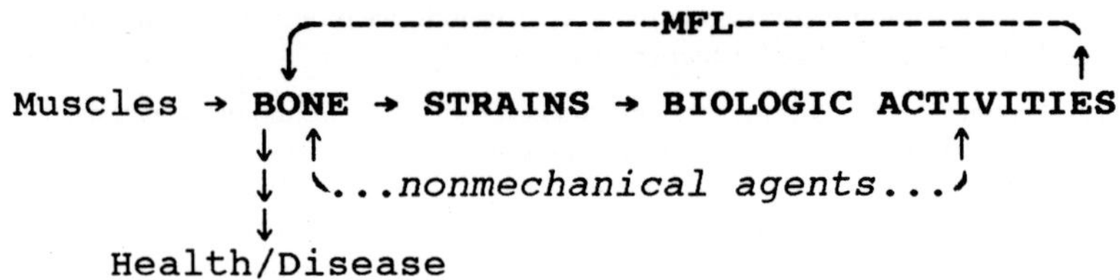

FIG. 3. Biomechanical interactions. Biologic activities include modeling and remodeling. Nonmechanical factors include systemic and local ones. Mechanically dedicated message traffic (and the bone's mechanostat) is shown in *bold-face capital letters*. *MFL*, mechanical feedback loop. Modified from [18]

Who "Drives" the Bone "Car"?

Most texts about the pathogenesis of osteoporosis emphasize nonmechanical causes [5], but this chapter does not. A reader might well ask "Why?" To explain, in the 1960 paradigm [1], effector cells mainly determine bone health and disease, so the causes and management of bone disorders will depend on those cells or their regulation by nonmechanical factors (hormones, vitamins, calcium, age, sex, race, cytokines, diet, genes, etc.). In that view, the effector cells known as osteoblasts and osteoclasts will "drive" the bone "car". Or: *stimulus → osteoblasts/osteoclasts → bone health/disease*.

That paradigm omitted things found after 1960 and reviewed earlier, in this chapter. In the newer paradigm the biologic mechanisms that establish bone health and disease need nonmechanical factors in order to work, as cars need wheels, motors, and fuel in order to move. But in a negative feedback arrangement, mechanical factors guide those mechanisms in time and anatomical space, as steering, brakes, and accelerators guide cars in time and space. Nonmechanical factors can help or hinder that guidance but cannot replace it; otherwise they could normalize bone strength and mass in paralyzed limbs.

Viewed in that context, the voluminous studies of osteoblasts and osteoclasts [22] focused on this "car's" wheels (sometimes under the illusion that they studied its "driver"?). Yet the real "driver" that can cause osteopenias and osteoporoses comprises modeling and remodeling working under the control of the mechanostat [2,23]. Figure 3 suggests some of the involved interactions.

In answer to the question "Why?" posed earlier, scientists and granting agencies need to know why systemic and local nonmechanical effects on modeling and remodeling responses to mechanical usage deserve systematic study. This chapter presents some reasons, Parenthetically, in the new paradigm, similar general ideas would apply to joints, tendons, ligament, and fascia [2,12].

Implications for Therapy

Because modeling could cure an osteopenia and conservation-mode remodeling could prevent one [20], research should seek agents that have such effects. (a) Intermittent parathyroid hormone administration and some prostaglandins can make modeling add impressive amounts of new bone [24,25]. But as the mechanostat hypothesis predicted, after those treatments stop, disuse-mode remodeling removes the added bone. (b) Estrogen and many bisphosphonates can depress remodeling, which depresses bone losses too. While often called "antiresorption agents," estrogen and bisphosphonates are antiremodeling agents that eventually depress both bone formation and resorption, and usually equally. (c) Using anabolic agents to add bone, and antiremodeling agents to keep it, Jee's Activate-Restore-Maintain (ARM) idea [26] had enough success in animal experiments to justify pursuing it.

Implications for Cell and Molecular Biologic Research

The cell and molecular biology that modeling, remodeling, and microdamage physiology depend on need but still lack systematic study. So does the mechanostat. Learning how to control the mechanostat poses an important problem for both osteoporosis research and general skeletal research. AM Parfitt emphasized that idea at the 1997 Hard Tissue Workshop [3].

The above material means that studies of osteoblasts and osteoclasts would mainly concern the skeletal "car's" wheels. At present at least, studying its "driver" should require studying the responses of modeling and remodeling to mechanical and non-mechanical factors in intact subjects. Those may be strong statements but others now agree with them (DB Burr, WSS Jee, AM Parfitt, G Rodan).

Implications for Genetic Effects on Bone Strength and Mass, and on Osteoporosis

This is a complex matter, but in brief: (a) Genetic effects might affect muscle strength, neuromotor functions, longitudinal bone growth, or the properties of bone as a material. (b) Genetic effects could change the thresholds for modeling, remodeling, or microdamage. (c) Genetic effects could affect the responsiveness of modeling and remodeling to systemic and local nonmechanical influences, or to mechanical ones. The latter responses could apply to bone strains or microdamage. (d) Genetic effects could alter the signals and signalling mechanisms that help to govern bone's biologic responses to its mechanical usage.

Each of those changes could affect bone strength, mass, and architecture in ways the Utah paradigm can predict [2,12], and which in some cases the natural experiments of disease verify (examples include, in part, muscular dystrophy, osteogenesis imperfecta, osteopetrosis, achondroplasia, progeria, pseudohypoparathyroidism, familial vitamin D resistant rickets, and Marfan's syndrome). This suggests that searches for the one gene that prevents or causes osteoporosis could be pursuing an illusion. Many genes should be considered in research of the matter.

Implications for Biomechanical Studies

Because of their effects on bone strength and mass, the strain thresholds for modeling, remodeling, and microdamage need more study [9,13]. The responses of modeling and remodeling to strains, like the signalling mechanisms that control them, need more study too, in humans as well as in laboratory animals.

While this chapter describes longitudinal strains as controlling modeling and remodeling, shear and strain gradients, rates, and frequencies might help in that control, and so could other factors [2,9]. Until their role is clarified longitudinal strains can provide good indices of the mechanical loads on bone.

Implications for Absorptiometry: Bone Strength Indices (BSIs)

Absorptiometry can provide noninvasive indices of bone strength [17,19]. Current DXA methods (dual energy X-ray absorptiometry) can determine bone mineral content and density at a given sampling site [21] to estimate the mass contribution to bone strength. But peripheral quantitative computed tomography (pQCT) can measure both that and the architectural contribution [17,27–32] to obtain bone strength indices (BSIs) that provide much better estimates of bone strength ($r > 0.95$, $P < 0.0001$) than bone mineral content or density alone ($r < 0.7$) [27]. Thus, pQCT-derived BSIs may see increasing use in osteoporosis work.

Implications for Muscle Strength

Early studies found impressive correlations between pQCT-derived BSIs and measured muscle strength ($r > 0.93$, $P < 0.0001$) [17,31,32]. Bone mineral content and mass correlate less well with measured bone strength and with things like estrogen, age, sex, height, race, dietary calcium, and vitamin D ($r < 0.7$).

Because it strongly influences bone strength and mass, muscle strength needs systematic study as a function of age, sex, race, diet, endocrine status, disease (including the above kinds of osteoporosis), genes, and medications. In humans, muscle strength is easily measured with grip testers, or as the Newton-meters of torque exerted around the elbow, hip, knee, or other joints [11,15,17].

On the Need for New Standards in Osteoporosis Work

By one definition osteoporosis exists when bone mineral density or mass falls more than 2.5 standard deviations below applicable norms [5,21], but that tells nothing about its cause, on which effective treatment should nevertheless depend. In that regard, comparing bone strength to muscle strength might help to distinguish physiologic osteopenias from true osteoporoses [19,29]. In physiologic osteopenias the BSIs should lie on or near the line that graphs bone strength on the vertical axis, against corresponding muscle strength on the horizontal, for people with normal bone-adaptive mechanisms. In true osteoporoses BSIs could lie below that line [33].

Thus, new noninvasive standards are needed for the relationships between bone and muscle strengths as functions of sex, age, race, endocrine and menopausal status, diet, vitamin and calcium intakes, disease, occupation, heredity, medications, etc.

A Role of Pathogenesis in the Choice of Treatment

The above physiology means that increased physical activities and muscle strength might benefit the common physiologic osteopenias, since their bone-adaptive mechanisms would work properly. But that might make patients with the less common true osteoporosis worse (in a situation in Munich it did [H Schiessl, personal communication]). Their disordered adaptive mechanisms could not very well strengthen already too-fragile bones in response to increased activities. This emphasizes the need to learn how to distinguish these conditions from each other.

Conclusion

As DB Burr noted [14], the growing evidence that muscle and physical activities are important determinants of bone strength and mass in health and disease injects a new dimension into the pathophysiology of osteoporoses, as well as into skeletal physiology in general [2,11,12,34]. As one might expect, that incites some controversy that will need time to resolve. The author suggests this should be welcomed rather than discouraged, since in the past controversies have fuelled much of the progress in science, and resolving them has made science better off than before.

References

1. McLean FC, Urist MR (1961) Bone (2nd edn). University of Chicago Press, Chicago
2. Frost HM (1995) Introduction to a new skeletal physiology. vol I, II. The Pajaro Group, Pueblo
3. Jee WSS (1997) Only publications—journals or books—can be entered on the Reference List. For WSS Jee, please add the name of a specific publication, with appropriate data. Alternatively, delete the entry and renumber all subsequent references on the list and citations in the text. Please delete the annotation shown here about Jee. If the information is considered essential, it can be inserted in the text where you consider most appropriate
4. Mosekilde L (1997) Osteoporosis—mechanisms and models. In: Whitfield JE, Morely P (eds) Anabolic treatments for osteoporosis. CRC Press, Boca Raton, pp 31–58
5. Marcus R, Feldman D, Kelsey J (eds) (1996) Osteoporosis. Academic, Orlando
6. Burr DB, Forwood MR, Fyrhie DP, Martin RB, Schaffler MB, Turner CH (1997) Bone microdamage and skeletal fragility in osteoporotic and stress fractures. J Bone Miner Res 12:6–15
7. Burr DB (1997) Microdamage in bone. Curr Opin Orthop 8:8–14
8. Kimmel DB (1993) A paradigm for skeletal strength homeostasis. J Bone Miner Res 8 (Suppl 2):515–522
9. Martin RB, Burr DB (1989) Structure, function and adaptation of compact bone. Raven, New York
10. Jee WSS (1989) The skeletal tissues. In: Weiss L (ed) Cell and tissue biology: a textbook of histology. Urban and Schwartzenberg, Baltimore pp 211–259
11. Schönau E (ed) (1996) Paediatric osteology. New trends and diagnostic possibilities. Elsevier Science, Amsterdam
12. Takahashi HE (1995) Spinal disorders and growth and aging. (Springer, Berlin Heidelberg New York Tokyo
13. Turner CH, Forwood MR (1995) Bone adaptation to mechanical forces in the rat tibia. In: Odgaard A, Weinans H (eds) Bone structure and remodeling. World Scientific, London, pp 65–78
14. Burr DB (1997) Muscle strength, bone mass, and age-related bone loss. J Bone Miner Res 12:1547–1551
15. Faulkner JA, Brooks SV, Zerva E (1990) Skeletal muscle weakness and fatigue in old age: underlying mechanisms. In: Cristofalo JV, Lawton MP (eds) Annual review of gerontology and geriatrics. Springer Berlin Heidelberg, New York, pp 147–166

16. Kannus P. Sievanen H, Vuori L (1996) Physical loading, exercise and bone. Bone 18 (Suppl 1):1–3
17. Schiessl H, Ferretti JL, Tysarczyk-Niemeyer G, Willnecker J (1996) Nonin vasive bone strength index as analyzed by peripheral quantitative computed tomography (pQCT). In: Schonau E (ed) Paediatric osteology: new developments in diagnostics and therapy. Elsevier, Amsterdam, pp 141–146
18. Frost HM (1996) Perspectives: a proposed general model of the mechanostat (suggestions from a new paradigm). Anat Rec 244:139–147
19. Frost HM (1997) On defining osteopenias and osteoporoses: Problems! Another view (with insights from a new paradigm). Bone 20:385–391
20. Frost HM (1997) "Osteoporoses": a rationale for further definitions? Calcif Tissue Int 62:89–94
21. Kanis JA (1994) Assessment of fracture risk and its application to screening for post-menopausal osteoporosis: synopsis of a WHO report. Osteoporosis Int 4:368–381
22. Bilezikian JP, Raisz LG, Rodan GA (1996) Principles of bone biology. Academic, Orlando
23. Frost HM, Ferretti JL, Jee WSS (1997) Perspectives: some roles of mechanical usage, muscle strength and the mechanostat in skeletal physiology, disease and research. Calcif Tissue Int 62:1–7
24. Takahashi HE, Tanizawa T, Hori M, Uzawa T (1991) Effect of intermittent administration of human parathyroid hormone (1–34) on experimental osteopenia of rats induced by ovariectomy. In: Jee WSS (ed) The rat model for bone biology studies. Cells and Mater (Suppl 1):113–118
25. Ma YF, Ferretti JL, Capozza RF, Cointry G, Alippi R, Zanchetta J, Jee WSS (1995) Effects of ON/OFF anabolic hPTH and remodeling inhibitors on metaphyseal bone of immobilized rat femurs. Tomographical (pQCT) description and correlation with histomorphometric changes in tibial cancellous bone. Bone 17 (Suppl):321–327
26. Jee WSS, Ma YF, Chow SY (1995) Maintenance therapy for added bone mass or how to keep the profit after withdrawal of therapy of osteopenia. Bone 17 (Suppl):309–319
27. Ferretti JL (1995) Perspectives of pQCT technology associated to biomech anical studies in skeletal research employing rat models. Bone 17 (Suppl):353–364
28. Ferretti JL, Capozza RF, Tysarczyk-Niemeyer G, Schiessl H, Steffens M (1995) Tomographic determination of stability parameters allows nonivasive estimation of bending or torsion strength. Osteoporosis Int 5:298–304
29. Frost HM (1997) Osteoporoses: Their nature, and therapeutic targets (insights from a new paradigm). In: Whitfield JF, Morely P (eds) Bone anabolic agents. CRC Press, Boca Raton pp 1–29
30. Gasser JA (1995) Assessing bone quantity by pQCT. Bone 17 (Suppl):145–154
31. Schönau E, Werhahn E, Schiedrmaier U, Mokow E, Schiessl H, Schiedhauer K, Michalk D (1996) Influence of muscle strength on bone strength during childhood and adolescence. Horm Res 45 (Suppl 1):63–66
32. Sievanen H, Heinonen A, Kannus F (1996) Adaptation of bone to altered loading environment: A biomechanical approach using X-ray absorptiometric data from the patella of a young woman. Bone 19:55–59
33. Schiessl H, Frost HM, Jee WSS (1997) Perspectives: estrogen and bone-muscle strength and "mass" relationships. Bone 22:1–6
34. Jee WSS, Frost HM (1992) Skeletal adaptations during growth. Triangle 31:77–88

The Present State and Future Prospects for Bone Mass Measurement

MASAO FUKUNAGA[1], TERUKI SONE[1], TATSUSHI TOMOMITSU[1], YOSHIYUKI IMAI[1], RIKA NOGAMI[1], NOBUAKI OTSUKA[1], KIYOHISA NAGAI[1], AKIRA KITAYAMA[2], and MICHINOBU ITAYA[2]

Summary. Many bone measurement techniques have been developed and used in the early detection of bone loss, the prediction of fracture, and the monitoring of therapeutical responses in osteoporosis. Each technique has its own principle and fundamental features such as the site of measurement (e.g., appendicular or axial bone), precision, accuracy, spatial resolution, data-acquisition time, and radiation dose. Each also differs in its performance in the clinical practice of osteoporosis. The purpose of this chapter is to review the present state and future prospects for the use of bone mass measurements clinically.

Key words. Bone mineral density, Microdensitometry, Dual-energy X-ray absorptiometry, Peripheral quantitative computed tomography, Quantitative ultrasound

Introduction

In Japan, the incidence of osteoporosis is increasing along with a rapid increase in the elderly population. This degenerative bone disease, which is frequently complicated by fractures, reduces the quality of life. Therefore, it is important not only medically but also socially to detect, prevent, and treat osteoporosis to reduce fracture risk. Since low bone mass and microarchitectural deterioration of bone tissue in osteoporosis lead to bone fragility and a consequent increase in fractures [1], it is essential to measure bone mass accurately, as bone quality cannot be properly assessed in vivo.

Recently, many bone densitometric techniques, including radiographic absorptiometry (RA) or microdensitometry (MD), single–energy X-ray absorptiometry (SXA), dual–energy X-ray absorptiometry (DXA), peripheral quantitative computed tomography (pQCT), and quantitative ultrasound (QUS), have been developed, and have contributed to a better understanding of osteoporosis both in research and

[1] Department of Nuclear Medicine, Kawasaki Medical School, 577 Matsushima, kurashiki 701-0192, Japan
[2] Department of Radiological Technology, Kawasaki College of Allied Health Professions, 577 Matsushima, Kurashiki 701–0192, Japan

clinically [2]. Each technique is based on a different principle, measurement site, and fundamental performance. In this chapter both the present state and future prospects for the clinical use of bone mass measurements in the detection, prevention and treatment of osteoporosis will be reviewed.

Microdensitometry

Microdensitometry (MD), also known as radiographic absorptiometry (RA), is a quantitative technique used to assess integral, trabecular and cortical bone mass by photodensitometry of X-ray film [3]. Since MD was developed in Japan in 1980, it has been widely used in the diagnosis of metabolic bone diseases, and the evaluation of therapeutic responses.

Although MD is a simple technique, it is time consuming to analyze the bone mass index, and there are a relatively high number of precision errors. Recently, to automate measurement procedures, speed up analysis, and improve precision, new MD methods such as digital image processing (DIP) and computed X-ray densitometry (CXD) employing digital imaging optical apparatus have been developed [4,5].

In MD, DIP and CXD, hand radiographs are made with an aluminum phantom placed between both hands, and bone mass indices, such as ΣGS/D, are made from the relative aluminum concentrations at the middle of the second metacarpal bone. The integral area under the absorption curve, ΣGS, represents the amount of bone mass, and ΣGS/D is an index in which ΣGS is divided by bone width to yield bone density. ΣGS/D is called the DIP value in DIP and the m–BMD (metacarpal bone mineral density) value in CXD. In addition, other parameters such as the metacarpal index (MCI), GS min, which corresponds to the peak of the middle position of the bone marrow, and GS max, which is equal to the mean peak height of the cortex in the radial and ulnar sites, are obtained.

With the DIP device (DIP–1000, Hamamatsu Photonix Co., Shizuoka Japan), X-ray films are photographed using a high-resolution charge-coupled device (CCD) camera and are analyzed using a high-resolution image processor. With the CXD device, the Bonalyzer (Teijin Ltd., Tokyo, Japan), the X-ray radiographs are scanned by light-emitting diodes and CCD sensors instead of the microdensitometer used with MD.

The percentage of operating errors has been reduced from 5% with MD to 1%–2% of the coefficient of variation (CV) with DIP and CXD. Data-processing time has been shortened from 20 min with MD to 1–2 min. In DIP, the non-dominant hand is applied to the measurement side, and an aluminum slope is used as the standard phantom, while in CXD, the dominant hand is applied, and an aluminum wedge is used.

The correlation between the DIP values (x) and the m-BMD values (y) in the second metacarpal is very high ($r = 0.984$, y $= 0.915$x $+ 0.141$, $P < 0.0001$, $n = 40$). As for accuracy, the correlation between m-BMD in the metacarpal cadaver measured by CXD and BMD measured by DXA, using the DCS-600, is also excellent ($r = 0.927$, $P < 0.001$, $n = 15$) [6]. The precision error in DIP was -1.13 of the percentage error for the inter-device, 0.57% of the CV for the inter-observer, 0.30% for the intra-assay, and 0.39% for the inter-assay. The metacarpal DIP values correlate with BMDs from radial DXA using the DCS-600 ($r = 0.890$), spinal DXA using the QDR-2000 ($r = 0.655$) and femoral DXA using the QDR-2000 ($r = 0.734$) (all $P < 0.001$, $n = 33$) (Table 1).

TABLE 1. Correlations between bone mass parameters in the metacarpals measured by digital image processing, and bone mineral densities (BMDs) in the radius, lumbar spine, and femoral neck measured by dual-energy X-ray absorptiometry (DXA)

	ΣGS/D	MCI	GSmin	GSmax
Radius	0.890	0.650	0.824	0.886
L_{2-4}	0.655	0.538*	0.653	0.628
Femoral Neck	0.734	0.706	0.766	0.700

ΣGS/D, DIP value (metacarpal BMD); MCI, metacarpal index; GSmin, peak of the middle position of the bone marrow; GSmax, mean peakheight of the cortex.

All P values < 0.001, except * (P < 0.002).

These data indicate that the correlation between DIP values from metacarpal DIP and BMDs from radial DXA is stronger than that of spinal or femoral DXA. The annual bone loss in normal Japanese women, aged 55–84 years, has been estimated from a cross-sectional study as 1.0% for metacarpal CXD, 1.0% for radial DXA using the DCS-600 (Aloka Co., Tokyo, Japan), 0.70% for spinal DXA using the QDR (Hologic Inc., Waltham, USA), and 0.87% for femoral DXA using the QDR [7]. The age-related bone loss rate in CXD is larger than that in spinal DXA. This probably can be attributed to measurement errors due to arthritic changes especially in the elderly, and to other artifacts. Several prospective studies have shown that RA measurement predicts the risk of spiral fractures [8,9]. In phalangeal RA, the probability for spinal fracture increases by approximately 1.5–1.8 times for each SD decrease in BMD.

It is essential in MD/RA to obtain X-ray films with an optimum constant density. Therefore, to avoid some sources of errors occurring in RA, the same kind of X-ray film, sensitizer, X-ray apparatus, exposure time, and standard phantom should be used, with the same developing conditions, and with accurate positioning of hands.

The advantages of MD/RA are that it is simple and inexpensive to perform, precision errors are low, the radiation dose is low, and it is especially sensitive in detecting bone loss in elderly persons. However, bones measured by MD/RA are mainly of the cortical component, and are not sites biologically relevant to osteoporotic fractures as are the distal radius, hip, and spine. Furthermore, there are few data to recommend the use of MD/RA in monitoring bone mass or therapeutic responses. Therefore, measurement of the bone mass index at the phalanges and metacarpals by MD/RA should be used for the screening of bone loss or as a supplemental method in the assessment of response to interventions.

Dual-energy X-ray Absorptiometry

DXA has been widely used in the clinical assessment of osteoporosis [10–13]. DXA has several advantages such as a short scan time, high precision, and improved spatial resolution with high photon fluence, and the ability to measure BMDs in the lumbar spine and femoral neck, which are common sites for osteoporotic fractures.

At present several kinds of DXA devices are commercially available in Japan: the DCS-600, -600E, DTX-200 (Osteometer, Rødovre, Denmark), pDXA (Stratec Medizintechnik GmbH, Pforzheim, Germany), DXA-70 (Mochida Pharmaceutical Co., Tokyo, Japan), and the Dexa Scan (Direx Medical Systems Ltd., Petah-Tikva, Israel) for radial BMD, the Heelscan (KDK Corp., Kyoto, Japan) for calcaneal BMD, and the QDR-1000, -1000 plus, -1500, -2000, -4500 (Hologic Inc., Waltham, USA), DPX, -α, -L, -IQ, EXP-5000 (Lunar Co., Madison, USA), XR-26, -36 (Norland Co., Fort Atkinson, USA), DCS-900, -3000 (Aloka Co., Tokyo, Japan), and BMD 1X (Hitachi Medico Co., Tokyo, Japan) for axial BMD.

Axial DXA devices in particular are considered standard for BMD measurements. They are used for the diagnosis of osteoporosis or osteopenia, to predict fracture risk, and to monitor therapeutic responses. Peripheral DXA is useful especially in elderly subjects and for screening for low bone mass. Axial DXA is preferred for detecting bone loss during early postmenopause and to evaluate therapeutic responses.

In 1994, the World Health Organization proposed a diagnostic category of osteoporosis in adult women, based on BMD measurements [14]. In 1996, the Japanese Society of Bone and Mineral Research collected normal BMD data from more than 5000 subjects from many institutions: lumbar BMDs by DXA (QDR, DPX, XR, and BMD 1X), radial BMDs by DXA (DCS-600, pDXA, and DTX-200), and pQCT (XCT-960 (Stratec Medizintechnik GmbH, Pforzheim, Germany), metacarpal BMDs by MD (CXD, and DIP), femoral BMDs by DXA (QDR, DPX, and XR), and calcaneal BMDs by DXA (Heelscan) in females, lumbar BMDs by DXA (QDR, and XR), and metacarpal BMDs by MD (CXD, and DIP) in males [7]. The reference values of BMD per 5 years from age 20 to 85+ (Table 2) as well as the young adult mean (YAM) of BMD from age 20 to 44 were determined. Among the diagnostic criteria, diagnosis of low bone mass is made on the basis of lateral X-ray films of the spine, and BMDs in the lumbar spine, radius, femoral neck, metacarpals, and calcaneus measured by DXA, pQCT, or MD.

These criteria are applicable only to females. If a patient shows any non-traumatic vertebral fracture with grade I radiographic osteopenia or BMD less than 80% of YAM, or BMD less than 70% of YAM without fracture, or grade II or more radiographic osteopenia, primary osteoporosis is diagnosed after a complete differential diagnosis to exclude other diseases associated with low bone mass [15]. Osteopenia is diagnosed in a patient without vertebral fractures with 70% to 80% of YAM or grade I radiographic osteopenia.

TABLE 2. Percent of young adult mean (YAM) of BMDs in Japanese women aged 50–54 and 60–64 years at various sites measured with different densitometric devices

	% YAM: Age 50–54	% YAM: Age 60–64
DXA		
Radius (DCS-600)	94	79
Lumbar spine (QDR)	91	79
Femoral neck (QDR)	94	81
Calcaneus (Heelscan)	94	83
MD		
Metacarpal (CXD)	95	83

MD, microdensitometry.

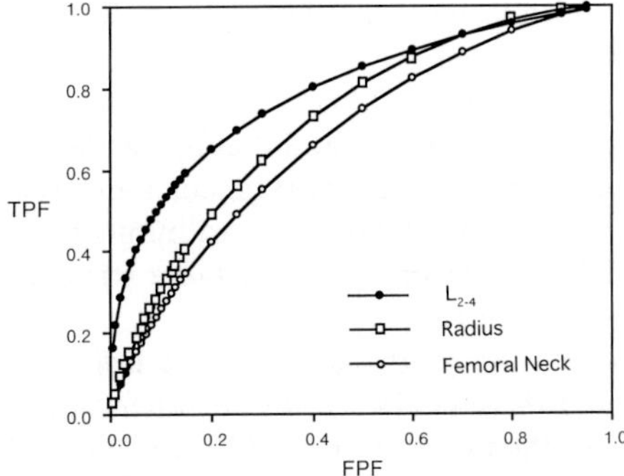

FIG. 1. Receiver operating characteristic curves used in predicting vertebral fractures from BMD measurements at different sites. *TPF*, true-positive fraction; *FPF*, false-positive fraction

Although peak bone mass and bone loss associated with menopause and aging are two major predictors of subsequent fracture, BMD measurement at the specific site of fracture, compared with BMD measurements at other sites, is superior in predicting fractures [16]. For example, a vertebral fracture is better predicted by lumbar BMD measurement than by radial and femoral BMD measurements (Fig. 1).

In newly developed DXA devices, some improvements in both hardware and software have been made including a shorter data-acquisition time with a fan beam and multidetectors, lateral vertebral scanning with the subject in the supine position employing a C arm, measurement of volumetric BMD by both anteroposterior and lateral projections, estimation of body composition with a whole-body scan mode, and measurement of geometry, such as hip axis length [17] and vertebral morphometry [18]. These advances in DXA will undoubtedly provide more information to clarify the pathophysiology of osteoporosis.

Peripheral Quantitative Computed Tomography

Tomographic images on X-ray CT represent the distribution of the attenuation coefficient of tissue. Therefore, with commercially available CT scanners and a cross-calibration phantom for bone mineral, BMD can be measured [19]. Spinal QCT has advantages such as separate measurements of trabecular and cortical BMD, acquisition not of areal BMD (g/cm^2) but of volumetric BMD (g/cm^3), and recognition of the trabecular arrangement to a certain degree. However, it also has some limitations, such as relatively high precision errors and radiation doses, and marrow fat affects the CT number when QCT is performed using a single energy source.

Using pQCT, where the peripheral bones such as the radius and tibia involving less marrow fat than the spine are employed as measurement sites, it has been possible to measure BMDs with high precision [20,21], with a CV of 0.5%, high accuracy [22], and using a low radiation dose. As pQCT devices, the XCT-960 and Densiscan-1000 (Scanco Medical, Zurich, Switzerland) are available commercially. With the XCT-960, measurements in the distal radius are performed at only one site with a single axial slice 2.5-mm thick. With the Densiscan-1000, measurements in both the distal radius and tibia are performed using multislices 1.0 mm thick (10 slices in the epiphysis and 6 slices in the diaphysis).

In a routine quantitative examination with the Densiscan-1000, three parameters are calculated (a) total bone (cortical and trabecular bone; 100%-volume D100), (b) trabecular bone; (50% volume-D50) at the epiphyseal region, and (c) cortical bone (P100) at the meta- and diaphyseal regions of radius and tibia. The measurement of the distal site reflects trabecular bone, and the measurement of the proximal site reflects cortical bone. In addition, high spatial resolution of 0.2 mm allows the qualitative examination of bone structure, e.g., the detection of microcalluses and microfractures.

With the Densiscan-1000, the D50- or D100-to-P100 ratios in the radius are 0.39 and 0.18, respectively. On the other hand, with the DCS-600, a peripheral DXA apparatus, the ratios of integral BMDs in the one-sixth or one-tenth of radial length to the BMD in the one-third are 0.82 and 0.68, respectively. Cortical BMD (P100, $n = 44$) is more closely related to the total BMD (D100, $r = 0.839$, $P < 0.001$) than is trabecular BMD (D50, $r = 0.698$, $P < 0.001$). In vivo correlations between D50, D100, or P100 in the radius measured by the Densiscan-1000 and BMD in the mid-radius, lumbar spine, or femoral neck measured by DXA are also shown in Table 3. Regarding the relationship between parameters obtained with the pQCT in the radius and BMD in the lumbar spine, with correlation coefficients ranging from 0.525 for P100, 0.730 for D100, and 0.833 for D50 (all $P < 0.001$, $n = 44$), it appears that BMD at the lumbar spine, composed mainly of trabecular bone, reflects trabecular BMD (D50) in the radius more than BMD at other sites (D100 and P100).

Cortical thickness can be measured with pQCT using high spatial resolution. The cortical thickness in the radius has been calculated by the Densiscan-1000 using the threshold algorithm and a circular ring model assumption [23]. The most prominent percent decrease in age-related change was found in cortical thickness (Table 4). More

TABLE 3. In vivo correlations between D50, D100, or P100 in the radius by Densiscan-1000, and BMD in the mid-radius, lumbar spine, and femoral neck

		DXA: mid-radius	DXA: L_{2-4}	DXA: femoral neck
pQCT	D50	0.811	0.833	0.854
	D100	0.812	0.730	0.800
	P100	0.802	0.525	0.632

pQCT, peripheral quantitative computed tomography.

TABLE 4. Age-related changes in cortical density, cortical area, cortical thickness, and total density in the radius from ages 40 to 70 years. Estimated from a linear (a) or square (b) regression model. Data from Sone et al.[23]

	% Decrease (a)	% Decrease (b)
Cortical density	4.9	5.0
Cortical area	29.3	38.1
Cortical thickness	29.3	55.9
Total density	21.7	38.7

than 80% of age-related bone loss in the radius is caused by decreased thickness of cortical bone.

The pQCT is a reliable procedure for precise separate quantitative BMD evaluation of trabecular and cortical bone for the prediction of fracture risk [24] and for monitoring the therapeutic effect on osteoporotic patients [25]. In addition, high resolution of pQCT can be used in the assessment of bone architecture. Combined analysis of both BMD and structure should help to clarify the pathophysiology of osteoporosis.

Quantitative Ultrasound

Skeletal status can be characterized by the transmission of ultrasound, non-ionizing radiation, through bone [26,27]. Speed of sound (SOS) is affected by the bone through which ultrasound waves pass, and is also dependent on the elastic property of the medium, i.e., the rigidity or stiffness of the material. The frequency spectra emitted by an ultrasound transducer are attenuated as they pass through bone. Broadband ultrasound attenuation (BUA) reflects the frequency dependence of ultrasound attenuation, and is influenced by the number, spacing, and orientation of trabeculae. Therefore, QUS can evaluate not only BMD but also the structure and quality of bone. Recently a number of QUS devices have become commercially available or have been developed (Table 5).

In QUS devices, some indexes other than SOS and BUA are also measured or calculated, i.e., Stiffness calculated from SOS and BUA, the transmission index (TI) defined as the full width at half maximum (FWHM) of the transmitted ultrasound wave, the osteosono-assessment index (OSI) obtained from $(SOS)^2 \times TI$, and the percent trabecular bone area constructed from the fractal dimension of the bone area ratio, which is the square of the ratio of the length of the bone tissue to the width of the calcaneus [27]. In QUS, transmitting or reflecting ultrasound is used. Among transmission techniques, either a water bath (a wet system) or the contact method (a dry system) is employed.

TABLE 5. Commercially available quantitative ultrasound devices

Device	Site	System	Index	Special feature
A-1000	Calcaneus	Wet	SOS, BUA, Stiffness	
AOS-100	Calcaneus	Dry	SOS, TI, OSI	
Benus	Calcaneus	Water bag	SOS, % Trabecular Area	
CUBA	Calcaneus	Dry	SOS	
CM-100	Calcaneus	Dry	SOS	
UBIS-3000	Calcaneus	Wet	SOS, BUA	BUA image
UXA-300	Calcaneus	Wet	SOS, AOS, V-BMD, EI	SXA image
Sound Scan-2000	Tibia	Dry	SOS	
Omnisense	Multiple	Dry	SOS	

SOS, speed of sound, BUA, broadband ultrasound attenuation, TI, transmission index, OSI, osteosono-assessment index, AOS, attenuation of sound, V-BMD, volumetric BMD, EI, elastic index, SXA, single-energy X-ray absorptiometry.

TABLE 6. Correlations between parameters in the calcaneus measured by the AOS-100 and those measured by the A-1000 or UXA-300

| | | AOS-100 | | |
		AOS-100: SOS	AOS-100: TI	AOS-100: OSI
A-1000	SOS	0.911	0.664	0.799
	BUA	0.539	0.725	0.715
	Stiffness	0.825	0.768	0.836
UXA-300	SOS	0.856	0.782	0.853
	AOS	0.587	0.650	0.665
	EI	0.767	0.792	0.825

TABLE 7. Correlations between SOS, BUA and Stiffness measured by the A-1000 and age, height, weight, body mass index (BMI), and lumbar BMD in 361 women

	SOS (m/s)	BUA (dB/MHz)	Stiffness (% YAM)
Age (yrs.)	*−0.687	*−0.559	*−0.725
Height (cm)	*0.358	*0.441	*0.446
Weight (kg)	0.030	*0.212	*0.111
BMI (kg/m^2)	*−0.178	−0.041	*−0.146
Lumbar BMD (g/cm^2)	*0.611	*0.523	*0.660

$*P < 0.001$.

The correlation between parameters in the calcaneus measured by the AOS-100 (Aloka Co., Tokyo, Japan) and those measured by the A-1000 (Lunar Co., Madison, USA) or UXA-300 (Aloka Co., Tokyo, Japan) are shown in Table 6. The SOS measured by the AOS-100 correlates highly with that measured by the A-1000 or UXA-300. The OSI measured by the AOS-100 also correlates closely with the SOS or Stiffness measured by the A-1000, and the SOS or the elastic index (EI) measured by the UXA-300.

In this cross-sectional study, QUS parameters moderately correlated with height (Table 7). They also negatively correlated with age, as in many previous reports [28,29]. In addition, there were significant negative correlations with SOS, BUA, and Stiffness for lumbar BMD.

Many QUS devices measure SOS across the bone, but the Sound Scan-2000 (Myriad Ultrasound Systems, Rehovot, Israel) measures SOS along a fixed longitudinal 5-cm distance of the cortical layer at the tibial shaft, its midportion [30]. With this device, a transmission wave with a center frequency of 0.25 MHz is used for the measurement of SOS, and a reflection wave of 1 MHz is used for correction of positioning. SOS in the cortical bone is influenced by material property and cortical thickness. Therefore, both quantitative and qualitative information regarding the tibia can be evaluated. Our preliminary studies indicate that tibial SOS correlates significantly with lumbar BMD (DXA), radial BMD (DXA), and calcaneal SOS (QUS) ($r = 0.351 − 0.514, P < 0.02 − 0.001, n = 29–72$) [31].

The UXA-300 is a hybrid QUS/SXA device for the assessment of EI of the calcaneus [32]. The width, SOS, and BUA (AOS) are measured by QUS, cross-sectional BMC (C-BMC) and BMD (C-BMD) are measured by SXA, and volumetric BMD (V-BMD, C-

BMD/width) are measured by both QUS and SXA. With this device, the SOS through a material depends on its modulus of elasticity and bone mass density. On this basis, EI is calculated by $(SOS)^2 \times$ V-BMD. The EI was found to correlate with lumbar BMD (DXA) ($r = 0.731$, $P < 0.001$, $n = 100$) and calcaneal stiffness (QUS) ($r = 0.827$, $P < 0.001$) [32]. In addition, correlation with lumbar BMD is better in EI than that in SOS or attenuation of sound (AOS).

The UBI 3000 (Diagnostic Medical Systems, Montpellier, France) is a unique QUS device able to demonstrate a high-resolution image of BUA in the calcaneus [33]. As the reproducibility of QUS mainly depends on the positioning of both the foot and the transducers, BUA imaging improves the reproducibility of QUS measurements.

Most QUS techniques measure the bone in transmission, and they are limited to a few sites. Omnisense (Sunlight Ultrasound Technology Ltd., Rehovot, Israel) measures SOS using a reflection mode at multiple sites [34] including the radius, ulna, metacarpals, and phalanges.

Bone strength and fracture risk are considered to be affected by BMD, bone structure, and bone quality. Therefore, QUS should provide more discriminative capacity regarding fracture risk. In fact, QUS parameters can be used to predict hip fracture in elderly women, independently of BMD [36,37].

Future Prospects

The architecture or structure of the trabecular network is another determinant of bone strength, independent of bone densitometry. Among many noninvasive techniques, QCT/pQCT, QUS and quantitative magnetic resonance have the potential for providing information about bone quality and structure [37–39]. Trabecular distribution obtained by these techniques is quantified by texture analysis including fractal dimension, frequency, and run-length analysis.

In the future, combined measurements of bone mass and bone architecture or bone quality should provide the diagnostic accuracy needed to identify patients with osteoporotic fracture risk.

Acknowledgments. This study was supported in part by a Research Project Grant (No. 9–403) from Kawasaki Medical School.

References

1. Consensus Development Conference (1993) Diagnosis, prophylaxis, and treatment of osteoporosis. Am J Med 94:646–650
2. Genant HK, Engelke K, Fuerst T, Glüer CC, Grampp S, Harris ST, Jergas M, Lang T, Lu Y, Majumdar S, Mathur A, Takada M (1996) Noninvasive assessment of bone mineral and structure: State of the art. J Bone Miner Res 11:707–730
3. Inoue T, Kushida K, Miyamoto S, Sumi Y (1983) Quantitative assessment of bone density on X-ray picture. J Jpn Orthop Assoc 57:1923–1936
4. Hayashi Y, Yamamoto K, Fukunaga M, Ishibashi T, Takahashi K, Nishii Y (1990) Assessment of bone mass by image analysis of metacarpal bone roentgenograms: A quantitative digital image processing (DIP) method. Radiat Med 8:173–178

5. Matsumoto C, Kushida K, Yamazaki K, Imose K, Inoue T (1994) Metacarpal bone mass in normal and osteoporotic Japanese women using computed X-ray densitometry. Calcif Tissue Int 55:324–329

6. Imai H, Watanabe R, Fukunaga M, Imai S, Miyake M, Takeda N (1994) Measurement of bone mineral density in metacarpal bone in cadavers: Comparison of BMD values measured using the Bonalyzer and DXA (in Japanese). J Jpn Soc Bone Morphom 4:33–37

7. Orimo H, Sugioka Y, Fukunaga M, Muto Y, Hotokebuchi T, Gorai I, Nakamura T, Kushida K, Tanaka H, Ikai T, Oh-ashi Y (1998) Diagnostic criteria of primary osteoporosis. J Bone Miner Metab 16:139–150

8. Takada M, Engelke K, Hagiwara S, Grampp S, Jergas M, Glüer CC, Genant HK (1997) Assessment of osteoporosis: Comparison of radiographic absorptiometry of the phalanges and dual X-ray absorptiometry of the radius and lumbar spine. Radiology 202:759–763

9. Ross PD (1997) Radiographic absorptiometry for measuring bone mass. Osteoporosis Int 7 (Suppl):S103–S107

10. Wahner HW, Fogelman I (1994) The evaluation of osteoporosis: dual energy X-ray absorptiometry in clinical practice. Martin Dunitz, London

11. Blake GM, Fogelman I (1997) Technical principle of dual energy X-ray absorptiometry. Semin Nucl Med 27:210–228

12. Inoue T, Yamazaki K, Kushida K (1997) Utility of dual X-ray absorptiometry and single X-ray absorptiometry as diagnostic tools for involutional osteoporosis. Osteoporosis Int 7 (Suppl 3):S117–S119

13. Adams JE (1998) Single- and dual-energy: X-ray absorptiometry, In: Genant HK, Guglielmi G, Jergas M (eds) Bone densitometry and osteoporosis. Springer, Berlin, pp 305–334

14. Kanis JA, Melton III LJ, Christiansen C, Johnston CC, Khaltaev NI (1994) The diagnosis of osteoporosis. J Bone Miner Res 9:1137–1141

15. Orimo H (1997) Diagnostic criteria of primary osteoporosis in Japan. Osteoporosis Int 7 (Suppl 2):S22

16. Jergas M, Glüer CC (1997) Assessment of fracture risk by bone density measurements. Semin Nucl Med 27:261–275

17. Faulkner KG, Cummings SR, Glüer CC, Palermo L, Black D, Genant HK (1993) Simple measurement of femoral geometry predicts hip fracture: The study of osteoporotic fractures. J Bone Miner Res 8:1211–1217

18. Steiger P, Cummings SR, Genant HK, Weiss H (1994) Morphometric X-ray absorptiometry of the spine: Correlation in vivo with morphometric radiography. Osteoporosis Int 4:238–244

19. Guglielmi G, Lang TF, Cammisa M, Genant HK (1998) Quantitative computed tomography at the axial skeleton. In: Genant HK, Guglielmi G, Jergas M (eds) Bone densitometry and osteoporosis. Springer, Berlin, pp 335–347

20. Tomomitsu T, Sone T, Fukunaga M, Ito M, Ishida Y, Hayashi K (1995) Fundamental study of peripheral QCT (Densiscan-1000) (in Japanese). J Jpn Soc Bone Morphom 5:147–153

21. Ito M, Tsurusaki K, Hayashi K (1997) Peripheral QCT for the diagnosis of osteoporosis. Osteoporosis Int 7 (Suppl 3):S120–S127

22. Imai Y, Sone T, Tomomitsu T, Imai H, Mikawa Y, Watanabe R, Fukunaga M (1997) Precision and accuracy for peripheral quantitative computed tomography evaluated using radial specimens. J Bone Miner Res 12 (Suppl 1):S263

23. Sone T, Imai Y, Tomomitsu T, Fukunaga M (1997) Age-related rarefaction and bone loss of cortical bone: Study with high-resolution pQCT instrument (in Japanese). Osteoporosis Jpn 5:194–196

24. Louis O, Boulpaep F, Willnecker J, Winkel PV, Osteaux M (1995) Cortical mineral content of the radius assessed by peripheral QCT predicts compressive strength on biomechanical testing. Bone 16:375–379
25. Rüegsegger P (1994) The use of peripheral QCT in the evaluation of bone remodeling. Endocrinologist 4:167–176
26. Glüer CC (1997) Quantitative ultrasound techniques for the assessment of osteoporosis: Expert agreement on current status. J Bone Miner Res 12:1280–1288
27. Morita R, Yamamoto I, Yuu I, Hamanaka Y, Ohta T, Takada M, Matsushita R, Masuda K (1997) Quantitative ultrasound for the assessment of bone status. Osteoporosis Int 7 (Suppl 3):S128–S134
28. Yamazaki K, Kushida K, Ohmura M, Sano M, Inoue T (1994) Ultrasound bone densitometry of the os calcis in Japanese women. Osteoporosis Int 4:220–225
29. Takeda N, Miyake M, Kita S, Tomomitsu T, Fukunaga M (1996) Sex and age patterns of quantitative ultrasound densitometry of the calcaneus in normal Japanese subjects. Calcif Tissue Int 59:84–88
30. Foldes AJ, Rimon A, Keinan DD, Popovtzer MM (1995) Quantitative ultrasound of the tibia: A novel approach for assessment of bone status. Bone 17:363–367
31. Nogami R, Sone T, Tomomitsu T, Fukunaga M (1998) Fundamental study of tibial ultrasound bone densitometry device, Sound Scan-2000. The 17th Annual Meeting of Japanese Society for Bone and Mineral Research, Tokyo
32. Takeda N, Miyake M, Kita S, Imai H, Tomomitsu T, Fukunaga M (1995) Fundamental and clinical study of ultrasound bone mineral quantifying equipment (UXA-300, Aloka) (in Japanese). J Jpn Soc Bone Morphom 5:53–59
33. Roux C, Fournier B, Laugier P, Chappard C, Kolta S, Dougados M, Berger G (1996) Broadband ultrasound attenuation imaging: A new imaging method in osteoporosis. J Bone Miner Res 11:1112–1118
34. Barkmann R (1997) A new reflection quantitative ultrasound device for measuring a large variety of bones: First in vivo investigations. The 12th International Bone Densitometry Workshop, Crieff, Scotland
35. Glüer CC, Cummings SR, Bauer DC, Stone K, Pressman A, Mathur A, Genant HK (1996) Osteoporosis: Association of recent fractures with quantitative US findings. Radiology 199:725–733
36. Hans D, Dargent-Molina P, Schott AM, Sebert JL, Cormier C, Kotzki PO, Delmas PD, Pouilles JM, Breart G, Meunier PJ (1996) Ultrasonographic heel measurements to predict hip fracture in elderly women: The EPIDOS prospective study. Lancet 348:511–514
37. Engelke K, Kalender W (1998) Beyond bone densitometry: Assessment of bone architecture by X-ray computed tomography at various levels of resolution. In: Genant HK, Guglielmi G, Jergas M (eds) Bone densitometry and osteoporosis. Springer, Berlin, pp 417–447
38. Genant HK, Majumdar S (1997) High-resolution magnetic resonance imaging of trabecular bone structure. Osteoporosis Int 7 (Suppl 3):S135–S139
39. Genant HK, Engelke K, Glüer CC, Lang T, Majumdar S (1995) Recent advances in the noninvasive assessment of bone density, quality and structure. J Jpn Soc Bone Morphom 5:93–108

Anisotropic Behavior in Viscoelasticity and Fracture Mechanics of Compact Bone

Yuji Tanabe

Summary. This chapter deals with the in vitro techniques for the determination of viscoelastic properties and fracture toughness of compact bone. The reliability and feasibility of these techniques have been validated through numerical simulation and experiments on bovine compact bone. The method using the split-Hopkinson pressure bar (SHPB) technique was able to sharply reduce the time required for computation to find viscoelastic parameters, and this could be an alternative method to conventional creep and stress relaxation experiments. Young's modulus of compact bone was experimentally determined as a function of orientation applying the dynamic mechanical analysis (DMA). Young's modulus is considered to be dominated by the microstructural arrangement of the mineral phase such as the directions of the c-axes of hydroxyapatite crystals in bone, and the previous model in terms of the unidirectional continuous fibre-reinforced composite theory was unable to obtain a good corresponding prediction to the experimental result. Fracture toughness tests have revealed anisotropic and rate-dependent behaviour in the critical stress intensity factor, K_C, of compact bone. The existence of a fracture process zone due to microcrack initiation ahead of the main crack front has been demonstrated. Its contribution to the improvement of the resistance to crack growth or fracture has been discussed also. These findings have helped us to understand the optimum microstructure of compact bone as well as to develop more sophisticated biomaterials such as bone-analogue materials.

Key words. Compact bone, Mechanical properties, Anisotropy, Viscoelasticity, Fracture toughness

Introduction

Evaluation of the mechanical properties of bone is necessary for the development of implanted materials with favourable mechanical compatibility with natural bone tissue [1]. Compact bone behaves as a viscoelastic, anisotropic and semi-brittle solid.

Department of Mechanical Engineering, Faculty of Engineering, Niigata University, Ikarashi Ni-nocho, Niigata 950-2181, Japan

Therefore, the stress or strain state in bone subjected to arbitrary external loads should be evaluated with the inclusion of such mechanical characteristics. Moreover, the microcrack initiations in bone matrix have been recently reported. Although these microcracks are easily initiated even at low stress level in our daily life, and are considered to be the one of contributory factors to bone remodelling, their accumulation could be the trigger of unstable macroscopic fracture. Fracture mechanics widely used in the assessment of integrity in engineering structural components should be a powerful approach to finding the solution to the mechanism of stable and unstable microcrack growth in bone.

Hence, in this chapter the principles and the in vitro techniques for the determination of viscoelastic properties and fracture toughness of compact bone are reviewed briefly. The reliability and feasibility of these techniques are demonstrated through numerical simulation and experiments on bovine compact bone. Anisotropic effects in viscoelastic characteristics, Young's modulus, and fracture toughness as well as rate-dependent behaviour in fracture toughness are identified, and the source of these characteristics are discussed also in conjunction with the microstructural aspects of compact bone.

Identification of Dynamic Properties of Compact Bone Using Split-Hopkinson Pressure Bar Technique

A novel method has been developed for the identification of the viscoelastic characteristics of compact bone using transient response information obtained from the split-Hopkinson pressure bar (SHPB) test [2]. The SHPB technique is one of the impact tests, and enables us to perform precise determination of dynamic or impact load to samples at high strain rates ranging between 10 and $1000\,s^{-1}$. Details of the principle of the SHPB technique can be found elsewhere [3], and the experimental apparatus in the compression version is illustrated schematically in Fig. 1.

The method combines the solution procedures of two problems. One is the identification (or inverse) problem and the other is the associated problem, namely the prediction (or direct) problem of stress wave propagation in the SHPB apparatus. The solutions are accomplished using Laplace transformation and the Gauss-Newton iterative scheme for non-linear least squares problems. The method was validated through numerical experiments, i.e., the final identified viscoelastic parameter values agreed well with the corresponding exact values indicating that maximum relative error was less than 5%.

The method was subsequently applied to the SHPB experiments on bovine femoral compact bone (plexiform bone), assuming that the mechanical behaviour of the bone could be represented by the three-element standard linear solid model as shown in Fig. 2a. The viscoelastic characteristics were determined as a function of orientation using the cylindrical bone specimens, 10 mm in diameter and 10 mm in length. Figure 2b shows the orientational-dependent behaviour with this viscoelasticity. It was found that the rigidity, E_1, and the internal frictional loss, η, of bovine plexiform bone under

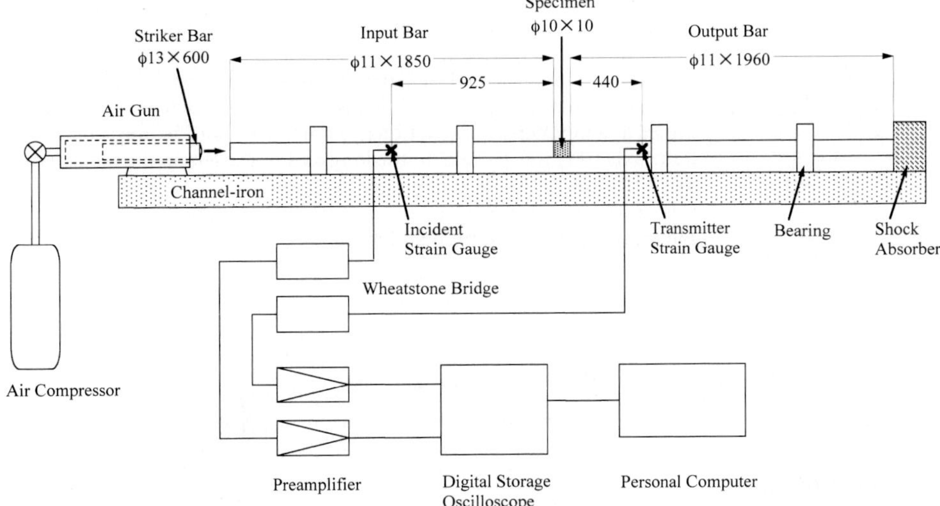

FIG. 1. Schematic illustration of split-Hopkinson pressure bar apparatus in compression version. The apparatus is composed of three cylindrical steel rods of input, output, and striker bars containing a cylindrical bone specimen sandwiched between the input and output bars. After an impingement of the striker bar fired through an air gun on the input bar, a compressive stress pulse is generated and travels down the input and output bars through the specimen. The stress pulse transmitted into the output bar is detected by a transmitter strain gauge and its record is utilised for the identification of viscoelastic characteristics of the specimen

impact compression are greatest in the direction parallel to the long axis of the bone. The advantage of the proposed method is that the time required for characterisation of the dynamic properties of bone can be sharply reduced.

Anisotropy in Young's Modulus of Compact Bone

Dynamic mechanical analysis (DMA) is another useful technique for the determination of viscoelastic properties of materials. Stress and strain histories under cyclic sinusoidal loading are usually measured, and loss tangent, tan δ, as a measure of viscosity in the DMA is calculated from the time lag or phase angle between them. This technique has been validated through its application to many high polymer materials so far, and could be applicable to compact bone. Therefore, a series of experiments on bovine tibial cortical bone has been completed using a commercial DMA apparatus [4]. Young's modulus under cyclic loading, or dynamic modulus, E', and tan δ were determined as a function of orientation using small specimens at loading frequencies of 1, 5, and 10 Hz, and at 37°C.

Rectangular beam specimens 1 mm by 3 mm by 22 mm were machined from the mid-diaphyseal medial cortices of bovine tibiae. The specimens were cut with their long axis at angles of 0° (longitudinal), 22.5°, 45°, 67.5°, and 90° (transverse) to the long axis of the bone. Specimens mainly consisted of primary bone, plexiform bone,

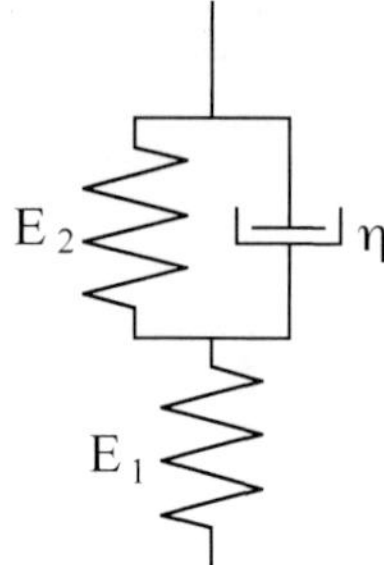

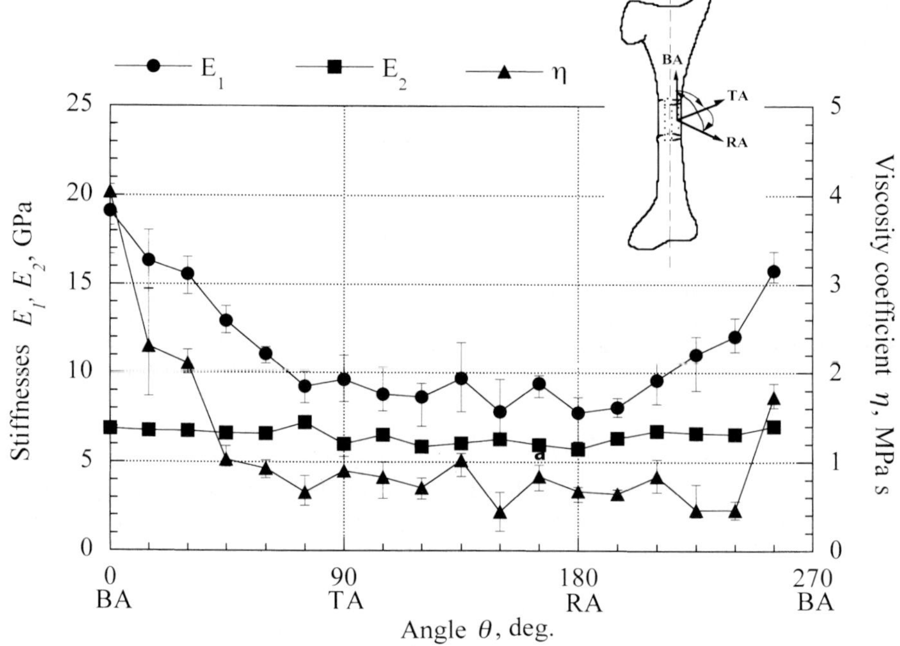

FIG. 2a,b. Three-element standard linear solid and variation in viscoelastic characteristics of bovine femoral plexiform bone with respect to orientation of specimen axis. **a** Three-element standard linear solid model can be represented by a parallel spring (E_2) and dashpot (η) in series with another spring (E_1). **b** Viscoelastic parameters were determined as a function of orientation in a Cartesian coordinate system. The bone axis (*BA*) was parallel to the long axis of the femur, the tangential axis (*TA*) was in the circumferential direction, and the radial axis (*RA*) was in the endosteal-periosteal direction. Each datum point represents the mean (with a maximum and minimum) of five specimens

and showed fewer haversian systems. The DMA apparatus (DMA7, Perkin Elmer, Norwalk, CT, USA) was used to perform cyclic three-point bending tests on the specimens with span length of 20 mm.

Figures 3 and 4 show the effect of orientation on E' and tan δ, respectively. E' smoothly decreases with an increase of angle up to 67.5° and then goes down remarkably at angles between 67.5° and 90° at all frequencies showing 23 GPa for the longitudinal (0°) direction at 10 Hz and 14 GPa for the transverse (90°) direction at 10 Hz. It is clear that a unidirectional continuous fibre-reinforced composite model [5] cannot be applied to the prediction of the orientational-dependent behaviour in dynamic modulus. E' in this study shows higher value than Young's modulus by the ultrasonic technique reported in a previous work [6]. Tan δ is almost constant at each loading frequency independent of orientation except for the slightly higher values at the transverse (90°) direction. This implies that anisotropic behaviour in

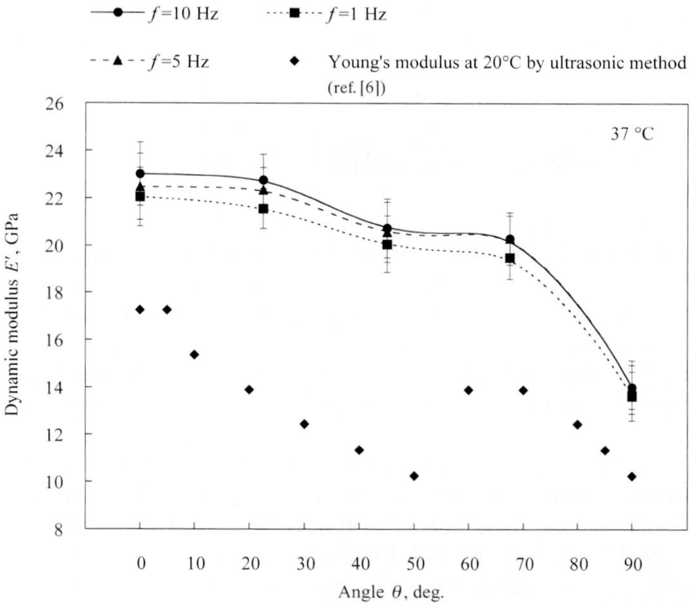

FIG. 3. Variation in dynamic modulus (E') of bovine tibial plexiform bone with the orientation of specimen axis to the long axis of the bone (θ) at various loading frequencies (f), compared with the orientational-dependent behaviour of Young's modulus obtained by the ultrasonic technique (*solid diamonds*). Each datum point represents the mean of five specimens

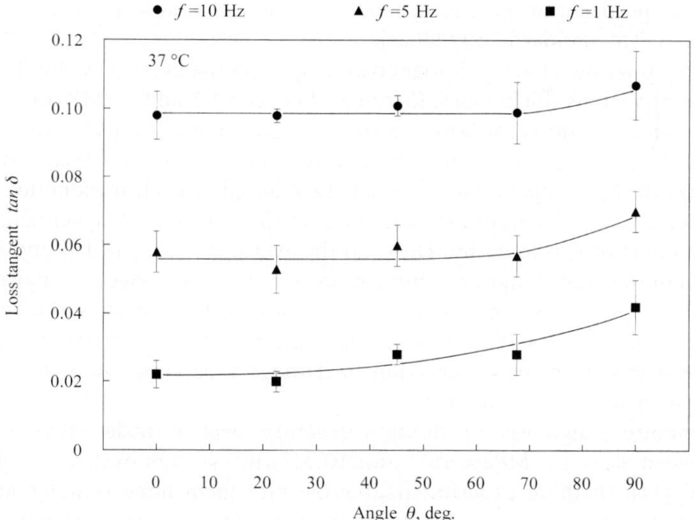

FIG. 4. Variation in loss tangent (tan δ) of bovine tibial plexiform bone with the orientation of the specimen axis to the long axis of the bone at various loading frequencies. Each datum point represents the mean of five specimens

mechanical properties of compact bone is dominated by the microstructural arrangement of the mineral phase such as the direction of the c-axes of hydroxyapatite crystals in bone [7].

Fracture Toughness of Compact Bone

Compact bone is a semi-brittle material. Hence stable crack growth or equivalent damage extension can exist before catastrophic fracture occurs, and it can affect the determination of fracture mechanics parameters, such as the critical stress intensity factor, K_C, and the critical strain energy release rate, G_C. Both K_C and G_C are usually referred to as fracture toughness. The effects of initial crack length and specimen thickness on K_C under mode I loading have been examined [8] in an attempt to establish the nature of micromechanical damage prior to unstable macroscopic fracture in bone.

Haversian bone samples were taken from the mid-diaphyseal anterior cortices of fresh bovine femurs. Compact tension specimens, specially designed and standardised for the fracture toughness test [9] were then wet-machined into thicknesses of 3, 5, 6, 7, and 8 mm, with overall dimensions 17.5 mm $\times$ 16.8 mm. The machined notches of 6, 7, 8, 9, 10, and 11 mm, with a notch tip radius of curvature of 50 μm and a tip angle of 30°, were introduced as initial cracks at angles of 0° and 90° to the bone axis (denoted T-L and L-T specimens, respectively). Side-grooves were introduced into the L-T specimens so that the crack path should be parallel to the initial crack direction. The test specimens, saturated in physiological saline, were loaded at 20°C at a cross-head speed of $3.3 \times 10^{-6}\,\mathrm{m\,s^{-1}}$, using an Instron-type materials testing machine (AG-25TD, Shimadzu, Kyoto, Japan). Load, P, and crack opening displacement, v, during crack propagation were recorded. K_C was determined from the $P - v$ curve following the ASTM standard E399-90 [9].

Figure 5 shows the effect of initial crack length on the average K_C for T-L and L-T specimens of various thicknesses. K_C ranges between 1.3 and 1.6 MPa m$^{1/2}$ in the T-L specimens and 2.5 and 4.2 MPa m$^{1/2}$ in the L-T specimens. These K_C values of haversian bone are approximately three times larger than that of industrially synthesised hydroxyapatite. K_C is dependent on initial crack length, i.e., clear reduction in K_C can be seen as initial crack length increases in both the L-T and T-L specimens. Figure 6 shows the effect of specimen thickness on the average K_C for the T-L and L-T specimens with initial crack length of 7 mm. Specimen thickness does not appear to affect K_C in the T-L specimens, while K_C clearly decreases with increasing thickness in the L-T specimens. These results shown in Figs. 5 and 6 could be interpreted according to a hypothesis based on the observation of damage accumulation, or microcracking ahead of the main crack front [10].

The fracture toughness in mode I fracture over a wide range of loading rates between $\dot{K}_I = 10^{-4}\,\mathrm{MPa\,m^{1/2}\,s^{-1}}$ and $10^{6}\,\mathrm{MPa\,m^{1/2}\,s^{-1}}$ has been subsequently investigated [11]. In these experiments, bovine plexiform bone samples taken from the mid-diaphyseal anterior cortices of fresh bovine femurs were used. Fracture toughness tests at high loading rates greater than $\dot{K}_I = 10^{3}\,\mathrm{MPa\,m^{1/2}\,s^{-1}}$ were performed using the SHPB technique mentioned earlier with the specially designed loading devices. Figure 7 shows K_C as a function of loading rate. The L-T specimens tend

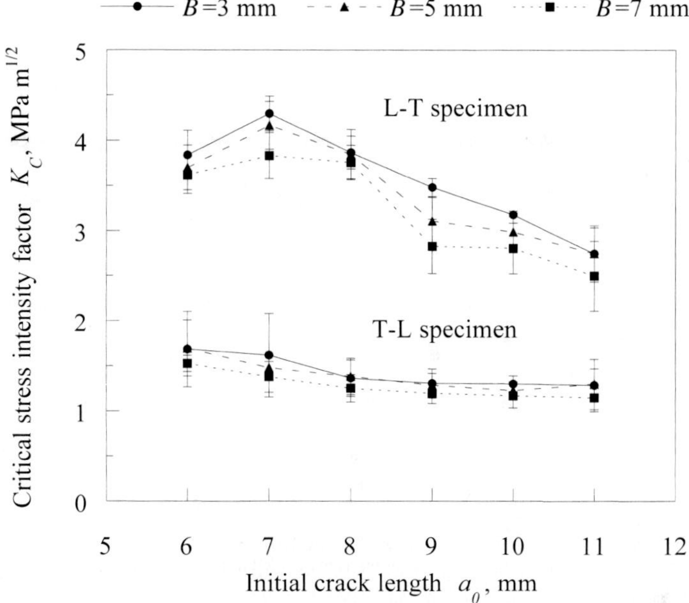

FIG. 5. Effect of the initial crack length (a_0) on the average critical stress intensity factor (K_C) of bovine femoral haversian bone for various thicknesses (B) of T-L and L-T specimens. The initial cracks were introduced into longitudinal and tangential directions to the long axis of the femur in the T-L and L-T specimens, respectively. Each datum point represents the mean of five specimens

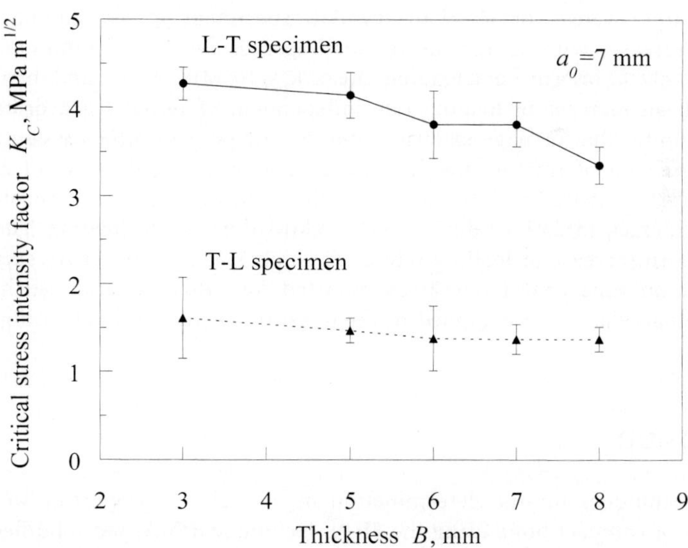

FIG. 6. Effect of thickness on the average critical stress intensity factor of bovine femoral haversian bone for the T-L and L-T specimens with initial crack length of 7 mm. Each datum point represents the mean of five specimens

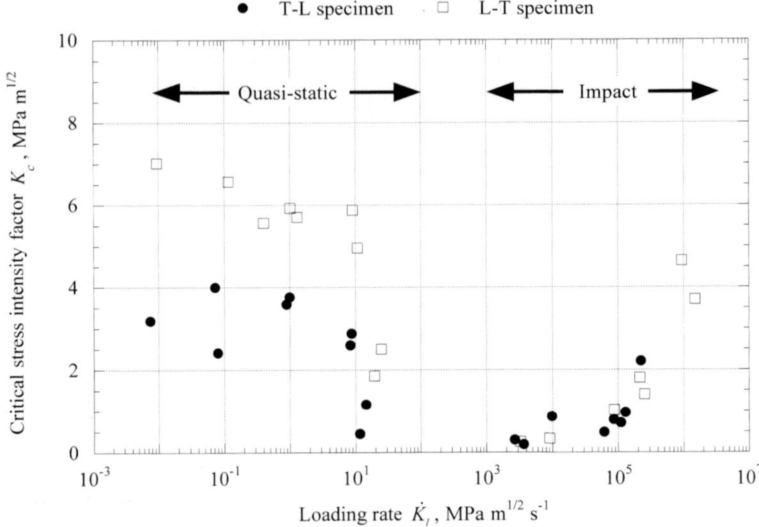

FIG. 7. Critical stress intensity factor of bovine femoral plexiform bone as a function of loading rate for the T-L and L-T specimens. The loading rate is represented in terms of stress intensity factor rate ($\dot{K}_I$). Fracture toughness tests were performed using a commercial materials testing machine at loading rates less than 10^2 MPa m$^{1/2}$ s^{-1} (*Quasi-static*) and the split-Hopkinson pressure bar technique at loading rates greater than 10^3 MPa m$^{1/2}$ s^{-1} (*Impact*)

to have larger values of K_C than the T-L specimens at all loading rates. K_C initially decreases with an increase of loading rate and has a minimum value of approximately 0.2 MPa m$^{1/2}$ at a loading rate of $\dot{K}_I \cong 10^3$ MPa m$^{1/2}$ s^{-1}, and then increases again with an increase of loading rate independent of initial crack orientation. It has been found that damage extension due to microcrack initiation contributes to the improvement of fracture toughness [10]. Relatively small values of K_C at high loading rates compared to those at low loading rates in Fig. 7 are probably due to fewer microcrack initiations during such a short duration of loading. The increase of K_C with an increase of loading rate in the high loading rate region suggests that the minimum time criterion [12] as reported for other materials such as polymethylmethacrylate can be applied to the onset of fracture in bone at high loading rates.

Conclusion

In vitro techniques for the determination of viscoelastic properties and fracture toughness of compact bone using the SHPB technique, DMA, and modified fracture toughness test have been briefly described. The reliability and feasibility of these techniques were validated through numerical simulation and experiments on bovine compact bone. Anisotropic and rate-dependent behaviour in viscoelastic parameters, Young's modulus, and the critical stress intensity factor were identified and discussed in conjunction with the microstructure and tendency for microscopic failure in bone. These findings should give us useful information for understanding the optimum microstructure of compact bone as well as contributing to the development of more sophisticated biomaterials such as bone-analogue materials. Construction or the reconstruction sequence of such novel microstructures is an exciting topic in bone biomechanics, and will be discussed in a future work.

References

1. Bonfield W (1991) Bioactive materials for bone replacement. Med Bio Eng Comput 29 (Suppl 1):47
2. Tanabe Y, Kobayashi K, Sakamoto M, Hara T, Takahashi HE (1994) Identification of the dynamic properties of bone using the split-Hopkinson pressure-bar technique. In: Kambic HE, Yokobori AT Jr (eds) Biomaterials' mechanical properties ASTM STP 1173. American Society for Testing and Materials, Philadelphia, pp 127–141
3. Lindholm US (1964) Some experiments with the split Hopkinson pressure bar. J Mech Phys Solids 12:317–335
4. Tanabe Y, Tanner KE, Bonfield W (1994) Dynamic mechanical analysis of bovine cortical bone (Abstract) Second World Cong Biomech, Amsteldam, The Netherlands, 1:45
5. Currey JD (1969) The relationship between the stiffness and the mineral content of bone. J Biomech 2:477–480
6. Bonfield W, Grynpas MD (1977) Anisotropy of Young's modulus of bone. Nature 270:453–454
7. Sasaki N, Matsushima N, Ikawa T, Yamamura H, Fukuda A (1989) Orientation of bone mineral and its role in the anisotropic mechanical properties of bone-transverse anisotropy. J Biomech 22:157–164
8. Komatsubara K, Tanabe Y, Hara T (1994) Effects of crack length and specimen thickness on fracture toughness of bone (Abstract) Second World Cong Biomech, Amsteldam, The Netherlands, 2:234
9. American Society for Testing and Materials (1993) Standard test method for plane strain fracture toughness testing of metallic materials. ASTM annual book of standards, section 3, designation E399-90, pp 509–539
10. Vashishth D, Trifonas J, Behiri JC, Bonfield W (1994) Secondary crack propagation in cortical bone. Proc 1994 Eng Sys Des Anal Conf 4:37–41
11. Tanabe Y, Tanner KE, Bonfield W (1996) Impact fracture toughness of bovine compact bone (in Japanese). J Jpn Soc Clin Biomech Relat Res 17:337–341
12. Homma H, Shockey DA, Murayama Y (1983) Response of cracks in structural materials to short pulse loads. J Mech Phys Solids 31:261–279

Development and Differentiation of Macrophages, Osteoclasts, and Dendritic Cells

MAKOTO NAITO, GO HASEGAWA, SHIGEO ITO, and YUSUKE EBE

Summary. Primitive macrophages appear in the yolk sac and fetal liver, migrate into other tissues, and differentiate into fetal macrophages. In adult mice, tissue macrophages are proliferating populations distinct from monocytes. After the depletion of macrophages by the administration of liposome-entrapped dichloro-methylene diphosphonate, the repopulation of affected macrophages appears to depend upon the increase of precursors in the liver and spleen. In mice homozygous for the osteopetrosis (*op*) mutation, the absence of macrophage colony-stimulating factor (M-CSF) activity results in various degrees of deficiency of monocytes, macrophages, and osteoclasts, but not of dendritic cells. The administration of M-CSF to *op/op* mice increased the number of macrophages and osteoclasts and induced bone remodeling. Dendritic cells were generated in cultures of bone marrow cells and mononuclear cells from peripheral blood in the presence of granulocyte/macrophage colony-stimulating factor. These results indicate that the development, differentiation, and proliferation of macrophages, osteoclasts, and dendritic cells are regulated by the tissue microenvironment, including the in situ production of macrophage growth factors in both fetal and adult life.

Key words. Macrophages, Osteoclasts, Dendritic cells, Macrophage colony-stimulating factor, Osteopetrotic mice

Introduction

It has been generally accepted that monocytes originate from precursor cells in the bone marrow, migrate into various tissues of the body, and differentiate into macrophages, osteoclasts, and dendritic cells [1]. It has been suggested that mono-cytes in the blood are direct precursors of macrophages and osteoclasts. Monocytes are differentiated via promonocytes from monoblasts originating in bone marrow [1]. Monoblasts are derived from macrophage colony-forming unit (CFU-M) originating from pluripotential myeloid hematopoietic stem cells. During ontogeny, however,

Second Department of Pathology, Niigata University School of Medicine, 1 Asahimachi-dori, Niigata 951-8510, Japan macrophages develop before the production of monocytes in the fetal hematopoietic tissues [2–4].

In adult animals, tissue macrophages are phenotypically and functionally heterogeneous populations and proliferate, suggesting that macrophages are a long-lived and self-proliferating population distinct from monocytes. Several macrophage growth factors have been shown to support the generation of heterogeneous macrophage populations in function and phenotypes. Osteopetrotic mice defective in the production of macrophage colony-stimulating factor (M-CSF) are a useful model with which to investigate the biological role of M-CSF in macrophage differentiation.

This chapter describes the development, differentiation, and proliferation of macrophages, osteoclasts, and dendritic cells based on studies of macrophage ontogeny, macrophage differentiation in *op/op* mice, and macrophage repopulation after macrophage depletion.

Macrophages in Ontogeny

In mammalian ontogeny, mononuclear cells showing immature ultrastructure and expressing macrophage antigen (designated as primitive macrophages) develop first in the yolk sac [2–7]. These immature cells rapidly differentiate into more mature macrophages (designated as fetal macrophages) [2–4]. Primitive macrophages migrate from the yolk sac to the hepatic hematopoiesis, colonize in the fetal liver [2–4], and differentiate into fetal macrophages in various tissues. The number of fetal macrophages increases with fetal days, and these cells gradually express peroxidase activity and antigens [2–4] corresponding to those of tissue macrophages in adult animals [8].

In the late stage of ontogeny, a few primitive/fetal macrophages enter the fetal thymus and express Ia antigens [9] and differentiate into interdigitating cells. Fetal macrophages also migrate to the subepidermal mesenchyme and enter the epidermis [10]. Such fetal macrophages express Ia antigens, exhibit a dendritic morphology, and differentiate into epidermal Langerhans cells [10]. These dendritic cell populations are considered to be a specifically differentiated subpopulation of the primitive/fetal macrophage population.

The yolk sac and fetal liver contain granulocyte/macrophage-colony-forming unit [CFU-GM], as well as mature macrophages. Although myeloid precursors are readily detectable during fetal development by colony-forming assays, the levels of granulopoiesis and monocytopoiesis are very low in the murine yolk sac. The development of the monocytic cell series is thought to be completed in the fetal mouse liver by the middle stage of hepatic hematopoiesis [2–4], suggesting that monocytes migrate into fetal tissues and differentiate into macrophages in the late fetal stage.

A number of growth factors appear to be responsible for regulating the macrophage differentiation and generation of heterogeneous populations in ontogeny. In the yolk sac and fetal liver, M-CSF is detected during fetal development [11]. The yolk sac and fetal liver may provide a microenvironment for the development, differentiation, and proliferation of macrophages by producing CSFs during the fetal period.

Macrophages, Osteoclasts, and Dendritic Cells in Adult Animals

Macrophage Heterogeneity and Growth Factors

Based on the mononuclear phagocyte system (MPS), monocyte-derived macrophages have no proliferative potential in tissues under a normal steady-state condition [1]. The lifespan of macrophages is 3.8–14.9 days in tissues [1]. In contrast, resident macrophages in adult as well as in fetal tissues share a proliferative capacity and survive by self-renewal in various experimental conditions [12–14]. In mice with monocytopenia induced by the administration of strontium-89 [14], the number of Kupffer cells was not reduced. The enhanced proliferation of Kupffer cells contributed to the maintenance of Kupffer cells. These results also support the notion that resident macrophages are an independent, self-sustaining, and slow-replicating cell population.

The production and differentiation of monocytes and macrophages are controlled by various growth factors, including interleukin (IL)-6, IL-3, GM-CSF, and M-CSF [15]. Among various CSFs, M-CSF is the most critical molecule for mediating the development and differentiation of macrophage populations. In colony-forming assays, a marked difference in morphological characteristics and in several functional properties has been recognized in each type of CSF-derived macrophage [15,16]. The in vivo roles of CSFs have been demonstrated clearly by producing mice with disrupted CSF genes. GM-CSF-deficient mice develop alveolar proteinosis in which surfactant lipids and proteins accumulate in the alveolar space [17], indicating defective alveolar macrophage differentiation and defective macrophage processing of surfactant in the lung. Mice with a homologous mutation in the coding region of the M-CSF gene (*op/op*) are characterized by an impairment in the differentiation of monocytes into macrophages and severe deficiencies of blood monocytes and tissue macrophages [18,19]. However, there are varying numbers of macrophages in different tissues. These M-CSF-independent macrophages are small and round in shape and ultrastructurally immature [19]. The development and differentiation of such M-CSF-independent macrophages are probably regulated by the effects of other factors, especially GM-CSF [20].

Osteoclasts

The *op/op* mouse was originally used as an animal model of osteopetrosis. The osteosclerotic changes in these mice are the result of the impairment of osteoclast development. The administration of M-CSF to *op/op* mouse improves or cures the osteosclerosis not only via differentiation and proliferation of the osteoclasts [21,22], but also via rapid proliferation, differentiation, and fusion of the preosteoclasts [23], indicating that M-CSF is a key factor for osteoclast differentiation.

In contrast to the biological significance of M-CSF in macrophage and osteoclast differentiation, it has been demonstrated that aged *op/op* mice undergo a hematopoietic recovery, progressive increases in the numbers of osteoclasts and macrophages, and a resolution of the osteopetrosis [24]. In our study, the bone marrow cavities were markedly reconstructed and marrow hematopoiesis was expanded in 1-year-old *op/op* mice [25]. Numbers of osteoclasts and bone marrow macrophages in aged *op/op* mice were increased. In contrast, the number of Kupffer cells in the liver did not increase with aging. These findings suggest that the bone marrow hematopoietic system has the capacity to use alternative osteoclast and macrophage differentiation mechanisms to compensate for the absence of M-CSF.

It was recently reported that osteopetrosis develops in mice in which the c-*fos* protooncogene was disrupted by homologous recombination. In these *fos*-knockout mice, however, the numbers of tissue macrophages were increased [26], indicating that *fos* is one of the key regulators of osteoclast and macrophage differentiation.

Dendritic Cells

Dendritic cells are a heterogeneous cell population exhibiting a dendritic morphology [27]. The nonlymphoid T cell-associated dendritic cell population includes Langerhans cells, interdigitating cells, indeterminate cells, and veiled cells. These cells are thought to participate in antigen transport to the skin, lymph nodes, and other lymphoid tissues. Indeterminate dendritic cells resemble Langerhans cells except that they are devoid of Birbeck granules. Langerhans cells, veiled cells, and interdigitating cells express major histocompatibility complex [MHC] class II [Ia] molecules, and function as antigen-presenting cells in the T cell-mediated immune response [27].

In the postnatal period, dendritic precursor cells are present in bone marrow [28] and circulate in peripheral blood [29]. GM-CSF appears to be an important cytokine for the viability, survival, and mobilization of dendritic cells [28–30]. It has been reported that bone marrow cell cultures containing GM-CSF and tumor necrosis factor-α generate dendritic cells with Birbeck granules [31].

As to the origin of dendritic cells, there are two conflicting views: (1) the dendritic cells are derived from monocytes [32] and (2) the precursor cells are not monocytic but derive from a pathway of myeloid cell differentiation [30]. Dendritic cells in the lymphoid tissues and skin are not defective in *op/op* mice with a total absence of functional M-CSF activity [33], whereas in cultures supplemented with GM-CSF and IL-4, dendritic cells were generated [34]. These findings support the possibility that dendritic cells under physiological conditions are differentiated from non-monocytic cells via a pathway distinct from that of MPS, and that their differentiation is not impaired by a lack of M-CSF activity. Monocyte-derived dendritic cells may play important roles in inflammatory conditions.

Conclusion

Macrophages, osteoclasts, and dendritic cells are thought to be derived from precursors in bone marrow and/or fetal hematopoietic organs (Fig. 1). The differentiation of these cell populations may be controlled by a complex mechanism including cytokines, CSFs, and adhesion molecules, leading to characteristic signal transduction for cell differentiation, proliferation, and activation.

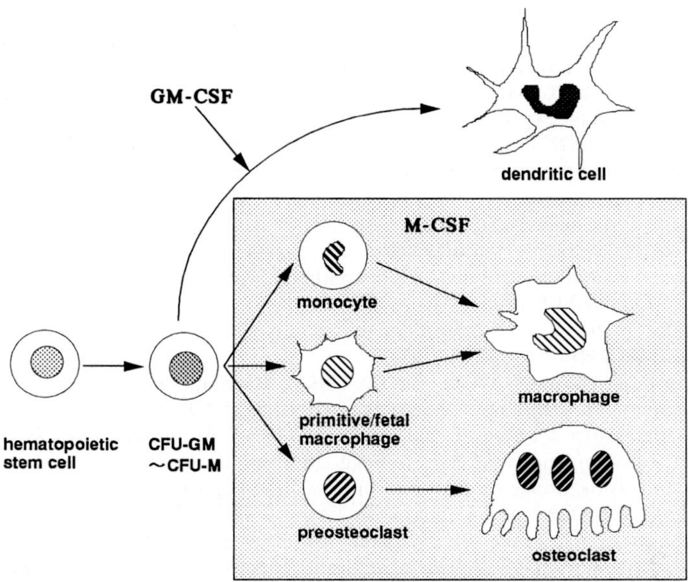

FIG. 1. Differentiation pathways of macrophages, osteoclasts, and dendritic cells. *CFU-GM*, granulocyte/macrophage colony-forming unit; *CFU-M*, macrophage colony-forming unit; *GM-CSF*, granulocyte/macrophage colony-stimulating factor; *M-CSF*, macrophage colony-stimulating factor

References

1. van Furth R (1989) Origin and turnover of monocytes and macrophages. Curr Top Pathol 79:125–147
2. Naito M, Takahashi K, Nishikawa S-I (1990) Development, differentiation, and maturation of macrophages in the fetal mouse liver. J Leukoc Biol 48:27–37
3. Naito M, Yamamura F, Nishikawa S-I, Takahashi K (1990) Development, differentiation, and maturation of fetal mouse yolk sac macrophages in cultures. J Leukoc Biol 46:1–10
4. Takahashi K, Yamamura F, Naito M (1989) Differentiation, maturation, and proliferation of macrophages in the mouse yolk sac: A light-microscopic, enzyme-cytochemical, immunohistochemical, and ultrastructural study. J Leukoc Biol 45:87–96
5. Cline MJ, Moore, MAS (1972) Embryonic origin of the mouse macrophages. Blood 39:842–849
6. Kelemen E, Calvo W, Fliedner TM (1979) Atlas of human hemopoietic development. Springer, Berlin, pp 1–224
7. Moore MAS, Metcalf D (1970) Ontogeny of the haemopoietic system: Yolk sac origin of in vivo and in vitro colony forming cells. Br J Haematol 18:279–296
8. Wisse E (1974) Observations on the fine structure and peroxidase cytochemistry of normal rat liver Kupffer cells. J Ultrastruct Res 46:393–426
9. Hsiao L, Takahashi K, Takeya M, Arao T (1991) Differentiation and maturation of macrophages into interdigitating cells and their multicellular complex formation in the fetal and neonatal rat thymus. Thymus 17:219–235

10. Hsiao L, Takeya M, Arao T, Takahashi K (1989) An immunohistochemical and immuno-electron microscopic study of the ontogeny of rat Langerhans cell lineage with anti-macrophage and anti-Ia monoclonal antibodies. J Invest Dermatol 93:780–786

11. Azoulay M, Webb CG, Sachs L (1987) Control of hematopoietic cell growth regulators during mouse fetal development. Mol Cell Biol 7:3361–3364

12. Rooijen NV, Kors N, Ende vd M, Dijkstra CD (1990) Depletion and repopulation of macrophages in spleen and liver of rat after intravenous treatment with liposome-encapsulated dichloromethylene diphosphonate. Cell Tissue Res 260:215–222

13. Yamamoto T, Naito M, Moriyama H, Umezu H, Matsuo H, Kiwada H, Arakawa M (1996) Repopulation of murine Kupffer cells after intravenous administration of liposome-encapsulated dichloromethylene diphosphonate. Am J Pathol 149:1271–1286

14. Naito M, Takahashi K (1991) The role of Kupffer cells in glucan-induced granuloma formation in the liver of mice depleted of blood monocytes by administration of strontium-89. Lab Invest 64:664–674

15. Rutherford MS, Witsell A, Schook LB (1993) Mechanisms generating functionally heterogeneous macrophages: chaos revisited. J Leukoc Biol 53:602–618

16. Morioka Y, Naito M, Sato T, Takahashi K (1994) Immunophenotypic and ultra-structural heterogeneity of macrophage differentiation in bone marrow and fetal hematopoiesis of mouse in vitro and in vivo. J Leukoc Biol 55:642–651

17. Dranoff G, Crawford AD, Sadelain M, Ream B, Rashid A, Bronson RT, Dickersin GR, Bachurski CJ, Mark EL, Whitsett JA, Mulligan RC (1994) Involvement of granulocyte-macrophage colony-stimulating factor in pulmonary homeostasis. Science 264:713–716

18. Yoshida H, Hayashi S-I, Kunisada T, Ogawa M, Nishikawa S, Okamura H, Sudo T, Shultz LD, Nishikawa S-I (1990) The murine mutation "osteopetrosis" (op) is a muta-tion in the coding region of the macrophage colony stimulating factor (Csfm) gene. Nature 345:442–443

19. Naito M, Hayashi S-I, Yoshida H, Nishikawa S-I, Shultz LD, Takahashi K (1991) Abnormal differentiation of tissue macrophage populations in "osteopetrosis" [op] mice defective in the production of macrophage colony-stimulating factor. Am J Pathol 139:657–667

20. Wiktor-Jedrzejczak W, Ansari AA, Sperl M, Urbanowska E (1992) Distinct in vivo func-tions of two macrophage subpopulations as evidenced by studies using macrophage-deficient op/op mouse. Eur J Immunol 22:1951–1954

21. Felix R, Cecchini MG, Fleisch H (1990) Macrophage colony stimulating factor restores in vivo bone resorption in the op/op osteopetrotic mouse. Endocrinology 127:2592–2594

22. Kodama H, Yamasaki A, Nose M, Nishida S, Ohgame Y, Abe M, Kumagawa M, Suda T (1991) Congenital osteoclast deficiency in osteopetrotic (op/op) mice is cured by injec-tions of macrophage colony-stimulating factor. J Exp Med 173:269–272

23. Umeda S, Takahashi K, Shultz LD, Naito M, Takagi K (1996) Effects of macrophage colony-stimulating factor (M-CSF) on macrophages and related cell populations in osteopetrosis (op) mouse defective in production of functonal M-CSF protein. Am J Pathol 149:559–574

24. Begg SK, Radley JM, Pollard JW, Chisholm OT, Stanley ER, Bertoncello I (1993) Delayed hematopoietic development in osteopetrotic (op/op) mice. J Exp Med 177:237–242

25. Umezu H, Hasegawa G, Takatsuka H, Ebe Y, Tokunaga K, Naito M, Shultz LD (1997) Bone reconstruction and crystal storage in bone marrow macrophages of aged osteopetrosis (op) mice. Dendritic Cells 7:43–46

26. Grigoriadis AE, Wang Z-Q, Cecchini MG, Hofstetter W, Felix R, Fleisch HA, Wagner EF (1994) c-Fos: A key regulator of osteoclast-macrophage lineage determination and bone remodeling. Science 266:443–448

27. Fossum S (1989) The life history of dendritic leukocytes (DL). Curr Top Pathol 79:101–124
28. Inaba K, Inaba M, Romani N, Aya H, Deguchi M, Ikehara S, Muramatsu S, Steinman RM (1992) Generation of large numbers of dendritic cells from mouse bone marrow cultures supplemented with granulocyte/macrophage colony-stimulating factor. J Exp Med 176:1693–1702
29. Inaba K, Steinman RM, Witmer-Pack M, Aya H, Inaba M, Sudo T, Wolpe W, Schler G (1992) Identification of proliferating dendritic cell precursors in mouse blood. J Exp Med 175:1157–1167
30. Steinman RM (1981) Dendritic Cells. Transplantation 31:151–155
31. Caux C, Dezutter-Dambuyant C, Schmitt D, Banchereau J (1992) GM-CSF and TNF-α cooperate in the generation of dendritic Langerhans cells. Nature 360:258–261
32. Hashimoto K, Tarnowski WM (1968) Some new aspects of the Langerhans cell. Arch Dermatol, 97:450–464
33. Takahashi K, Naito M, Shultz LD, Hayashi H, Nishikawa S (1993) Differentiation of dendritic cell populations in macrophage colony stimulating factor-deficient mice homozygous for the osteopetrosis (op) mutation. J Leukoc Biol 53:19–28
34. Akagawa KS, Takasuka N, Nozaki Y, Komuro I, Azuma M, Ueda M, Naito M, Takahashi K (1996) Generation of CD1+RelB+ dendritic cells and tartrate-resistant acid phosphatase-positive osteoclast-like multinucleated giant cells from human monocytes. Blood 88:4029–4039

Histomorphometric and Node-Strut Analysis of Effects of Exercise or Incadronate Disodium on hPTH (1–34)-Induced Bone Mass in Ovariectomized Rats

HIDEAKI E. TAKAHASHI, NORIAKI YAMAMOTO, YUICHI TAKANO,
TASUKU MASHIBA, TATSUHIKO TANIZAWA, NAOTO ENDO,
TORU UCHIYAMA, and AKEMI ITO

Summary. Intermittent administration of human parathyroid hormone (hPTH) (1–34) activates bone formation and increases cancellous bone mass in ovariectomized (OVX) rats. However, PTH-induced increases in cancellous bone volume rapidly decrease to the original levels after withdrawal of hPTH(1–34). Besides confirming that intermittent PTH administration increases cancellous bone mass, this study determined whether PTH-induced cancellous bone mass could be maintained by running exercise after PTH treatment was discontinued, whether a bisphosphonate, incadronate disodium (YM-175), could also maintain that bone, and, if so, whether that maintenance effect persisted after YM-175 withdrawal. Eleven-week-old Sprague-Dawley rats were OVX and hPTH (1–34), 30 μg/kg, was injected subcutaneously three times per week for 12 weeks, beginning 1 week after OVX in experiment 1, and for 8 weeks beginning 4 weeks after OVX in experiment 2. After withdrawal of PTH, treadmill exercise was done for the next 8 weeks (15.7 m/min, 1 h/day, 5 days/week), or YM-175, 10 μg/kg, was injected subcutaneously three times per week for 4 weeks. In the proximal tibial metaphysis, histomorphometric analysis with standard bone histomorphometry and node-strut analyses revealed that hPTH administration partially prevented OVX-induced cancellous bone loss. Eight weeks after PTH administration stopped, PTH-induced increases in cancellous bone mass had returned to the OVX/V (vehicle injection) level. Treadmill exercise helped to maintain the PTH-induced bone mass but did not increase bone mass in OVX control rats. YM-175 administration maintained the PTH-induced additions to tibial cancellous bone mass after PTH treatment stopped and even for 8 weeks after treatment with YM-175 had also stopped.

Key words. Ovariectomized rat, Human PTH (1–34), Physical exercise, Incadronate disodium, Histomorphometry

Department of Orthopedic Surgery, Niigata University School of Medicine, Niigata 951-8510, Japan

Introduction

Loss of bone occurs in involutional osteoporosis with aging and in disuse osteo-porosis due to mechanical unloading. The bone losses in these osteopenias depend on imbalances between bone formation and resorption that occur during bone modeling and remodeling. It has been shown that intermittent administration of human PTH (1–34) can increase bone formation and cancellous bone mass and prevent bone loss after ovariectomy in rats [1–8], dogs [9,10], and humans [11,12]. However, bone mass tends to fall to the original level several weeks or months after treatment with PTH stops [13]. We previously reported some effects of physical exercise [14] and a bisphosphonate, incadronate disodium (YM-175) [15], on the hPTH (1–34)-induced increase in bone mass, using standard his-tomorphometry. However the effects of physical exercise and of bisphosphonate on the microstructure of the hPTH-induced cancellous bone have not yet been studied.

Accordingly, this study compared the effects of ovariectomy, exercise, and the bis-phosphonate, incadronate disodium, on the maintenance of hPTH (1–34)-induced bone mass after treatment with PTH and bisphosphonate had stopped, using standard bone histomorphometry and node-strut analysis.

Materials and Methods

Animal Care and Study Protocol

One hundred forty-one 11-week-old Sprague-Dawley female rats (Charles River Japan Laboratories, Kanagawa, Japan) were used for the two experiments. The rats weighed approximately 250 g at the beginning of the experiments. They were housed in indi-vidual cages and fed a commercial standard diet (Oriental Yeast, Tokyo, Japan) that contained 1.2% calcium, 0.85% phosphorus, and 80 IU of vitamin D_3/100 g of diet. All rats were given food and water ad libitum throughout the experiments. Synthetic human PTH (1–34) at 30 μg/kg (Asahi Chemicals, Tokyo, Japan) was injected subcu-taneously three times per week. The hormone was prepared in a vehicle of acidified saline containing 0.1% bovine serum albumin (BSA). Vehicle injection was performed in the same manner.

Figure 1 outlines the design of both experiments.

Experiment 1

Fifty-three rats were divided into eight groups as follows: Group 1, OVX/V: ovariec-tomy (OVX), then vehicle (V) injection for 12 weeks. Group 2, OVX/PTH: OVX, then PTH injection for 12 weeks. Group 3, sham/V: sham operation, then vehicle injection for 12 weeks. Group 4, OVX/V/ex(−): OVX, then vehicle injection for the initial 12 weeks and no exercise for the final 8 weeks. Group 5, OVX/V/ex(+): OVX, then vehicle injection for the initial 12 weeks, and then treadmill exercise for the final 8 weeks. Group 6, OVX/PTH/ex(−): OVX, then PTH injection for initial 12 weeks, and no exer-cise for the final 8 weeks. Group 7, OVX/PTH/ex(+): OVX, then PTH injection for the initial 12 weeks, followed by treadmill exercise for the final 8 weeks. Group 8,

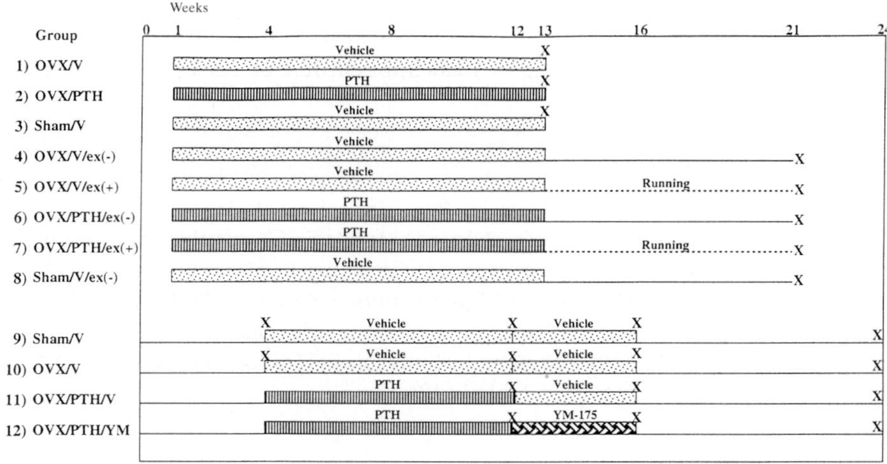

FIG. 1. Experimental design. Osteopenia was induced by ovariectomization (OVX) in the *OVX/V*, *OVX/PTH*, and *OVX/PTH/YM* groups. Ex(+) signifies treadmill exercise, and ex(−) means without it. Injection of PTH or vehicle was started 1 week after OVX in experiment 1 and 4 weeks after OVX in experiment 2. X shows time of sacrifice.

sham/V/ex(−): sham operation, vehicle injection for the initial 12 weeks, and no exercise for the final 8 weeks.

Both vehicle and PTH injections were started 1 week after ovariectomy or sham operation. The treadmill exercises were done at a speed of 15.7 m/min, 1 h/day, 5 days/week for 8 weeks in a motor-drive wheel treadmill with a wheel diameter of 0.5 m. The rats in groups 1–3 and 4–8 were sacrificed at 13 and 21 weeks after surgery, respectively. These rats were doubly labelled with calcein (3,3′-bis[N, N-di(carboxymethy)aminomethyl]-fluorescein; Wako Pure Chemical, Osaka, Japan), using 10 mg/kg administered subcutaneously according to a labeling schedule of 1-4-1-1 before sacrifice (Fig. 1).

Experiment 2

Eighty-eight rats were divided into four groups, which were numbered as sequential additions to the eight groups in experiment 1. Ovariectomy was performed in 60 rats and sham operation in 28 rats. All treatments started 4 weeks after sham operation or ovariectomy. The groups were as follows: Group 9, sham/V: sham operated, then vehicle was injected for the first 12 weeks and then stopped for the next 8 weeks. Group 10, OVX/V: OVX, then vehicle was injected for 12 weeks and stopped for the next 8 weeks. Group 11, OVX/PTH/V: OVX, then PTH was injected for the first 8 weeks, vehicle only was injected for the next 4 weeks, and no treatment was given for the final 8 weeks. Group 12, OVX/PTH/YM: OVX, then PTH was injected for the first 8 weeks, YM-175 was injected for another 4 weeks, and no treatment was given for the final 8 weeks. Incadronate disodium (YM-175), 10 μg/kg (Yamanouchi Pharmaceutical, Tokyo, Japan), was injected subcutaneously three times per week. Groups of 6 or 7 rats were sacrificed at 4, 12, 16, and 24 weeks after surgery after double labeling with subcutaneous injections of 20 mg/kg of oxytetracycline (Pfizer Laboratories, New York, NY, USA) and 6 mg/kg of calcein (Wako Pure Chemical, Osaka, Japan) according to a labeling schedule of 1-5-1-2 before sacrifice (Fig. 1).

Specimen Preparation

The left tibiae were removed, fixed in 70% ethanol for 1 day, and immersed in Villanueva bone staining solution for 7 days. Undecalcified 7-μm-thick sections in the frontal planes of the proximal tibiae were cut with a Jung-K microtome (Reichert Jung, Heidelberg, Germany). The standard bone histomorphometry [16] and node-strut analysis [17,18] were done, aided by a semiautomatic digitizing system (System Supply, Nagano, Japan). Standard bone histomorphometric nomenclatures, symbols, and units were used, as shown in Table 1 [19].

Statistics

All data are expressed as means ± standard error of the mean. In each experiment, a one-way analysis of variance (ANOVA) was performed among the group means within each time period. When the analysis of variance indicated significant differences among means, the differences were evaluated using the Fisher protected least significant difference (PLSD) test. A probability of less than 0.05 was considered significant.

Results

Effects on parameters of the standard bone histomorphometry and node-strut analysis of proximal tibial metaphysis were examined.

TABLE 1. Nomenclature and abbreviations of bone histomorphometric and node-strut analysis

Nomenclature	Variables	Unit
Bone volume	BV/TV	%
Osteoid surface	OS/BS	%
Eroded surface	ES/BS	%
Bone formation rate	BFR/BV	%
Bone formation rate	BFR/TV	%/year
Trabecular thickness	Tb.Th	μm
Trabecular number	Tb.N	N
Trabecular separation	Tb.Sp	μm
Node-to-node strut length	NdNd/TSL	%
Number of nodes	N.Nd/TSL	N/mm
Cortex-to-node strut length	CtNd/TSL	%
Terminus-to-terminus strut length	TmTm/TSL	%
Total strut length per tissue volume	TSL/TV	mm/mm^2
Number of nodes	N.Nd/TV	N/mm^2

Experiment 1 (Tables 2 and 3)

Effects of OVX. The BV/TV of the OVX/V group and the OVX/V/ex(−) group was significantly lower than that of the sham/V and sham/V/ex(−) groups at 13 and 21 weeks, respectively. The OS/BS of the OVX/V group and the OVX/V/ex(−) group was higher than that of the sham/V and sham/V/ex(−) groups, but the ES/BS of the OVX/V group was significantly higher than that of the sham/V group. The BFR/TV of the OVX/V group was significantly higher than that of the sham/V group. The Tb.Th and Tb.N of the OVX/V group were significantly lower than those of the sham/V group. The NdNd/TSL, N.Nd/TSL, TSL/TV, and N.Nd/TV of the OVX/V group were significantly lower than those of the sham/V group. The N.Nd/TSL, TSL/TV, and N.Nd/TV of the OVX/V/ex(−) group were significantly lower than those of the sham/V/ex(−) group.

Effects of PTH. The BV/TV of the OVX/PTH, OVX/PTH/ex(−), and OVX/PTH/ex(+) groups was significantly lower than that of the sham/V and sham/V/ex(−) groups at both 13 and 21 weeks. The OS/BS of the OVX/PTH group was significantly higher than that of the sham/V group at 13 weeks, but the values for the OVX/PTH/ex(−) group did not differ significantly from the values for the OVX/V/ex(−) group. The ES/BS of the OVX/PTH group was significantly higher than that of the sham/V group at 13 weeks, but did not differ significantly from the values for the OVX/V/ex(−) and OVX/PTH/ex(−) groups. The BFR/TV of the OVX/PTH was significantly higher than that of the OVX/V and sham/V groups. The Tb.Th and Tb.N of the OVX/PTH group were significantly higher than those of the OVX/V group. The NdNd/TSL, N.Nd/TSL,

TABLE 2. Data from 13-week groups in experiment 1

Group (N)		1 (6)	2 (6)	3 (6)	ANOVA
Variables	Unit	OVX/V	OVX/PTH	Sham/V	
BV/TV	%	10.4 ± 1.9**	18.0 ± 2.1**	30.2 ± 2.8	<0.0001
OS/BS	%	19.1 ± 2.3**	32.5 ± 1.9**	9.3 ± 2.0	<0.0001
ES/BS	%	9.8 ± 1.5**	10.2 ± 1.0*	3.3 ± 0.5	<0.0005
BFR/BV	%	435.0 ± 39.0**	599.8 ± 79.9**#	76.0 ± 14.8	<0.0001
BFR/TV	%/y	42.0 ± 5.2*	103.3 ± 11.4**	21.7 ± 3.5	<0.0001
Tb.Th	μm	100.2 ± 15.8**	131.5 ± 12.8##	132.0 ± 8.7	<0.001
Tb.N	N	3.7 ± 0.4**	4.9 ± 0.2**##	5.7 ± 0.24	<0.0001
Tb.Sp	μm	200.7 ± 37.1**	114.4 ± 8.9**	84.0 ± 8.5	<0.0001
NdNd/TSL	%	15.6 ± 3.8*	18.1 ± 4.2*	34.7 ± 7.2	NS‡
N.Nd/TSL	N/mm	0.8 ± 0.2*	0.6 ± 0.1**	1.5 ± 0.2	<0.01
CtNd/TSL	%	2.4 ± 1.1	6.3 ± 1.7#	5.8 ± 0.6	NS
TmTm/TSL	%	39.1 ± 6.8	40.1 ± 10.7	20.2 ± 4.7	NS
TSL/TV	mm/mm²	1.3 ± 0.2**	1.8 ± 0.2**	4.4 ± 0.4	<0.0001
N.Nd/TV	N/mm²	1.2 ± 0.4**	1.1 ± 0.3**	6.8 ± 1.5	<0.005

Values are means ± SE.

Different from the sham/V group: * $P < 0.05$. ** $P < 0.01$ ANOVA followed by post hoc (Fisher's PLSD) test.

Different from the OVX/V group: # $P < 0.05$. ## $P < 0.01$.

‡ Not significant.

TABLE 3. Data from 21-week groups in experiment 1

Group(N)		4 (7)	5 (7)	6 (7)	7 (7)	8 (7)	ANOVA
Variables	Unit	OVX/V/ex (−)	OVX/V/ex (+)	OVX/PTH/ex (−)	OVX/PTH/ex (+)	Sham/V/ex (−)	
BV/TV	%	9.1 ± 1.7**	11.4 ± 1.3**	12.9 ± 1.0**#	$17.8 \pm 1.0^{\#\#\S\S}$**††	26.5 ± 1.6	<0.0001
OS/BS	%	14.6 ± 1.6**	14.5 ± 1.6**	17.6 ± 1.3**	$29.3 \pm 2.2^{\#\#\S\S}$**††	8.0 ± 1.9	<0.0001
ES/BS	%	7.8 ± 0.6**	8.2 ± 0.7**	8.6 ± 1.6**	9.4 ± 0.8**	4.4 ± 0.8	<0.01
BFR/BV	%	197.0 ± 26.6*	264.4 ± 20.0**	$354.1 \pm 28.2^{\#\#\S}$	$485.7 \pm 48.1^{\#\#}$††	86.3 ± 19.0	<0.0001
BFR/TV	%/y	15.7 ± 1.2	29.9 ± 5.4	$45.1 \pm 4.7^{\S\S}$*	$88.1 \pm 13.4^{\#\#\S\S}$**†	20.6 ± 7.1	<0.0001
Tb.Th	μm	105.4 ± 13.6**	115.5 ± 15.2**	119.1 ± 16.8**	$126.0 \pm 19.5^{\#}$**	141.2 ± 12.3	<0.01
Tb.N	N	3.8 ± 0.4**	3.7 ± 0.4**	3.9 ± 0.5**	$4.6 \pm 0.3^{\#\#\S\S}$**††	5.5 ± 0.5	<0.0001
Tb.Sp	μm	192.3 ± 25.3**	195.2 ± 23.2**	175.9 ± 37.4**	$130.6 \pm 10.8^{\#\#\S\S}$**††	83.2 ± 13.0	<0.0001
NdNd/TSL	%	6.9 ± 2.3**	5.6 ± 3.2**	5.0 ± 4.0*	$19.5 \pm 4.2^{\#\#}$†**§	34.3 ± 4.8	<0.0001
N.Nd/TSL	N/mm	0.5 ± 0.1**	0.5 ± 0.2**	0.4 ± 0.2**	$0.9 \pm 0.1^{\#\#\S\S}$**††	2.0 ± 0.1	<0.0001
CtNd/TSL	%	2.0 ± 2.0	7.0 ± 3.5	5.8 ± 2.8	8.2 ± 1.9	5.3 ± 1.2	NS
TmTm/TSL	%	38.1 ± 5.7*	53.5 ± 9.7**	50.7 ± 7.0**	33.5 ± 5.0*§	13.4 ± 2.4	<0.05
TSL/TV	mm/mm^2	1.2 ± 0.2**	1.1 ± 0.3**	0.9 ± 0.2**	$2.1 \pm 0.2^{\#\#\S\S}$**††	4.1 ± 0.2	<0.0001
N.Nd/TV	N/mm^2	0.5 ± 0.1**	0.6 ± 0.3**	0.3 ± 0.1**	$2.0 \pm 0.3^{\#\#\S\S}$**††	6.6 ± 0.6	<0.0001

Values are means ± SE.

Different from OVX/V/ex (−): # $P < 0.05$, ## $P < 0.01$.

Different from OVX/V/ex (+): $^{\S} P < 0.05$, $^{\S\S} P < 0.01$.

Different from OVX/PTH/ex (−): † $P < 0.05$, †† $P < 0.01$.

Different from sham/V/ex (−): * $P < 0.05$, ** $P < 0.01$.

TSL/TV, and N.Nd/TV of the OVX/PTH group were significantly lower than those of the sham/V group but did not differ significantly in the OVX/PTH and OVX/V groups or in the OVX/PTH/ex(−) and OVX/V/ex(−) groups.

Effects of Exercise. The BV/TV, OS/BS, ES/BS, BFR/TV, Tb.Th, Tb.N, TSL/TV, and N.ND/TSL values did not differ significantly in the OVX/V/ex(−) and OVX/V/ex(+) groups.

Effects of PTH and Exercise. Eight weeks after PTH administration stopped, the BV/TV decreased significantly in the OVX/PTH/ex(−) group, but it was maintained in the OVX/PTH/ex(+) group as compared with the OVX/PTH group. The OS/BS and BFR/TV values were also maintained in the OVX/PTH/ex(+) group, but they decreased to the level of the OVX/V group in the OVX/PTH/ex(−) group. The Tb.Th and Tb.N values of the OVX/PTH/ex(+) group were significantly higher than those for the OVX/PTH/ex(−) group. The TSL/TV, N.Nd/TSL, and NdNd/TSL values were maintained in the OVX/PTH/ex(+) group, but they decreased to the level of the OVX/V group in the OVX/PTH/ex(−) group.

Experiment 2 (Tables 4–7)

Effects of OVX. The BV/TV of the OVX group was significantly lower than that of the sham group, and the OS/BS of the OVX group was significantly higher than that of the sham group at 4, 8, 12, and 24 weeks after OVX. The BFR/BV was significantly higher than that of the sham group at 4, 12, and 24 weeks. The Tb.N of the OVX/V group was significantly lower than that of the sham/V group at 4, 12, 16, and 24 weeks. The TSL/TV of the OVX group was significantly lower than that of the sham group at

TABLE 4. Data from 4-week groups in experiment 2

Group (N)		9 (7)	10 (6)	ANOVA
Variable	Unit	Sham/V	OVX/V	
BV/TV	%	17.1 ± 2.1	6.8 ± 0.8**	<0.001
OS/BS	%	18.0 ± 3.6	43.7 ± 3.0**	<0.0001
ES/BS	%	7.2 ± 2.0	12.4 ± 2.9	NS§
BFR/BV	%/yr	212.5 ± 49.5	781.4 ± 165.4**	<0.01
BFR/TV	%/yr	34.9 ± 10.1	50.3 ± 7.4	NS
Tb.Th	μm	56.3 ± 2.8	51.4 ± 3.4	NS
Tb.N	N	3.0 ± 0.3	1.3 ± 0.1**	<0.0005
Tb.Sp	μm	310.5 ± 55.4	749.0 ± 61.5**	<0.0005
NdNd/TSL	%	19.2 ± 2.3	4.2 ± 1.6**	<0.01
N.Nd/TSL	N/mm	1.0 ± 0.1	0.3 ± 0.1**	<0.0001
Ct.Nd/TSL	%	6.1 ± 2.9	6.1 ± 2.8	NS
TmTm/TSL	%	35.6 ± 2.4	60.9 ± 5.7**	<0.01
TSL/TV	mm/mm²	3.0 ± 0.2	1.2 ± 0.1**	<0.0001
N.Nd/TV	N/mm²	2.8 ± 0.2	0.3 ± 0.1**	<0.0001

Values are means ± SE.

Different from the sham/V group: * $P < 0.05$, ** $P < 0.01$ ANOVA followed by post hoc (Fisher's PLSD) test.

§ Not significant.

TABLE 5. Data from 12-week groups in experiment 2

Group (N)		9 (7)	10 (6)	11 (7)	ANOVA
Variable	Unit	Sham/V	OVX/V	OVX/PTH/V	
BV/TV	%	29.5 ± 2.1	9.0 ± 1.9**	25.3 ± 2.9[##]	<0.001
OS/BS	%	5.8 ± 1.9	31.3 ± 7.4**	41.1 ± 4.2**	<0.0005
ES/BS	%	5.2 ± 1.4	9.9 ± 2.1*	7.7 ± 0.7	NS
BFR/BV	%/yr	38.4 ± 13.9	219.6 ± 70.2*	592.0 ± 67.1**[##]	<0.0001
BFR/TV	%/yr	10.4 ± 3.7	14.4 ± 4.5	153.0 ± 28.6**[##]	<0.0001
Tb.Th	μm	68.5 ± 2.4	62.1 ± 4.6	85.8 ± 3.6**[##]	<0.001
Tb.N	N	4.4 ± 0.4	1.5 ± 0.3**	2.9 ± 0.3**[##]	<0.0001
Tb.Sp	μm	176.4 ± 22.0	847.7 ± 207.4*	272.3 ± 31.9[##]	<0.005
NdNd/TSL	%	44.5 ± 6.1	9.0 ± 3.0**	26.3 ± 6.4[#]*	<0.005
N.Nd/TSL	N/mm	1.7 ± 0.2	0.6 ± 0.2**	1.0 ± 0.2*	<0.005
Ct.Nd/TSL	%	2.8 ± 1.3	3.8 ± 1.3	4.6 ± 2.2	NS
TmTm/TSL	%	12.8 ± 3.9	49.4 ± 10.9*	31.1 ± 7.9	<0.05
TSL/TV	mm/mm^2	4.6 ± 0.5	1.3 ± 0.3**	2.6 ± 0.4[#]	<0.0005
N.Nd/TV	N/mm^2	8.3 ± 1.6	0.9 ± 0.3**	2.7 ± 2.7*	<0.01

Values are means ± SE.
Different from the sham/V group: * $P < 0.05$, ** $P < 0.01$.
Different from the OVX/V group: [#] $P < 0.05$, [##] $P < 0.01$.

4, 8, 12, and 24 weeks after OVX. The N.Nd/TSL and Tm.Tm/TSL of the OVX group were significantly lower than those of the sham group.

Effects of PTH. During PTH administration, the BV/TV of the OVX/PTH group significantly increased as compared with the OVX group. The OS/BS of the OVX/PTH group at 12 weeks maintained the same level as that of the OVX group at 4 weeks but was higher than that at 12 weeks. The BFR/TV of the OVX/PTH group at 12 weeks was significantly higher than that of any other group at 12 weeks. The Tb.Th and Tb.N of the OVX/PTH/V group were significantly higher than those of the OVX/V group at 12, 16, and 24 weeks. The TSL/TV of the OVX/PTH group increased during PTH administration and decreased after treatment with the drug stopped, at the same rate as in the sham group. N.Nd/TSL revealed the same trend as TSL/TV during and after PTH administration.

Effects of YM-175. The BV/TV of the OVX/PTH/YM group was maintained at 16 weeks as compared with that of the OVX/PTH group before administration of YM-175 at 12 weeks. The OS/BS and BFR/TV of the OVX/PTH/YM group decreased nearly to zero at 16 weeks. No significant difference in Tb.Th, Tb.N, and Tb.Sp was shown between the OVX/PTH/V and OVX/PTH/YM groups at 16 weeks. The TSL/TV and N.Nd/TSL of the OVX/PTH/YM group revealed no significant changes when compared with the OVX/PTH group at 16 weeks.

Effects at 24 Weeks of Withdrawal of PTH and YM-175. The BV/TV in the OVX/PTH/YM group (this was 8 weeks after treatment with YM-175 stopped) was maintained. Its values were significantly higher than in the OVX/V and OVX/PTH/V groups.

TABLE 6. Data from 16-week groups in experiment 2

Group (N)		9 (7)	10 (6)	11 (7)	12 (7)	ANOVA
Variable	Unit	Sham/V	OVX/V	OVX/PTH/V	OVX/PTH/YM	
BV/TV	%	30.6 ± 3.2	$8.7 \pm 1.5^{**}$	$19.9 \pm 1.7^{**\#\#}$	$22.5 \pm 3.1^{*\#\#}$	<0.0001
OS/BS	%	10.1 ± 3.5	$26.5 \pm 3.6^{**}$	$15.4 \pm 3.7^{\#}$	$0.7 \pm 0.1^{*\#\#\dagger\dagger}$	<0.0001
ES/BS	%	8.8 ± 0.9	$15.1 \pm 1.4^{*}$	$14.1 \pm 1.4^{**}$	$9.4 \pm 1.0^{\#\#\dagger}$	<0.05
BFR/BV	%/yr	66.2 ± 30.6	$142.2 \pm 23.7^{*}$	81.4 ± 24.3	$1.5 \pm 0.6^{\#\#\dagger}$	<0.01
BFR/TV	%/yr	17.6 ± 7.3	13.5 ± 3.8	15.2 ± 4.3	$0.3 \pm 0.1^{*\dagger}$	NS
Tb.Th	μm	63.7 ± 3.4	70.1 ± 3.8	$82.7 \pm 2.9^{**\#\#}$	$80.6 \pm 4.1^{**\#}$	<0.005
Tb.N	N	4.8 ± 0.3	$1.2 \pm 0.2^{**}$	$2.4 \pm 0.2^{**\#\#}$	$2.6 \pm 0.3^{**\#\#}$	<0.0001
Tb.Sp	μm	151.0 ± 14.5	$889.7 \pm 178.0^{**}$	$366.0 \pm 44.0^{\#\#}$	$340.6 \pm 51.7^{\#\#}$	<0.0001
NdNd/TSL	%	40.7 ± 6.8	$6.8 \pm 4.2^{*}$	30.8 ± 9.6	24.5 ± 8.3	<0.05
N.Nd/TSL	N/mm	1.7 ± 0.7	$0.7 \pm 0.2^{**}$	$1.1 \pm 0.2^{*}$	$0.9 \pm 0.2^{*}$	<0.05
Ct.Nd/TSL	%	4.6 ± 1.7	1.7 ± 1.1	7.9 ± 3.9	$10.8 \pm 2.9^{\#\dagger\dagger*}$	<0.01
TmTm/TSL	%	15.1 ± 42.1	$42.1 \pm 8.0^{**}$	$19.7 \pm 5.6^{\#}$	27.0 ± 7.0	<0.05
TSL/TV	mm/mm^2	4.1 ± 0.9	$0.89 \pm 0.1^{**}$	$2.2 \pm 0.4^{\#\#}$	$2.2 \pm 0.55^{**}$	<0.01
N.Nd/TV	N/mm^2	7.5 ± 1.9	$0.7 \pm 0.3^{*}$	$2.5 \pm 1.0^{*}$	$2.3 \pm 1.3^{*}$	<0.01

Values are means $\pm$ SE.
Different from the sham/V group: $^{*} P < 0.05$, $^{**} P < 0.01$.
Different from the OVX/V group: $^{\#} P < 0.05$, $^{\#\#} P < 0.01$.
Different from the OVX/PTH/V group: $^{\dagger} P < 0.05$, $^{\dagger\dagger} P < 0.01$.

TABLE 7. Data from 24-week groups in experiment 2

Group (N)		9 (7)	10 (6)	11 (7)	12 (7)	ANOVA
Variable	Unit	Sham/V	OVX/V	OVX/PTH/V	OVX/PTH/YM	
BV/TV	%	24.9 ± 1.1	$8.4 \pm 1.0^{**}$	$12.6 \pm 1.5^{**}$	$24.9 \pm 2.3^{\#\#\dagger\dagger}$	<0.0001
OS/BS	%	5.1 ± 0.9	$17.2 \pm 2.6^{**}$	$23.1 \pm 3.3^{**}$	$1.1 \pm 0.4^{\#\#\dagger\dagger}$	<0.0001
ES/BS	%	3.8 ± 0.2	$11.3 \pm 1.4^{**}$	$9.9 \pm 1.0^{**}$	$9.1 \pm 1.5^{**}$	<0.0005
BFR/BV	%/yr	42.0 ± 3.7	$178.8 \pm 41.3^{**}$	$117.9 \pm 30.5^{**}$	$1.5 \pm 0.9^{\#\#\dagger\dagger}$	<0.0005
BFR/TV	%/yr	10.3 ± 0.9	14.0 ± 2.5	13.5 ± 3.7	$0.3 \pm 0.2^{**\#\#\dagger\dagger}$	<0.0005
Tb.Th	µm	57.1 ± 0.8	$67.9 \pm 3.0^{**}$	$76.5 \pm 3.8^{**\#}$	$82.3 \pm 2.7^{**\#\#}$	<0.0001
Tb.N	N	4.4 ± 0.2	$1.2 \pm 0.1^{**}$	$1.5 \pm 0.1^{**}$	$3.0 \pm 0.3^{**\#\#\dagger\dagger}$	<0.0001
Tb.Sp	µm	176.0 ± 11.8	$802.5 \pm 115.1^{**}$	$591.1 \pm 52.9^{**\#}$	$263.2 \pm 35.6^{\#\#\dagger\dagger}$	<0.0001
NdNd/TSL	%	30.7 ± 5.6	$1.7 \pm 1.7^{**}$	15.0 ± 7.8	18.5 ± 6.9	<0.05
N.Nd/TSL	N/mm	1.2 ± 0.1	$0.2 \pm 0.1^{**}$	$0.6 \pm 0.2^{*}$	$1.0 \pm 0.3^{\#\#}$	<0.01
Ct.Nd/TSL	%	6.9 ± 1.9	10.0 ± 6.0	0.6 ± 0.6	6.3 ± 3.1	NS
TmTm/TSL	%	26.4 ± 5.7	52.2 ± 11.5	48.3 ± 10.8	25.7 ± 7.5	NS
TSL/TV	mm/mm^2	3.1 ± 0.1	$0.8 \pm 0.2^{**}$	$1.5 \pm 0.3^{\#\#**}$	2.7 ± 0.3	<0.0001
N.Nd/TV	N/mm^2	4.0 ± 0.6	$0.2 \pm 0.2^{**}$	$0.9 \pm 0.4^{**}$	$2.8 \pm 0.9^{\#\#}$	<0.01

Values are means ± SE.
Different from the sham/V group: $^*P < 0.05$, $^{**}P < 0.01$.
Different from the OVX/V group: $^{\#}P < 0.05$, $^{\#\#}P < 0.01$.
Different from the OVX/PTH/V group: $^{\dagger}P < 0.05$, $^{\dagger\dagger}P < 0.01$.

The OS/BS and BFR/TV of the OVX/PTH/YM group remained nearly at zero. The Tb.Th and Tb.N of the OVX/PTH/YM group were significantly higher than those of the OVX/PTH/V group. The TSL/TV and N.Nd/TSL values for the OVX/PTH/YM group were maintained and were higher than those of the OVX/V and OVX/PTH/V groups.

Discussion

Intermittent administration of hPTH (1–34) increases bone formation and cancellous bone mass in animals [1–10] and humans [11,12]. Yet, continuous infusion of hPTH (1–34) caused a dose-dependent decrease in dry-weight bone mass and a hyperparathyroid-like condition in the high-dose group [20].

The effective dose and frequency ranges of hPTH (1–34) administration in rats are 1.5–6.0 µg/kg/day three times per week [4,7] and 40–80 µg/kg/day [1,6,8,21–23]. We selected intermittent administration of 30 µg/kg/day three times per week in both experiments, since the dose and frequency were known to increase the cancellous bone mass of the proximal tibia of the rats [14,15].

Although intermittent administration of hPTH(1–34) markedly increased trabecular bone mass, the bone mass rapidly decreased to the original level after PTH treatment stopped [14,15,22]. The same phenomenon occurred after the withdrawal of prostaglandin E_2 (PGE_2) treatment of bone [24].

Physical exercise can maintain and sometimes even increase bone mass [25,26]. In experiment 1, after 8 weeks of treadmill exercise in the OVX/V/ex(+) group, trabecular bone volume did not increase as compared with the OVX/V group. Perhaps our exercise program was relatively mild, although the heart rate of the rats increased immediately after exercise. The treadmill exercise did help to maintain the bone volume in the OVX/PTH/ex(+) group. It also seemed to help to maintain increased bone formation, trabecular number, and trabecular connectivity after treatment with hPTH (1–34) stopped. More intense exercise increased bone mass in OVX rats, and gymnasts exhibited higher bone mass than runners [26], although they had a similar prevalence of amenorrhea and oligomenorrhea [27], just as weight lifters had more bone than marathon runners [28]. The intensity (speed) of experiment 1 may not increase bone modeling, which responds to the largest bone strains and only helps to keep existing bone, which was induced by hPTH (1–34).

Existing bone volume may be maintained by suppressing BMU-based bone remodeling. The bisphosphonate, incadronate disodium (YM-175), did maintain PTH-induced increases in tibial cancellous bone volume, and it did markedly decrease both bone formation and resorption at 16 and 24 weeks after ovariectomy. Estrogen and diphosphonate treatment prevented cancellous bone loss in OVX rats by decreasing bone remodeling [5,29,30]. The tibial cancellous bone volume was maintained with decrease of both bone resorption and bone formation. The bone formation rate in the OVX/PTH/YM group was almost zero at 16 and 24 weeks. Since BV/TV, trabecular number, and connectivity showed no change from 16 to 24 weeks, that means the bone resorption was almost completely suppressed.

Bone remodeling is essential in the repair of microcracks and microfractures, both of which presumably represent effects of microscopic fatigue damage or micro-damage in bone. The protective effect on bone mass of the bisphosphonate persisted for at least 8 weeks after it was stopped. Further study of the dose, dose interval, and duration of bisphosphonate administration are needed to evaluate any effects on that repair.

In summary, our results indicate that intermittent treatment with hPTH (1–34) can fully restore tibial cancellous bone volume in female rats after ovariectomy. After that treatment stops, the added bone is removed, but both bisphosphonate YM-175 and treadmill running could minimize that loss and help to keep the added bone in OVX rats.

Acknowledgments. We thank Dr. Masayuki Hori of Asahi Chemical (Tokyo, Japan) for providing hPTH (1–34) and Dr. Ryuhei Fujimoto of Yamanouchi Pharmaceutical (Tokyo, Japan) for providing YM175. We also thank Mr. Hideki Akazawa for embedding and sectioning the bone specimens and Ms. Takako Homma for preparing this manuscript.

References

1. Gunness-Hey M, Hock JM (1984) Increased trabecular bone mass in rats treated with human synthetic parathyroid hormone. Metab Bone Dis Rel Res 5:177–181
2. Hefti E, Trechsel U, Bonjour JP, Fleisch H, Shenk R (1982) Increase of whole body calcium and skeletal mass in normal and osteopenic adult rats treated with parathyroid hormone. Clin Sci 62:389–396
3. Hock JM, Gera I, Fronseca J, Raisz LG (1988) Human parathyroid hormone-(1–34) increases bone mass in ovariectomized and orchidectomized rats. Endocrinology 122:2899–2904
4. Hori M, Uzawa T, Morita H, Noda T, Takahashi H, Inoue J (1988) Effect of human parathyroid hormone [(PTH(1–34)] on experimental osteopenia of rats induced by ovariectomy. Bone Miner 3:193–199
5. Shen V, Dempster DW, Mellish RW, Birchman R, Horbert W, Lindsay R (1992) Effects of combined and separate intermittent administration of low-dose human hormone fragment (1–34) and 17β estradiol on bone histomorphometry in ovariectomized rats with established osteopenia. Calcif Tissue Int 50:214–220
6. Tada K, Yamamuro T, Okumura H, Kasai R, Takahashi H (1990) Restoration of axial and appendicular bone volumes by h-PTH (1–34) in parathyroidectomized and osteopenic rats. Bone 11:163–169
7. Takahashi HE, Tanizawa T, Hori M, Uzawa T (1991) Effect of intermittent administation of human parathyroid hormone (1–34) on experimental osteopenia of rats induced by ovariectomy. Cells Mater (Suppl)1:113–117
8. Wronski TJ, Yen CF, Qi H, Dann LM (1993) Parathyroid hormone is more effective than estrogen or bisphosphonates for restoration of lost bone mass in ovariectomized rats. Endocrinology 132:823–831
9. Inoue J (1985) Bone changes with long term administration of low dose 1–34 human PTH on adult beagles. J Jpn Orthop Assoc 59:409–427
10. Podbesek R, Edouard C, Meunier PJ, Parsons JA, Reeve J, Stevenson RW, Zanelli JM (1983) Effects of two treatment regimes with synthetic human parathyroid hormone fragment on bone formation and the tissue balance of trabecular bone in greyhounds. Endocrinology 112:1000–1006
11. Hesch RD, Bruch U, Prokop M, Delling G, Rittinghaus EF (1989) Increase of vertebral density by combination therapy with pulsatile 1–38hPTH and sequential

addition of calcitonin nasal spray in osteoporotic patients. Calcif Tissue Int 44:176–180

12. Slovik D, Rosenthal DI, Doppelt SH, Potts JT Jr, Daly MA, Campbell JA, Neer RM (1986) Restoration of spinal bone in osteoporotic men by treatment with human parathyroid hormone (1–34) and 1,25-dihydroxyvitamine D. J Bone Miner Res 1:377–381

13. Gunness-Hey M, Hock JM (1989) Loss of the anabolic effect of parathyroid hormone on bone after discontinuation of hormone in rats. Bone 10:447–452

14. Yamamoto N, Takahahashi HE, Tanizawa T, Fujimoto R, Hara T, Tanaka S (1993) Maintenance of bone mass by physical exercise after discontinuation of intermittent hPTH (1–34) administration. Bone Miner 23:333–342

15. Takano Y, Tanaizawa T, Mashiba T, Endo N, Nishida S, Takahashi HE (1996) Maintaining bone mass by bisphosphonate incadronate disodium (YM175) sequential treatment after discontinuation of intermittent human parathyroid hormone (1–34) administration in ovariectomized rats. J Bone Miner Res 11:169–177

16. Frost HM (1983) Bone histomorphometry: choice of marking agent and labeling schedule. In: Recker RR (ed) Bone histomorphometry: techniques and interpretation. CRC Press, Boca Raton, FL, USA, pp 37–52

17. Garrahan NJ, Mellish RW, Compston JE (1986) A new method for the two-dimensional analysis of bone structure in human iliac crest biopsies. J Microsc 142:341–349

18. Mellish RW, Ferguson-Pell MW, Cochran GV, Lindsay R, Dempster DW (1991) A new manual method for assessing two-dimensional cancellous bone structure: comparison between iliac crest and lumbar vertebra. J Bone Miner Res 6:689–696

19. Parfitt AM, Drezner MK, Glorieux FH, Kanis JA, Malluche H, Meunier PJ, Ott SM, Recker RR (1987) Bone histomorphometry: standardization of nomenclature symbols, and units. Report of the ASBMR Histomorphometry Nomenclature Committee. J Bone Miner Res 6:595–610

20. Malluche HH, Sherman D, Meyer W, Ritz E, Norman AW, Massry SG (1982) Effects of long-term infusion of physiologic doses of 1–34 PTH on bone. Am J Physiol 242:F197–F201

21. Gera I, Hock JM, Gunness-Hey M, Fonseca J, Raisz LG (1987) Indomethacin does not inhibit the anabolic effect of parathyroid hormone on the long bones of rats. Calcif Tissue Int 40:206–211

22. Gunness-Hey M, Gera I, Fonseca J, Raisz LG, Hock JM (1988) 1,25 dihydroxyvitamin D_3 alone or in combination with parathyroid hormone does not increase bone mass in young rats. Calcif Tissue Int 43:284–288

23. Liu CC, Kalu DN, Salerno E, Echion R, Hollis BW, Ray M (1991) Preexisting bone loss associated with ovariectomy in rats is reversed by parathyroid hormone. J Bone Miner Res 6:1071–1080

24. Jee WSS, Lin BY, Ke HZ (1995) Extra cancellous bone induced by combined prostaglandin E_2 and risedronate administration is maintained after their withdrawal in older female rats. J Bone Miner Res 10:963–970

25. Yeh JK, Liu CC, Aloia JF, Foto A (1991) Effect of treadmill exercise and ovariectomy on femoral and lumbar vertebrae in young and adult rats. Cell Mater (Suppl) 1:159–166

26. Iwamoto J, Takeda T, Ichimura S (1998) Effect of exercise on tibial and lumbar vertebrae bone mass in mature osteopenic rats: bone histomorphometry study. J Orthop Sci 3:257–263

27. Robinson TL, Snow-Harter C, Taaffe DR, Gillis D, Shaw J, Marcus R (1995) Gymnasts exhibit higher bone mass than runners despite similar prevalence of amenorrhea and oligomenorrhea. J Bone Miner Res 10:26–35

28. Frost HM (1997) Why do marathon runners have less bone than weight lifters? A vital-biomechanical view and explanation. Bone 20:183–189

29. Wronski TJ, Dann LM, Scott KS, Crooke LR (1989) Endocrine and phamacological suppressors of bone turnover protect against osteopenia in ovariectomized rats. Endocrinology 125:810–816
30. Wronski TJ, Yen CF, Scott KS (1991) Estrogen and diphosphonate treatment provide long-term protection against osteopenia in ovariectomized rats. J Bone Miner Res 6:387–394

Human Parathyroid Hormone (1–34) Increases Cortical Bone Mass by Activating Bone Modeling in the Formation Mode in Ovariectomized Rats

Liu Zhang, Hideaki E. Takahashi, Tatsuhiko Tanizawa, Naoto Endo, and Noriaki Yamamoto

Summary. The purpose of this study was to determine the efficacy of human parathyroid hormone, hPTH (1-34), in augmenting cortical bone mass in ovariectomized (OVX) growing rats. Thirty 11-week-old female Sprague-Dawley rats were divided into five groups of six animals each. Ovariectomy was performed on 18 rats and 12 rats were subjected to sham surgery. All rats were left untreated for the 4 weeks postsurgery. At the end of pretreatment period, groups of baseline sham (Group 1) and OVX (Group 2) rats were killed. The remaining rats were divided into three groups and each treated as follows. Sham-operated rats (Group 3) and ovariectomized rats (Group 4) were injected with saline vehicle. Ovariectomized rats (Group 5) were injected with hPTH (1-34), $30\,\mu\text{g/kg}$, five times per week. All treatments were initiated at 4 weeks postsurgery for a 4-week period. To classify the effects of PTH on cortical bone modeling and remodeling during the treatment period, the PTH-treated group was injected subcutaneously with oxytetracycline just prior to the initiation of the PTH treatment. All animals were double-labeled with subcutaneous injections of calcein on day 6 and day 2 before euthanization. Cross sections of the tibial diaphysis were subjected to quantitative bone histomorphometry. PTH treatment of OVX rats (Group 5) increased cortical bone area and width, tended to decrease the bone marrow area, and did not significantly increase the endocortical resorbing surface compared to the vehicle-treated OVX rats. PTH administration in the OVX rats increased cortical bone by the addition of new circumferential bone on both the periosteal and endocortical surfaces by stimulating osteoblastic recruitment; the newly formed bone was lamellar in nature. PTH administration activated cortical bone modeling in the formation mode (activation-formation) on either the periosteal or endocortical envelopes. The present data indicate that PTH stimulated cortical bone modeling in the formation mode and augmented cortical bone mass in the tibial diaphysis of OVX rats. These findings are in agreement with previous observations

Department of Orthopaedic Surgery, Niigata University School of Medicine, 1 Asahimachi-dori, Niigata 951-8510, Japan that dogs and humans respond similarly to PTH, suggesting that PTH administration may be a useful anabolic agent in the prevention and treatment of postmenopausal osteoporosis.

Key words. Parathyroid hormone, Cortical bone, Modeling, Remodeling, Bone formation

Introduction

It has been reported that intermittent administration of PTH stimulated bone formation and increased cancellous bone mass in experimental animals [1–7] and osteoporotic patients [8,9,10]. These studies have demonstrated the anabolic effects of PTH on cancellous bone. However, the effect of PTH on cortical bone is still not well understood. In osteoporotic humans, PTH substantially stimulates iliac and vertebral trabecular bone formation, but it causes a small but significant loss of cortical bone [11,12]. Other studies in hyperparathyroid- and PTH-treated patients have not demonstrated a reduction in cortical bone [8,9,13]. Cortical bone loss was not observed in animals treated with high doses of PTH [14–16].

There is general agreement that the tibial shaft of a rat is a reproducible site for histomorphometry [16–19]. The periosteal envelope provides a site for evaluation of bone modeling in the formation mode (formation drift). The endocortical envelope is much more complex with parts modeling in the formation mode (formation drift) and parts modeling in the resorption mode (resorption drift) [20]. It is important to understand the effect of PTH administration on the tissue activities of modeling and remodeling in these two envelopes.

The objectives of the present study were (1) to clarify the modeling and remodeling effect of PTH on the periosteal and endocortical envelopes, (2) to determine the amount of newly added cortical bone at subperiosteal and subendocortical area by PTH administration, (3) to identify the quality of PTH-induced new bone (lamellar or woven), and (4) to determine whether PTH treatment induces cortical osteopenia.

Materials and Methods

Animal Care and Study Protocol

Thirty 11-week-old female Sprague-Dawley rats (Charles River Japan Laboratories, Kanagawa, Japan) were used in the experiment. The animals weighed approximately 250 g at the beginning of the experiment. They were acclimatized to local vivarium conditions (at 22°C with a 12-hour light/12-hour dark cycle) for two weeks. The rats were housed in individual cages and were fed a pelleted commercial standard diet which contained 1.2% calcium and 0.85% phosphorus and 80 IU vitamin D_3/100 g (Oriental Yeast, Tokyo, Japan). All rats were given food and water ad libitum during the experimental period.

Synthetic human PTH (1-34) (Asahi Chemical Industry, Shizuoka, Japan) was prepared in a vehicle of acidified saline containing 0.1% bovine serum albumin.

The animals were divided into five groups of six animals each (Fig. 1). Bilateral ovariectomies (OVX) were performed on 18 rats through a dorsal approach. Twelve

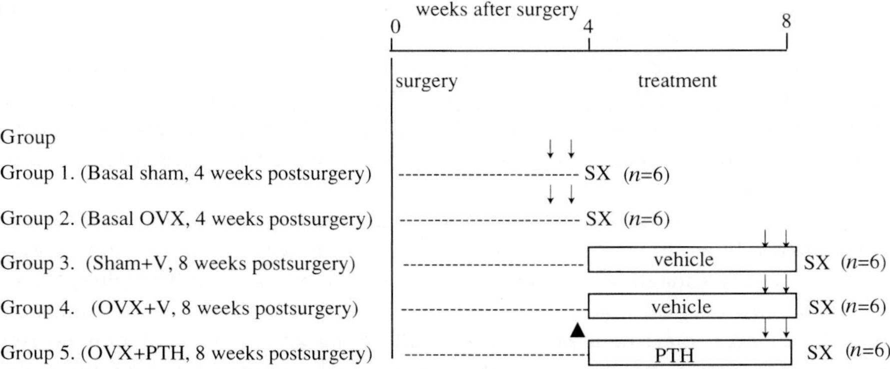

FIG. 1. Experimental protocol: All animals were left untreated for the first 4 weeks after surgery. The rats in Groups 1 and 2 were killed at pretreatment (4 weeks postsurgery). The rats in Group 3 (sham + V), Group 4 (OVX + V), and Group 5 (OVX + P) were subcutaneously injected with vehicle or human parathyroid hormone (hPTH) (1-34) (30 μg/kg/day, 5 days/week) respectively, initiated at 4 weeks postsurgery and continued for a period of 4 weeks (8 weeks postsurgery). All animals were double-labeled with a subcutaneous injection of calcein (10 mg/kg, body-weight) 6 and 2 days before being killed. The PTH-treated rats (Group 5) were subcutaneously injected with oxytetracycline (10 mg/kg, bodyweight) at the begining of the treatment period. *OVX*, ovariectomized; *SX*, time when killed; *arrows*, calcein administered; *solid triangle*, tetracycline administered

rats were subjected to sham surgery in which the ovaries were exposed but not removed. All animals were left untreated for the 4 weeks postsurgery. At the end of pretreatment period, groups of baseline sham (Group 1) and OVX (Group 2) rats were killed. The remaining rats were divided into three groups based and treated as follows. Sham-operated rats (Group 3) and ovariectomized rats (Group 4) were injected with saline vehicle. Ovariectomized rats (Group 5) were injected with PTH, 30 μg/kg, five times per week. All treatments were initiated at 4 weeks postsurgery for a 4-week period.

To determine the amount of the PTH-induced new bone during the experiment period, the rats in the PTH-treated group were injected subcutaneously with oxytetracycline (Pfizer Laboratories, New York, NY, USA) at a dose of 10 mg/kg bodyweight just before the PTH treatment start. All animals were double-labeled with subcutaneous injections of 10 mg/kg of calcein (Wako Pure Chemical, Osaka, Japan) on day 6 and day 2 before euthanization. All rats were killed by exsanguination from the abdominal aorta under ether ketamine hydrochloride and xylazine anesthesia.

Specimen Preparation and Bone Histomorphometry

The left tibia of each animal was removed and fixed with 70% ethanol, then cut in half cross-sectionally with a low-speed metallurgical saw. The distal half of the tibia was then dehydrated in ascending grades of ethanol, defatted in an acetone/ethanol mixture (1:1), and embedded in methyl-methacrylate without decalcification. Cross sections 200 μm thick were cut with a precision bone saw. Two sections 1 mm from the tibiofibular junction were mounted on plastic slides and ground to a thickness of 50 µm using a precision lapping machine (Maruto, Tokyo, Japan).

Histomorphometric measurements were performed using a semi-automatic digitizing system (System Supply, Nagano, Japan). To identify whether PTH-induced new bone was lamellar or woven, we viewed the sections of PTH-treated rats under polarized light and under magnification (Fig. 4). Cortical bone tissue area (bone + bone marrow) and bone marrow area were measured in one section per animal at a magnification of 10×. Cortical bone area was calculated by subtracting marrow area from cortical bone tissue area. Fluorochrome-based indices of bone formation were measured at 100× magnification using a fluorescence microscope (Optiphot, Nikon, Tokyo, Japan). Cortical bone parameters measured at the tibial diaphysis included total tissue area, marrow area, cortical width, bone area, periosteal mineralizing surface, endocortical mineralizing surface, periosteal bone formation rate, and endocortical bone formation rate. Periosteal new bone area was calculated by subtracting total tissue area of the control animals from that of the treated animals. Endocortical new bone area was calculated by subtracting marrow area from that of the treated animals. Additionally, we also calculated, according to the methods recommended by Jee et al. [18–20], the endocortical resorbing bone area (accumulative) by using the following formula:

Endocortical resorbing bone area = marrow porosity area of final treated bone − (marrow porosity area of initial untreated bone + new intramedullary bone area).

Whenever possible, we employed the histomorphometric terminology recommended by Parfitt et al. [21].

Statistical Analysis

Data are expressed as the mean ± standard error of the means (SEM) for each group. Group differences were subjected to analysis of variance (ANOVA), with the Fisher protected least-significant-difference test. P values less than 0.05 were considered to be significant.

Results

Effect of Ovariectomy on the Tibial Diaphysis

In static parameters, there were no significant differences in cortical bone tissue area, cortical bone area, bone marrow area, and cortical width between the untreated OVX rats (Group 2) and the untreated sham-operated control rats (Group 1) at the end of the pretreatment period (4 weeks postsurgery; Table 1). Similarly, there were no significant differences in cortical bone tissue area, cortical bone area, bone marrow area, and cortical width between the OVX (Group 4) and the sham control rats (Group 3) after four weeks of the vehicle-treatment, (8 weeks postsurgery, Table 2).

In dynamic parameters, periosteal mineralizing surface and periosteal bone formation rate were significantly greater in the untreated OVX rats (Group 2) compared to the untreated sham rats (Group 1) at the end of the pretreatment period (4 weeks postsurgery, Table 1). There were no significant differences in endocortical mineralizing surface and endocortical bone formation rate between the Group 1 and

TABLE 1. Effect of ovariectomy on histomorphometric indices of the tibial diaphysis (4 weeks postsurgery)

Group	Ct.TAr (mm^2)	Ct.BAr (mm^2)	Ma.Ar (mm^2)	Ct.Wi (mm)	Ps.MS/BS (%)	Ps.BFR/BS (μm^3/μm^2/d)	Ec.MS/BS (%)	Ec.BFR/BS (μm^3/μm^2/d)
Group 1 (sham: 4 w)	4.61 ± 0.16	4.04 ± 0.07	0.66 ± 0.06	0.79 ± 0.05	26.39 ± 4.47	0.31 ± 0.05	15.88 ± 4.61	0.13 ± 0.08
Group 2 (OVX: 4 w)	5.05 ± 0.19	4.17 ± 0.26	0.69 ± 0.05	0.76 ± 0.03	49.85 ± 6.72*	0.84 ± 0.13*	19.27 ± 5.23	0.21 ± 0.09

(Bone histomorphometric variables from the diaphysis are abbreviated as follows Ct.TAr, cortical bone tissue area; Ct.BAr, cortical bone area; Ma.Ar, bone marrow area; Ct.Wi, cortical width; Ps.MS/BS, periosteal mineralizing surface; Ps.BFR/BS, periosteal bone formation rate; Ec.MS/BS, endocortical mineralizing surface; Ec.BFR/BS, endocortical bone formation rate.)
Data are expressed as the mean ± SEM of six values per group.
* $P < 0.05$, significant difference from sham control (Group 1).

TABLE 2. Effect of parathyroid hormone (PTH) administration on histomorphometric indices of the tibial diaphysis in ovariectomized rats (8 weeks postsurgery)

Group	Ct.TAr (mm^2)	Ct.BAr (mm^2)	Ma.Ar (mm^2)	Ct.Wi (mm)	Ps.MS/BS (%)	Ps.BFR/BS (μm^3/μm^2/d)	Ec.MS/BS (%)	Ec.BFR/BS (μm^3/μm^2/d)
Group 3 (sham + V)	4.68 ± 0.10	3.99 ± 0.07	0.69 ± 0.05	0.83 ± 0.03	13.80 ± 5.6	0.17 ± 0.06	7.93 ± 1.4	0.03 ± 0.01
Group 4 (OVX + V)	4.83 ± 0.07	4.08 ± 0.08	0.72 ± 0.07	0.81 ± 0.02	40.21 ± 7.6*	0.42 ± 0.09*	11.09 ± 2.9*	0.05 ± 0.01*
Group 5 (OVX + PTH)	5.16 ± 0.22*†	4.51 ± 0.12*†	0.63 ± 0.05	0.92 ± 0.02*†	65.23 ± 9.6*†	0.95 ± 0.12*†	56.08 ± 9.7*†	0.68 ± 0.11*†

(Bone histomorphometric variables from the diaphysis are abbreviated as follows Ct.TAr, cortical bone tissue area; Ct.BAr, cortical bone area; Ma.Ar, bone marrow area; Ct.Wi, cortical width; Ps.MS/BS, periosteal mineralizing surface; Ps.BFR/BS, periosteal bone formation rate; Ec.MS/BS, endocortical mineralizing surface; Ec.BFR/BS, endocortical bone formation rate.)
Data are expressed as the mean ± SEM of six values per group.
* $P < 0.05$, significant difference from sham control (Group 3).
† $P < 0.05$, significant difference from OVX control (Group 4).

Group 2 (4 weeks postsurgery, Table 1). However, the endocortical mineralizing surface and endocortical bone formation rate were significantly greater in the OVX rats (Group 4) compared to the sham control rats (Group 3) after four weeks of treatment with the vehicle only (8 weeks postsurgery; Table 2).

Effect of PTH Treatment on the Tibial Diaphysis of Ovariectomized Rats

PTH administration in OVX rats (Group 5) for 4 weeks (8 weeks postsurgery) significantly increased the cortical bone tissue area (+7%), cortical bone area (+11%), and cortical width (+14%) over the vehicle-treated OVX rats (Group 4). PTH administration markedly stimulated bone formation activity by elevating osteoblastic recruitment and osteoblastic activity (mineralizing surface and mineral apposition rate), and bone formation rate in either periosteal or endocortical surfaces over group 4. In Group 5 the bone formation rate with PTH treatment was markedly increased compared to the vehicle-treated OVX rats (Group 4) 8 weeks after surgery. The largest response was in the bone formation rate at the endocortical bone envelope.

PTH treatment in the OVX rats for 4 weeks (Group 5) added a significant amount of new periosteal bone mass (mean $0.32\,\text{mm}^2$) and new endocortical bone mass (mean $0.09\,\text{mm}^2$), compared to the OVX vehicle-treated rats in group 4 (Table 3). There were no significant differences in endocortical resorbing surface between Group 4 and Group 5 (Table 3). Intracortical porosity was not observed as a consequence of ovariectomy or PTH treatment.

Figure 4 shows that lamellar-type bone was formed after PTH therapy ($30\,\mu\text{g/kg/day}$). No woven bone formation was observed at this doseage of PTH.

TABLE 3. Effect of PTH administration on periosteal and endocortical new bone mass, and endocortical resorption in ovariectomized rats (8 weeks postsurgery)

Group	PsNB.Ar (mm^2)	EcNB.Ar (mm^2)	EcR.Ar (mm^2)
Group 4 (OVX + V)	0.000	0.000	0.037 ± 0.01
Group 5 (OVX + PTH)	$0.32 \pm 0.08^\dagger$	$0.09 \pm 0.02^\dagger$	0.061 ± 0.01

Static histomorphometric abbreviations are: PsNB.Ar, periosteal new bone area; EcNB.Ar, endocortical new bone area; EcR.Ar, endocortical resorbing bone area (accumultive).

Calculations can be applied using the following formula as recommended by Jee et al. [17–19].

PsNB.Ar = cortical bone tissue area (treated)—cortical bone tissue area (control)

EcNB.Ar = Bone marrow area (control)—bone marrow area (treated)

EcR.Ar = bone marrow area (final treated)—[bone marrow area (initial untreated) + (new intramedullary bone area)]

Data are the mean $\pm$ SEM of six values per group.

$^*P < 0.05$, significant difference from OVX control (Group 4).

Discussion

This study has demonstrated that ovariectomized rats treated with PTH had an increase in cortical bone mass through the addition of new circumferential bone on the endocortical and periosteal surfaces. PTH appeared to stimulate osteoblastic recruitment and activity at the periosteal and endocortical bone envelopes. Thus, PTH administration activated cortical bone modeling in the formation mode (activation-formation), but did not significantly increase endocortical bone resorption, and resulted in a positive bone balance by the addition of new lamellar bone.

The increment in cortical bone appeared to be due to the stimulatory effect of PTH on either periosteal or endocortical bone formation. The anabolic effect of PTH was more pronounced on the endocortical surface, since PTH induced nearly a four-fold increase in endocortical mineralizing surface, but only a two-fold increase in periosteal mineralizing surface. These results are in agreement with those of other investigators who used a higher dose of PTH than in the present study [14,16].

In the current study, PTH administration did not succeed in activating cortical bone remodeling in rats whose age range was three to five months. There were no significant differences in the resorbing area of endocortical bone between the PTH-treated and the vehicle-treated OVX rats in the present study. Jee and co-workers demonstrated that activation of cortical bone remodeling is an age-related phenomenon in rats, and that it occurs only at a very old age and not in the age range of 3–8 months [18]. It was postulated that PTH treatment in old rats may activate bone remodeling on both the intracortical and endocortical surfaces.

Another interesting observation in the current study was that PTH led to an increase in cortical bone mass by the addition of new circumferential bone on the endocortical and periosteal surfaces (compare Fig. 3C with 3A and 3B). This newly added subendocortical and subperiosteal bone was lamellar in nature (Fig. 4). In the current study, we found that newly formed bone tissue is fully mineralized and normal in appearance. Woven bone formation was not observed with this dosage of PTH (30 µg/kg/day). This is in agreement with the findings of Gasser and Jerome [22], who demonstrated that with doses of PTH 100 µg/kg/day or less, newly formed bone is in a lamellar pattern. This contrasts with woven bone formation and fibrosis that can be observed at high doses of PTH (i.e., 200 µg/kg/day). In the present study where OVX rats were treated with PTH for 4 weeks, there was a significant increase in the net tibial shaft bone mass, contributed by new subperiosteal and subendocortical bone. The remarkable point here is that subperiosteal bone contributes more significantly to diaphyseal structure strength than does subendocortical bone [23–26].

The results of the curren study in an estrogen-depleted animal model do not support the previous findings that PTH augments cancellous bone at the expense of cortical bone [11,12]. The PTH-treated rats in the present study exhibited a significant increase in cortical bone mass. This is in agreement with a study previously reported by Wronski et al. [16], who treated young adult rats with a higher dose of PTH (80 µg/kg/day, 6 days/week) for a longer period of time (15 weeks). They also did not observe cortical bone loss. It should be noted that the present study and the study by Wronski et al. used young adult rats that lacked intracortical remodeling. Therefore, the possibility that cortical bone loss in PTH-treated patients is due to perturbations

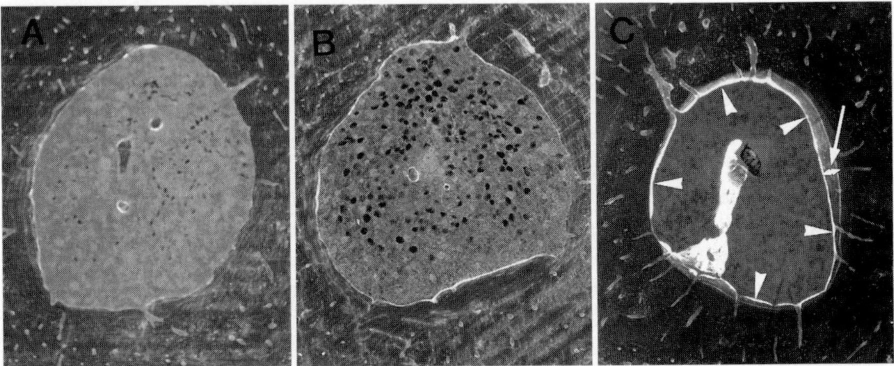

FIG. 2A–C. Fluorescent micrographs of representative endocortical regions of the cross sections of tibial shafts. **A** Sham-operated control rats with vehicle treatment (Group 3). **B** OVX control animals with vehicle treatment (Group 4). **C** OVX rats with PTH treatment (Group 5). A well-mineralized layer of subendocortical bone (*arrowheads*) can be observed in the PTH-treated tibiae. Virtually 100% of the endocortical surface was labeled with calcein and tetracycline in the PTH-treated OVX rats. In PTH-treated rats, almost visible is the formation draft in the endocortical surface (*arrowheads*). The new endocortical bone (*arrow*) appeared to be well-mineralized bone which is lining the cortex. ×40

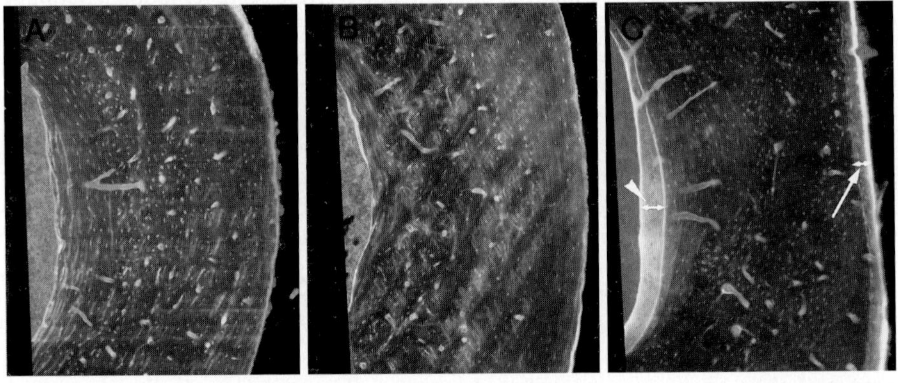

FIG. 3A–C. Fluorescent micrographs of periosteal and endocortical surfaces in the tibial shafts: **A**, Group 3; **B**, Group 4; **C**, Group 5. The newly added subperiosteal (*arrow*) and subendocortical bone (*arrowhead*) were added circumferentially, and the new bone was well-mineralized layer bone and thickened the cortex. The faint yellow tetracycline label administered before the initiation of therapy helped to identify the newly formed bone and the previous location of the subendocortical and subperiosteal surfaces (**C**). ×60

in intracortical remodeling cannot be ruled out. However, the cortical deficit in these patients may be a consequence of increased remodeling space induced by PTH. Such a cortical deficit would be reversible upon withdrawal of PTH treatment [27]. More recently, several investigators have reported the effects of PTH treatment in large remodeling animals with a Haversian system. They found that there was no loss in cortical bone mass in canine [28,29] and monkey [30] models during the half-year experimental period.

FIG. 4. Polarized light of a tibial shaft from OVX rats treated with PTH (Group 5): the newly added cortical bone was in a lamellar pattern in both endocortical (*arrowhead*) and periosteal (*arrow*) regions. ×60

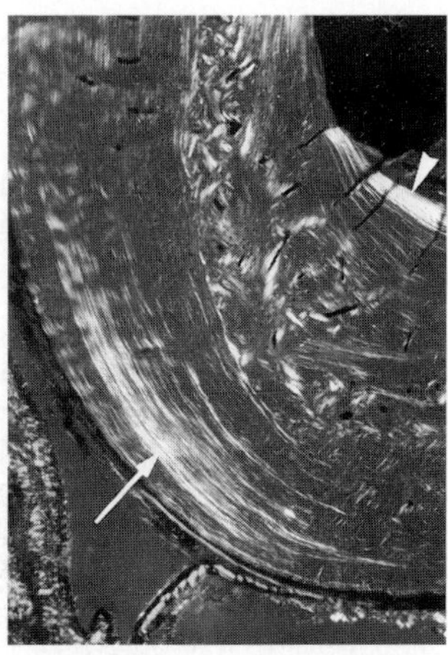

The current study indicates that PTH is a powerful bone-forming agent. It stimulates bone formation at the periosteal and endocortical surfaces through activation of modeling in the formation mode (formation drift) without significantly increasing resorption at endocortical surface. Frost [31] demonstrated that formation drift progressively adds bone to another bone surface without any associated resorption. In the present study, our results showed that PTH-treated OVX rats over a four-week period showed significant increase in cortical bone mass and thickness, mainly stimulated by modeling-dependent bone gain. The stimulation of bone formation on the endocortical surface by PTH treatment in the present study (Fig. 2) is most relevant to the prevention or treatment of osteoporosis. In osteoporosis, there is a loss of cortical bone from the medullary cavity resulting in a negative bone balance in the subendocortical region. The addition of more bone during growth, and the addition rather than subtraction of endocortical bone during adulthood by PTH administration, can prevent age-related cortical bone loss by increasing growth-related peak cortical bone mass and preventing and reversing age-related cortical bone loss. These findings, together with other observations that PTH administration induces similar changes in rats, dogs, monkeys, and humans [1,9–11,14–16,27–30,31], indicate that administration of PTH without side effects may be useful in the prevention and treatment of postmenopausal osteoporosis.

In summary, our results have indicated that PTH increases cortical bone mass and activates cortical bone modeling in the formation mode from either the periosteal or endocortical envelopes of the tibial diaphysis of growing ovariectomized rats. The newly formed bone on the endocortical and periosteal surfaces is lamellar in nature.

References

1. Hock JM, Gera I, Fonseca J, Raisz LG (1988) Human parathyroid hormone (1–34) increases bone mass in ovariectomized and orchidectomized rats. Endocrinology 122:2899–2904
2. Hori M, Uzawa T, Morita K, Noda T, Takahashi HE, Inoue J (1988) Effect of human parathyroid hormone (PTH 1–34) on experimental osteopenia of rats induced by ovariectomy. Bone Miner 3:193–199

3. Kimmel DB, Bozzato RP, Kronis KA, Coble T, Sindrey D, Kwong P, Recker RR (1993) The effect of recombinant human (1–84) or synthetic human (1–34) parathyroid hormone on the skeleton of adult osteopenic ovariectomized rats. Endocrinology 132:1577–1584

4. Liu CC, Kalu DN, Salerno E, Echon R, Hollis BW, Ray M (1991) Preexisting bone loss associated with ovariectomy in rats is reversed by parathyroid hormone. J Bone Miner Res 6:1071–1080

5. Nishida S, Yamaguchi A, Tanizawa T, Endo N, Mashiba T, Uchiyama Y, Suda, T, Yoshiki S, Takahashi HE (1994) Increased bone formation by intermittent parathyroid hormone administration is due to the stimulation of proliferation and differentiation of osteoprogenitor cells in bone marrow. Bone 15:717–723

6. Shen V, Dempster DW, Mellish RWE, Birchman R, Horbert W, Lindsay R (1992) Effects of combined and separate intermittent administration of low-dose human parathyroid hormone fragment (1–34) and 17β–estradiol on bone histomorphometry in ovariectomized rats with established osteopenia. Calcif Tissue Int 50:214–220

7. Wronski TJ, Yen CF, Qi H, Dann LM (1993) Parathyroid hormone is more effective than estrogen or bisphosphonates for restoration of lost bone mass in ovariectomized rats. Endocrinology 132:823–831

8. Slovik DM, Rosenthal DI, Doppelt SH, Potts JT, Daly MA, Campbell JA, Neer RM (1986) Restoration of spinal bone in osteoporotic men by treatment with human parathyroid hormone (1–34) and 1, 25-dihydroxyvitamin D. J Bone Miner Res 1:377–381

9. Reeve J, Davies UM, Hesp R, Mcnally E, Katz D (1990) Treatment of osteoporosis with human parathyroid peptide and observations on effect of sodium fluoride. Br Med J 301:314–318

10. Lindsay R, Nieves J, Formica C, Henneman E, Woelfert L, Shen V, Dempster D (1997) Randomised controlled study of effect of parathyroid hormone on vertebral bone mass and fracture incidence among postmenopausal women on oestrogen with osteoporosis. Lancet 350:550–555

11. Hesp R, Hulme P, Williams D, Reeve J (1981) The relationship between changes in femoral bone density and calcium balance in patients with involutional osteoporosis treated with parathyroid hormone fragment (hPTH1-34). Metab Bone Dis Relat Res 2:331–334

12. Pariesan M, Slilverberg SJ, Shane E, Cruz LDL, Lindsay R, Bilezikian JP, Dempster DW (1990) The histomorphometry of bone in primary hyperparathyroidism: preservation of cancellous bone structure. J Clin Endocrinol Metab 70:930–938

13. Christiansen P, Steiniche T, Brockstedt H, Mosekilde L, Hessov I, Melsen F (1993) Primary hyperparathyroidism: iliac crest cortical thickness, structure, and remodeling evaluated by histomorphometric methods. Bone 14:755–762

14. Ibbotson KJ, Orcutt CM, D'Souza SM, Paddock CL, Arthur JA, Jankowsky ML, Boyce RW (1992) Contrasting effects of parathyroid hormone and insulin-like factor I in an aged ovariectomized rat model of postmenopausal osteoporosis. J Bone Miner Res 7:425–432

15. Oxlund H, Ejersted C, Andreassen TT, Torring O, Nilsson MHL (1993) Parathyroid hormone (1–34) and (1–84) stimulate cortical bone formation both from periosteum and endosteum. Calcif Tissue Int 53:394–399

16. Wronski TJ, Yen CF (1994) Anabolic effects of parathyroid hormone on cortical bone in ovariectomized rats. Bone 15:51–58

17. Bagi CM, Mecham M, Weiss J, Miller SC (1993) Comparative morphometric changes in rat cortical bone following ovariectomy and/or immobilization. Bone 14:877–883

18. Jee WSS, Mori S, Li XJ, Chan S (1990) Prostaglandin E_2 enhances cortical bone mass and activates intracortical bone remodeling in intact and ovariectomized female rats. Bone 11:253–266

19. Jee WSS, Ke HZ, Li XJ (1992) Loss of prostaglandin E_2-induced extra cortical bone after its withdrawal in rats. Bone Miner 17:31–47
20. Jee WSS, Li XJ, Inoue J, Jee KW, Haba T, Ke HZ, Setterberg RB, Ma YF (1997) Histomorphometric assay of the growing bones. In: Takahashi H (ed) Handbook of bone morphology. Nishimula, Niigata City, Japan, pp 87–112
21. Parfitt AM, Drezner MK, Glorieux FH, Kanis JA, Malluche H, Meunier PJ, Ott SM, Recker RR (1987) Bone histomorphometry: standardization of nomenclature, symbols, and units. J Bone Miner Res 6:595–610
22. Gasser JA, Jerome CP (1992) Parathyroid hormone: a cure for osteoporosis? Triangle 31:111–121
23. Martin RB, Atkinson PG (1977) Age and sex-related changes in the structure and strength of human femoral shaft. J Biomechanics 10:223–231
24. Keller TS, Spengler DM, Carter DR (1985) Geometric, elastic, and structural properities of maturing rat femora. J Orthop Res 4:57–67
25. Frost HM (1988a) Structural adaptations to mechanical usage: a three-way rule for lamellar bone modeling. Comp Vet Orthop Trauma 1:7–17 and 2:80–85
26. Frost HM (1988b) Vital biomechanics: General concepts for structural adaptations to mechanical usage. Calcif Tissue Int 42:145–156
27. Inoue J (1985) Bone changes with long term administration of low dose 1–34 human PTH on adult beagles. J Jpn Orthop Assoc 59:409–427
28. Ma YF, Chen YY, Ijiri K, Jee WSS, Li XJ, Mcosker J, Gibson GW, Phipps R (1997) PTH in combination with risedronate in aged beagle dogs resulted in bone balances similar to PTH alone. Bone 20 (Suppl):99S
29. Zhang L, Takahashi HE, Inoue J, Tanizawa T, Endo N, Yamamoto N, Hori M (1997) Effects of intermittent administration of low dose human PTH(1–34) on cancellous and cortical bone of lumbar vertebral bodies in adult beagles. Bone 21:501–506
30. Jerome CP, Johnson CS, Lees CJ (1995) Parathyroid hormone (PTH) increases axial and appendicular bone mass without cortical bone loss in ovariectomized cynomolgus monkeys. J Bone Miner Res 10 (Suppl):416S
31. Frost HM (1995) Introduction To A New Skeletal Physiology Volume I Bone and Bones. Pajaro Group. Pueblo, Colorado, pp 45–47

Osteoporotic Vertebral Pseudarthrosis: Another Instability of the Spine

Kazuhiro Hasegawa

Summary. Idiopathic osteoporotic vertebral collapse or pseudarthrosis is reviewed in reference to clinical features, radiological characteristics, and recommended surgical treatment with a discussion of the pathomechanism proposed to date. Intravertebral instability derived from avascular necrosis and the resultant pseudarthrosis is considered a cause of incapacitating back pain or late neurological compromise. Although surgical treatments increasingly have been performed for patients with neurological deficit or prolonged incapacitating back pain, the surgery is still challenging in severe osteoporosis. An anterior procedure is more appropriate than a posterior one because the nature of the lesion is that of an anterior column deficiency with preserved posterior elements. The limitations of instrumentation surgery should be taken into account when assessing patients with severe osteoporosis. A less invasive and more effective procedure may become available in the future.

Key words. Intravertebral instability, Osteoporosis, Surgical treatment, Vertebral pseudarthrosis

Introduction

For several postulated pathomechanisms, such as bone ischemia idiopathic vertebral collapse or Kümmell disease is rarely reported. Following the first report by Kempinsky et al. [1], there has been an increase in published reports of cases of vertebral collapse with neurological deficit [2–14]. Most of these cases involved spinal osteoporosis. Vertebral collapse and resultant spinal kyphosis with osteoporosis sometimes lead to disability in daily activity due to chronic back pain [15–17]. Moreover, the disability may be serious if the patient has neurological deficit.

Typical clinical signs exhibited by these patients are abnormal movement at the intravertebral cleft in flexion-extension X-ray and prolonged back pain and/or paraparesis aggravated by standing or walking and improved on resting. While most of

Department of Orthopaedic Surgery, Niigata Cancer Center Hospital, 2-15-3 Kawagishi-cho, Niigata 951-8566, Japan this vertebral collapse involves the thoraco-lumbar junction, the lesions have been found distributed in the lower lumbar area [2,14,18–22].

Vertebral collapse with cleft formation has been called the *intravertebral vacuum phenomenon*, similar to the vacuum phenomenon in the intervertebral disc [23–26]. It is presumed that intraosseous vacuum cleft results from the release of gas within cracks in the subchondral bone after vertebral fracture [2,18–21,27–30]. It must be noted, however, that the vacuum phenomenon does not always result from osteoporotic vertebral collapse. Malignant disease involving the spine can also show this radiological phenomenon [31]. Typically on intravertebral lesion was demonstrated in a low-intensity area in a T1 weight image and in a high-intensity area in T2 weight image using MR imaging [14,32–35]. These findings suggest that the content within the vertebral lesion is fluid rather than the gas. Some researchers have suggested that this phenomenon represents an ununited vertebral fracture with possible formation of a pseudarthrosis [2,14,19]. Direct evidence of the pathology is, however, yet to be confirmed.

One of the biomechanical characteristics of pseudarthrosis is instability at the lesion. White and Panjabi defined "clinical instability" as the loss of the ability of the spine under physiologic loads to maintain its pattern of displacement so that there is no initial or additional neurological deficit, no major deformity, and no incapacitating pain. Trauma, tumor, surgery, degenerative changes, and developmental changes were given as causative pathologic conditions [36]. Whatever the condition is, they considered "instability" to be segmental (intervertebral) instability (Fig. 1a). The author has reported that osteoporotic pseudarthrosis could be an example of spinal instability [14]. Intravertebral instability resulting from vertebral pseudarthrosis is an another functional deficiency of the anterior column of the spine with preserved posterior elements (Fig. 1b).

In this chapter, the author will present a representative case of osteoporotic vertebral pseudarthrosis, discuss the mechanism of the pathology, and summarize surgical treatment proposed to date.

Case Report and Summary of the Clinical Features

Case Report

An 80-year-old woman experienced acute back pain when she was getting up. Although conservative treatment had been maintained for 6 months following a diagnosis of spinal osteoporosis, back pain on motion had been prolonged. On physical examination, she complained of severe motion pain and tenderness on her back around the thoracolumbar junction, and could not lie down on her back, nor could she walk more than 50 m without rest. She had thoracolumbar kyphosis with mild lower extremity weakness and numbness.

Radiographs showed multiple compression fractures and abnormal movement of the T12 vertebral body in flexion-extension view (Fig. 2). Magnetic resonance (MR) imaging showed an intravertebral lesion extended into the spinal canal with a very low intensity on T1-weighted and a very high intensity on T2-weighted scans. The intravertebral radiolucent area the so-called intravertebral vacuum phenomenon has been considered gas accumulated within the vertebra [2,18,19,26]. In a study by

FIG. 1. Schema of segmental (intervertebral) instability **a** and intravertebral instability due to vertebral pseudarthrosis **b** *Asterisks* indicate pseudarthrosis of the vertebra

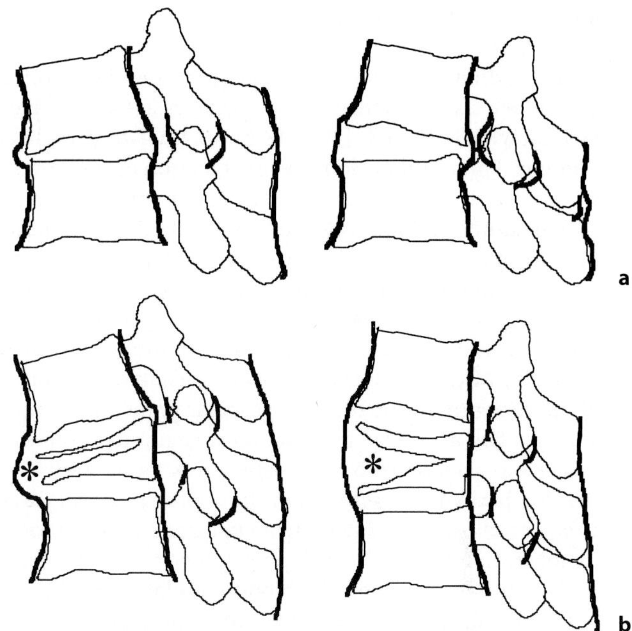

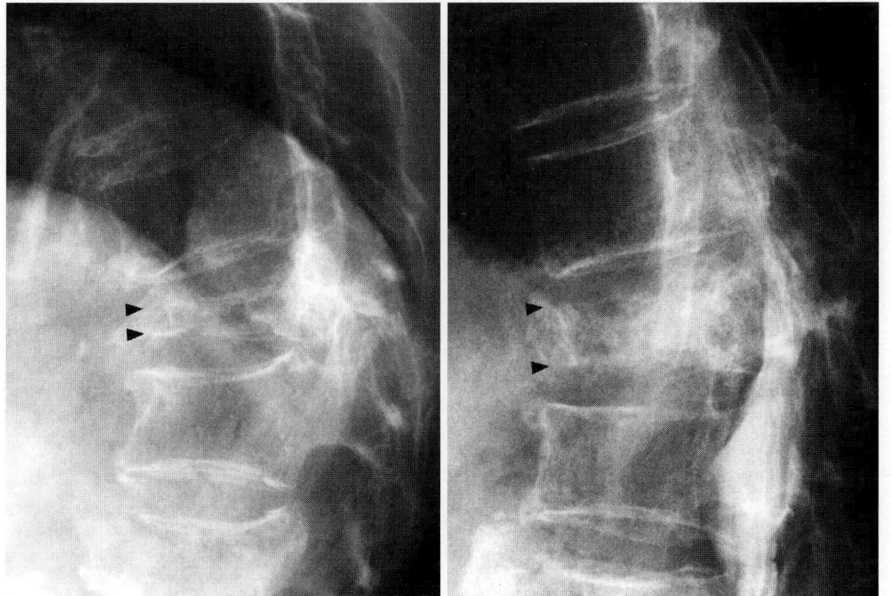

FIG. 2. Radiographs of **a** preoperative flexion and **b** extension flexion. Change of vertebral height indicates intravertebral instability (*arrowheads*)

Malghem et al., X-ray and MR imaging in nine patients was suggestive of vertebral avascular necrosis. This clearly showed that the progressive disappearance of a gaslike area of radiolucency on stress radiographs and the concurrent appearance of an area of fluidlike signal intensity on MR images are suggestive of a slow replacement of gas by fluid within the cleft [33]. MR findings of the present case are consistent with these findings. Three-dimensional reconstruction of the computed tomography (CT) image showed an intravertebral horizontal cleft with a preserved lateral wall.

The author and his colleagues performed osteosynthesis without instrumentation [14]. At operation the T12 vertebra was exposed through the transpleural approach. A hypertrophic membranous structure covered the lateral aspect of the vertebra. When lordotic stress was applied manually on the patient's back, abnormal movement was observed at the lesion. The serous fluid beneath the hypertrophic membrane shown by MRI was aspirated before excision of the soft tissue. The cavity of the body of the vertebra was lined with avascular granulation tissue resembling a pseudarthrosis [37]. The avascular granulation was curetted, the kyphosis was reduced, and the defect was packed with a tricortical iliac bone graft and cancellous chips. The pain that the patient had suffered in the supine position disappeared when she recovered from anesthesia. The T12 vertebra became stabilized with mild collapse 5 months after the operation (Fig. 3).

The author examined the blood circulation at the site of the affected vertebra in two other cases using MRI with and without enhancement using gadolinium. In both cases, MRI showed circumferential enhancement around the false joint preoperatively. Postoperatively, the enhanced areas were progressively enlarged into the grafted bone site. This suggests that opening the membrane of the false joint could induce revascularization into the avascular region from the circumference [14].

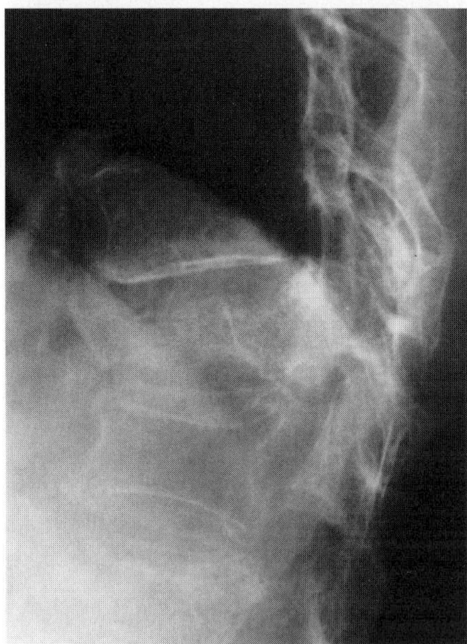

FIG. 3. The unstable T12 vertebra underwent osteosynthesis without instrumentation and stabilized with mild collapse

The characteristics of the pathology of the vertebral pseudarthrosis can be summarized as anterior column deficiency, also known as intravertebral instability, leading to unstable kyphotic deformity (Fig. 2) and back pain on walking or lying supine with or without neurological deficit.

Mechanism of Vertebral Pseudarthrosis

One of the possible mechanisms of osteoporotic vertebral deformity is the accumulation of microdamage at lower strains than those of normal vertebrae near the vertebral endplate, leading to flattened or codfish vertebra [38,39]. The greater accumulation of microcracks in vertebrae of functional spinal units with disc lesions, and more microcracks adjacent to rather than further from the lesions support the hypothesis that disc degeneration contributes to vertebral fragility by causing microdamage accumulation [40]. It is considered possible that microdamage in vertebral bodies could be repaired in patients with normal fracture healing ability. The possibility of bone formation for repairing microdamage in the bone may, however, be decreased in elderly patients with severe spinal osteoporosis.

Previous histological examination in vertebral collapse revealed nonspecific findings with trabecular bone necrosis with or without bone formation and fibrosis of the marrow. These findings were thought to be compatible with avascular necrosis of the vertebra [2,21,32]. Intraoperative findings of the author's cases showed that the intravertebral cleft was lined by smooth fibrocartilagenous membrane, with a great degree of motion between the fracture ends that is consistent with the pathology of pseudarthrosis [14,37]. Other authors have suggested that fibrous granulation tissue and necrotic bone found within collapsed vertebral bodies may alter vascularity of the lesion and result in impaired healing [12,13].

Ratcliffe investigated the arterial anatomy of the adult human lumbar vertebral body using microarteriography and identified three types of intraosseous arteries branched from segmental arteries: equatorial, metaphyseal, and peripheral. Each artery supplies a separate zone [41]. In most cases of vertebral collapse, the damaged portion is the anterior vertebra which is supplied by anterior metaphyseal arteries and peripheral arteries. Progressive collapse of the vertebra may further jeopardize vertebral vascularity, leading to a vicious cycle.

While no patients had symptoms at rest preoperatively, motion induced severe back pain. In addition, operative stabilization of pseudarthrosis immediately relieved the pain. These observations suggest that intravertebral instability due to pseudarthrosis is a cause of back pain in supine posture or walking. Therefore, intravertebral instability should be categorized as a cause of "spinal instability" proposed by White and Panjabi [36].

Surgical Treatment

The pathomechanism of vertebral pseudarthrosis will lead us to a rationale for surgical treatment. A goal of surgery for vertebral pseudarthrosis is restabilization of the anterior column and decompression of the nerve, if necessary. Surgical treatment is indicated when the patient presents neurological deficit or incapacitating back pain not responsive to any conservative treatment.

Shikata et al. reported seven cases of paraplegia secondary to osteoporotic vertebral fractures treated by decompression and Harrington stabilization. In all seven cases, substantial improvement was achieved through early decompression and firm stabilization [10]. Baba et al. treated 27 patients with osteoporotic vertebral collapse by an anterior or a posterior spinal decompression with or without spinal instrumentation. They recommended transpedicular posterolateral decompression and stabilization using a screw-rod construct. They had good to excellent results in 78% of the patients. Although a satisfactory result was achieved overall, they reported a 15% implant failure in their series [12]. Posterior instrumentation surgery usually involves several segments above and below the lesion even though the posterior elements are intact. Furthermore, using such stiff instrumentation on the osteoporotic spine, sequential compression fracture of adjacent vertebra is inferred after intervertebral fusion.

The posterior element at the level of vertebral collapse in an osteoporotic spine usually remains intact. This validates the efficacy of an anterior approach rather than a posterior one which unnecessarily destroys the posterior element. Kaneda et al. reported 51 cases treated by anterior stabilization using a Kaneda device (Acro Med Corp., Cleveland, OH, USA) and bone graft or AW-glass ceramics for osteoporotic vertebral collapse with excellent clinical results [13]. They stressed the significant validity of their anterior extrapleural-retroperitoneal approach and decompression followed by the solid stabilization rarely with complications even in the elderly series. However, in severe osteoporosis patients, sinking of the vertebral prosthesis was found in 11.8% [13].

Since instrumentation cannot achieve enough stability in the case of severe osteoporosis the author has been seeking an alternative to instrumentation surgery for vertebral reconstruction. I have considered conventional bone grafting a possibility to consolidate the vertebral lesion without instrumentation as described earlier [14]. Adjacent discs remain intact in this procedure; therefore, stress concentration to the adjacent vertebra can be avoided. The author has seen five elderly patients who had severe osteoporosis with pseudarthrosis who were treated by osteosynthesis without instrumentation. There were four women and one man, ranging from 68 to 86 years of age (average 76.8 years). Affected vertebral levels were one T12, one L1, two L2, and one L4. All patients had severe motion pain in the back or leg which was initiated with no traumatic episode and was prolonged for more than half a year notwithstanding conservative treatment with medication and the wearing of a corset. No patients could walk more than 50 m due to pain in the back or the leg, or lie down on their back. There was no history of steroid administration or other medication related to secondary osteoporosis. All patients underwent radiographic evaluation with flexion-extension X-ray and preoperative MRI study.

All patients realized that back pain due to supine posture was dramatically improved on the day of the operation, and pain on walking also decreased. In two cases, the graft bone collapsed during the follow-up period. Fragility of the graft bone in the osteoporosis patient is a weakness of the procedure. Both of the collapsed cases, however, obtained bone union at 4 months and 10 months postoperatively. The author believes that other materials, e.g., biodegradable bone cement [42], should be used for osteosynthesis instead of fragile autogenous bone in severe cases of osteoporosis.

Acknowledgment. The author thanks Hideaki E. Takahashi, MD, Takao Homma, MD, and Seiji Uchiyama, MD, for their helpful discussions and comments on this subject.

References

1. Kempinsky WH (1958) Osteoporotic kyphosis with paraplegia. Neurology 8:181–185
2. Maldague BE, Noel HM, Malghem JJ (1978) The intravertebral vacuum cleft: a sign of ischemic vertebral collapse. Radiology 129:23–29
3. Brower AC, Downey EF (1981) Kümmell disease: Report of a case with serial radiographs. Radiology 141:363–364
4. Kaplan PA, Orton DF, Asleson RJ (1987) Osteoporosis with vertebral compression fractures, retropulsed fragments, and neurologic compromise. Radiology 165:533–535
5. Maruo S, Takekawa F, Nakano K (1987) Paraplegie infolge von Wirbelk compression strakturen bei seniler Osteoporose. Z Orthop 125:320–323
6. Feldmann JL, Alcalay M, Queinnec JY, deBray JM (1988) Spinal cord compression related to vertebral osteonecrosis. Clin Exp Rheumatol 6:297–300
7. Harverson G (1988) Intravertebral vacuum phenomenon. Clin Radiol 39:69–72
8. Salomon C, Chopin D, Benoist M (1988) Spinal cord compression: an exceptional complication of spinal osteoporosis. Spine 13:222–224
9. Arciero RA, Leung KYK, Pierce JH (1989) Spontaneous unstable burst fracture of the thoracolumbar spine in osteoporosis: a report of two cases. Spine 14:114–117
10. Shikata J, Yamamuro T, Iida H, Shimizu K, Yoshikawa J (1990) Surgical treatment for paraplegia resulting from vertebral fracture in senile osteoporosis. Spine 15:487–488
11. Tanaka S, Kubota M, Fujimoto Y, Hayashi J, Nishikawa K (1993) Conus medullaris syndrome secondary to an L1 burst fracture in osteoporosis: a case report. Spine 18:2131–2134
12. Baba H, Maezawa Y, Kamitani K, Furusawa N, Imura S, Tomita K (1995) Osteoporotic vertebral collapse with late neurological complications. Paraplegia 33(5):281–289
13. Kaneda K, Ito M, Taneichi H, Sato S, Abumi K, Asano S (1996) Osteoporotic posttraumatic vertebral collapse with neurological deficits of the thoracolumbar spine; anterior decompression and reconstruction (in Japanese). Rinsho Seikei Geka (in Japanese) 31:463–470
14. Hasegawa K, Homma T, Uchiyama S, Takahashi HE (1997) Osteosynthesis without instrumentation for vertebral pseudarthrosis in the osteoporotic spine. J Bone Joint Surg 79B:452–456
15. Kanis JA, McCloskey EV (1992) Epidemiology of vertebral osteoporosis. Bone 13:S1–S10
16. Silverman SL (1992) The clinical consequences of vertebral compression fracture. Bone 13:S27–S31
17. Ryan PJ, Blake G, Herd R, Fogelman I (1994) A clinical profile of back pain and disability in patients with spinal osteoporosis. Bone 15(1):27–30
18. Larde D, Mathieu D, Frija J, Gaston A, Vasile N (1982) Spinal vacuum phenomenon: CT diagnosis and significance. J Comput Assist Tomogr 6:671–676
19. Kumpan W, Salomonowitz E, Seidl G, Wittich GR (1986) The intravertebral vacuum phenomenon. Skeletal Radiol 15:444–447
20. Lafforgue PF, Chagnaud CJ, Daumen-Legre V, Daver LM, Kasbarian M, Acquaviva P (1997) The intravertebral vacuum phenomenon ("vertebral osteonecrosis") Migration of intradiscal gas in a fractured vertebral body? Spine 22:1885–1891
21. Hashimoto K, Yasui N, Yamagishi M, Kojimoto H, Mizuno K, Shimomura Y (1989) Intravertebral vacuum cleft in the fifth lumbar vertebra. Spine 14:351–354

22. Chou LH, Knight RQ (1997) Idiopathic avascular necrosis of a vertebral body. Case report and literature review. Spine 22:1928–1932
23. Knutsson F (1942) The vacuum phenomenon in the intervertebral discs. Acta Radiol 23:173–179
24. Marr JT (1953) Gas in intervertebral discs. Am J Roentgenol 70:804–809
25. Ford LT, Gilula LA, Murphy WA, Gado M (1977) Analysis of gas in vacuum lumbar disc. Am J Radiol 128:1056–1057
26. Resnick D, Niwayama G, Guerra J, Vint V, Usselman J (1981) Spinal vacuum phenomena: Anatomical study and review. Radiology 139:341–348
27. Bretz W, Jenkins RG (1981) Gas density in an ununited fracture of a vertebral body. A case report. J Bone Joint Surg 63A:1183–1184
28. Golimbu C, Firooznia H, Rafii M (1986) The intravertebral vacuum sign. Spine 11:1040–1043
29. Lafforgue PF, Chagnaud CJ, Daver LMH, Daumen-Legre VMS, Peragut J, Kasbarian MJ, Volot F, Acquaviva P (1994) Intervertebral disk vacuum phenomenon secondary to vertebral collapse: prevalence and significance. Radiology 193:853–858
30. Modena V, Maiocco I, Bosio C, Bianchi A, DeFilippi PG, Daneo V (1985) Intravertebral vacuum cleft: Notes on five cases. Clin Exp Rheumatol 3:23–27
31. Gagnerie F, Taillan B, Euller-Ziegler L, Ziegler G (1987) Intravertebral vacuum phenomenon in multiple myeloma. Clin Rheumatol 6:597–599
32. Naul LG, Peet GJ, Maupin WB (1989) Avascular necrosis of the vertebral body: MR imaging. Radiology 172:219–222
33. Malghem J, Maldague B, Labaisse M, Dooms G, Duprez T, Devogelaer J, Berg BV (1993) Intravertebral vacuum cleft: Changes in content after supine positioning. Radiology 187:483–487
34. Dupuy DE, Palmer WE, Rosenthal DI (1996) Vertebral fluid collection associated with vertebral collapse. Am J Radiol 167:1535–1538
35. Harvey CJ, Saifuddin A, Nordeen MH, Taylor BA (1997) Sagittal vertebral body fractures: magnetic resonance imaging features. Br J Radiol 70:645–649
36. White AA, Panjabi MM (1990) Clinical Biomechanics of the Spine. J.B. Lippincott, Philadelphia, pp 278–362
37. Milgram JW (1990) Nonunion and pseudarthrosis of fracture healing. In: Milgram JW (ed) Radiologic and histologic pathology of nontumorous diseases of bone and joints, 1st ed. Northbrook IL, USA, pp 385–390
38. Hasegawa K, Takahashi HE, Koga Y, Kawashima T, Hara T, Tanabe Y, Tanaka S (1993) Mechanical properties of osteopenic vertebral bodies monitored by acoustic emission. Bone 14:737–743
39. Hasegawa K, Takahashi HE, Koga Y, Kawashima T, Hara T, Tanabe Y, Tanaka S (1993) Failure characteristics of osteoporotic vertebral bodies monitored by acoustic emission. Spine 18:2314–2320
40. Hasegawa K, Turner CH, Chen J, Burr DB (1995) Effect of disc lesion on microdamage accumulation in lumbar vertebrae under cyclic compression loading. Clin Orthop 311:190–198
41. Ratcliffe JF (1980) The arterial anatomy of the adult human lumbar vertebral body: a microarteriographic study. J Anat 131:57–79
42. Moore DC, Maitra RS, Farjo LA, Graziano GP, Goldstein SA (1997) Restoration of pedicle screw fixation with an in situ setting calcium phosphate cement. Spine 22:1696–1705

Part 2
Mechanical Loading and Its Regulation in Bone

The Mechanics of Bone Adaptation

Charles H. Turner[1] and Mohammed P. Akhter[2]

Summary. The skeleton's primary mechanical function is to provide rigid levers for muscles to act against as they hold the body upright in defiance of gravity. Many bones are exposed to thousands of repetitive loads each day. During growth and development, the skeleton adds mass to the weight-bearing bones to adapt them to their mechanical role, thus reducing the risk of fracture. The determinant of bone adaptation is the daily loading stimulus, which is a function of the magnitude, frequency, and duration of mechanical signals engendered within the bone. The processes of bone remodeling and modeling are affected by the magnitude of the daily loading stimulus. If the stimulus falls below a lower threshold, remodeling will be increased and bone mass will be lost, and if the stimulus surpasses an upper threshold, bone mass will be increased due to increased bone formation on modeling surfaces. These thresholds form surfaces in three-dimensional space defined by loading frequency, magnitude, and duration. There is also another threshold above which loading causes damage in the bone tissue, thus increasing bone remodeling and repair. The damage threshold is defined by loading magnitude and duration, but not frequency.

Mechanical signals within the bone are detected by a cellular network that responds by producing signaling molecules such as prostaglandins and nitric oxide. There are at least two intracellular pathways by which mechanical forces are translated into cellular responses, one involving constitutive enzymes near the cell membrane and another involving the integrin-actin cytoskeletal complex. The details of these pathways are discussed.

Key words. Bone density, Mechanotransduction, Mechanical stress, Biomechanics

[1] Departments of Orthopaedic Surgery Biomechanics and Biomaterials Research Center and Indiana University School of Medicine, IUPUI, Indianapolis, IN 46202, USA
[2] Department of Medicine, Creighton University, Omaha, NE 68131, USA

Introduction

The skeleton has two major functions: to provide a reservoir for essential minerals and to provide rigid levers for the muscles to act against. Although the role of the bones in maintaining mineral homeostasis is clearly important, the skeleton's mechanical function is certainly of equal importance in the regulation of bone cell biology. Bone cells begin with the genetic blueprint for the skeleton and sculpt it during growth and development until the skeletal design meets the loading requirements. This process, termed bone adaptation, requires bone cells to detect mechanical signals in situ and integrate these signals into appropriate changes in the bone architecture. For this to occur, the mechanical loading from many different types of daily activities must be integrated into a signal, the daily loading stimulus, that the bone cells detect and respond to. Based upon experimental evidence, the daily loading stimulus can be described mathematically in terms of the magnitude, frequency, and duration of mechanical signals engendered within the bone.

In this chapter, we outline the accumulated experimental evidence and theoretical development that provides a basic understanding of how bone adapts to mechanical signals.

Early Theories of Bone Adaptation

Over a hundred years ago, Roux [1] and Wolff [2] proposed that bone architecture is determined by mathematical laws: the thickness and number of trabeculae, i.e., the distribution of mass, must correspond to the quantitative distribution of mechanical stresses, and the trabeculae must be stressed axially in compression or tension. Pauwels furthered this work to describe the effects of mechanical stresses on long bone cross-sectional shape and fracture healing [3]. These laws describe the propensity of bone structure to achieve optimum balance between the cost of excessive bone mass and the cost of excessive bone fragility. However, they do not elucidate the mechanisms by which bone adapts to mechanical forces. Most importantly, they do not provide a clear mathematical description of the mechanical signal that initiates adaptation.

Defining the daily loading stimulus for bone adaptation has involved numerous studies over the last one hundred years. Wolff originally proposed that the stresses in the bone tissue determined the bone architecture. Later, Thompson [4] and Frost [5] pointed out that strain, the result of stress, was the direct stimulus on bone cells. Principal tensile or compressive strains are considered most important for bone adaptation, and shear strains seem to have little effect [6]. Cancellous structures tend to be arranged to minimize shear strains by placing struts in the direction of predominant loads [7].

Frost's Theory of Mechanical Usage Windows

Frost defined two fundamental processes in bone biology, called modeling and remodeling. Modeling is the process by which bone changes its shape or sculpts itself to adapt to its loading environment. The sculpting process takes place by "activation" of bone cells at a specific site, followed directly by bone formation or bone resorption. Bone remodeling is the process by which bone is resorbed and replaced in situ by new bone. Remodeling repairs microcracks and replaces aged bone. Bone modeling can increase the size or change the shape of bones in response to changes in mechanical usage. Rapid modeling responses often involve woven bone formation. Bone remodeling typically maintains bone mass, but if resorption cavities are underfilled with new bone, bone mass will decrease.

Frost proposed that the processes of bone modeling and remodeling are controlled by a feedback system in which changes in peak mechanical strain drive each of the processes and adjust bone mass and structure accordingly [5,8,9]. Frost's theory describes a control system in which bone structure is maintained such that ordinary mechanical strains do not exceed a minimum effective strain (MES), which Frost speculated to be 1500 to 2500 microstrain. If the local strains within the bone surpass the MES, bone will undergo modeling and change its structure to reduce the local strains to below the MES. This theory also incorporates another effective strain level of 50 to 200 microstrain, below which bone tissue will be resorbed until the local strains are increased. This latter process occurs in disuse or spaceflight. Furthermore, Frost proposed a third strain threshold of about 4000 microstrain that defined the minimum strain for the initiation of microdamage within the bone. Strains above the "damage threshold" would increase bone remodeling to repair the damage [9] and induce woven bone formation to cause a rapid increase in bone mass and protect against bone fracture.

Frost's bone adaptation model is summarized in Fig. 1, which shows a "physiological window" for bone that falls between the MES and the lower effective strain. When mechanical strains remain in the physiological window, there is subtle modulation of

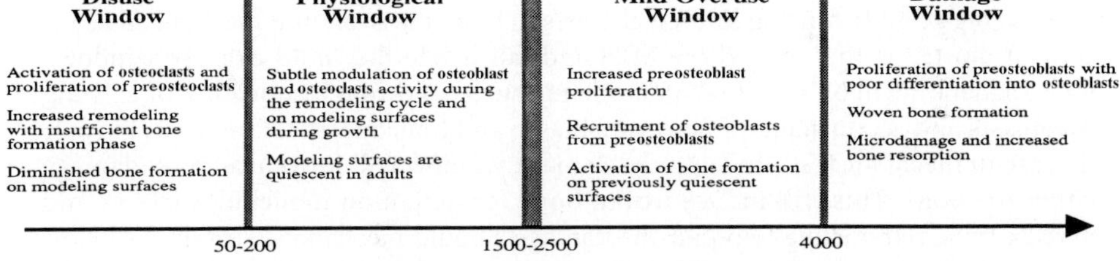

Mechanical Strain (microstrain)

FIG. 1. Frost's mechanical usage windows describe the response of bone tissue to mechanical loading magnitude (mechanical strain). The predominant mechanical strains engendered by the bone tissue determine its cellular activity and modulate the processes of modeling and remodeling at bone surfaces. Disuse is characterized by increased bone resorption on both modeling and remodeling surfaces and decreased bone formation on modeling surfaces, leading to rapid bone loss. Homeostasis is attained within the physiological window where there is, in general, a balance between bone resorption and bone formation. Slight gains in bone mass are achieved by mild overuse, which can activate osteoblasts on bone modeling surfaces. Greater gains in bone mass are achieved with very high loads, but these gains result from poorly organized, woven bone formation, and the high mechanical strains cause microdamage within the bone tissue and stimulate bone remodeling to repair the microcracks

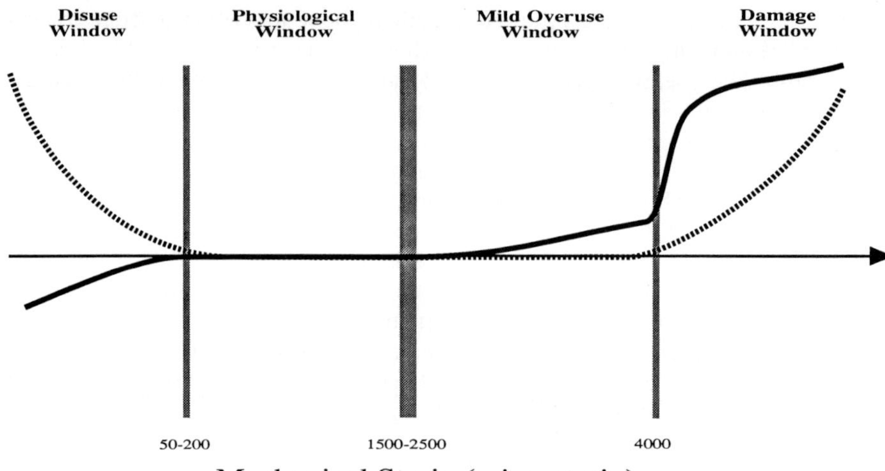

Mechanical Strain (microstrain)

FIG. 2. Effect of mechanical strain on bone modeling (*solid line*) and remodeling (*dashed line*). Frost's model dictates that mechanical usage affects modeling and remodeling processes differently. Disuse increases bone remodeling on trabecular and endocortical surfaces and a mismatch between bone resorption and formation, leading to bone loss. Bone formation on modeling surfaces is inhibited by disuse. Bone remodeling is minimal for mechanical strains in the physiological and mild overuse windows, but increases to repair microdamage within the bone matrix when the damage threshold is surpassed. Bone formation on modeling surfaces is slightly increased when the MES (1500–2500 microstrain) is surpassed. A large increase in bone formation occurs when woven bone formation is activated by large overloads within the damage window (see [14])

osteoblast and osteoclast activity during the remodeling cycle and on modeling surfaces during growth, causing limited changes in bone mass. Should mechanical usage cause strain levels that exceed the MES and fall inside the "mild overuse window," bone formation will be activated on modeling surfaces through activation of existing osteoblasts and recruitment of new osteoblasts, and bone mass will increase. Further increase in mechanical strains into the damage window will introduce microdamage within the bone. This will induce woven bone formation on modeling surfaces and increase bone remodeling to repair the damage. Should mechanical strains fall below the lower effective strain to within the disuse window, bone remodeling will be activated and bone formation will be diminished, leading to decreased bone mass.

Frost's theory of mechanical usage effects on bone modeling and remodeling is summarized graphically in Fig. 2. Bone remodeling is activated within the damage window, possibly by microcracks [10,11], and by disuse [12], but is maintained at only a low level in the physiological and mild overuse windows. Bone formation on modeling surfaces is decreased during disuse and increased during overuse, provided that the MES is surpassed [13]. A dramatic increase in modeling is seen when woven bone formation is activated by high strains [14].

Frost's theory provides a good starting point from which one can begin to understand bone adaptation. However, the model oversimplifies the mechanical strain stimulus by presenting it only in terms of mechanical strain magnitude, since it is known that strain rate, loading frequency, and loading duration also affect the tissue response. What follows is a further theoretical development of Frost's theory that incorporates the entire character of the daily loading stimulus.

Expanding upon Frost's Theory

There is a growing body of evidence demonstrating that fluid flow within the canaliculae and lacunae of bone is primarily responsible for mechanochemical signal transduction in bone cells [15]. If true, this suggests that hydrostatic stress gradients within the bone must develop to initiate bone adaptation. Hydrostatic fluid stress is generated by dynamic dilatational strains (i.e., volume changes in the tissue), but not by shear strains, suggesting that adaptation is controlled by loading rate. This mechanism is supported by experimental studies that showed dynamic, but not static, strains increased bone formation in animals [16–18].

Increased duration of skeletal loading does not yield proportional increases in bone mass. As the duration of loading is increased, the cumulative effects on bone mass diminish. This phenomenon is demonstrated in the study by Rubin and Lanyon [19] using the isolated avian ulna loading model. They applied mechanical loading of different durations daily and found that increasing loading duration past 36 cycles/day was not very effective for causing further increases in bone mass. In the study of Umemura et al. [20], in which rats were trained to jump various numbers of times per day and changes in their tibial and femoral bone mass, were measured, 5 jumps/day were sufficient to increase bone mass, but increasing numbers of jumps gave diminishing returns with respect to bone mass.

These experimental results tell us the following: dynamic strains drive bone adaptation, and increasing the number of loading cycles (duration) gives diminishing returns with respect to bone adaptation. These observations can be incorporated into a mathematical formula as follows:

$$S \propto \sum_{j=1}^{k} \log(1 + N_j)E_j \qquad (1)$$

where
$$E_j \propto \varepsilon_j f_j$$

and S is the daily loading stimulus, k represents the number of daily loading conditions, N is the number of daily loading cycles for each loading condition, and E represents the strain stimulus for each loading condition i.e., the product of the peak-to-peak principal strain (ε) and the loading frequency (f). The product εf is proportional to the peak strain rate in the bone. Equation 1 gives E for a sinusoidal loading waveform. However, the result can be generalized using the Fourier method that allows any periodic loading waveform to be expanded into a series of sine waves at different amplitudes and frequencies. So in the general case, the strain stimulus is defined as

$$E \propto \sum_{i=1}^{n} \varepsilon_i f_i \qquad (2)$$

Equation 1 predicts the results observed by ourselves and others using the rat tibiabending model. In this model, bending loads are applied to the tibiae of adult rats to induce bone adaptation [13]. New bone formation is influenced by loading frequency

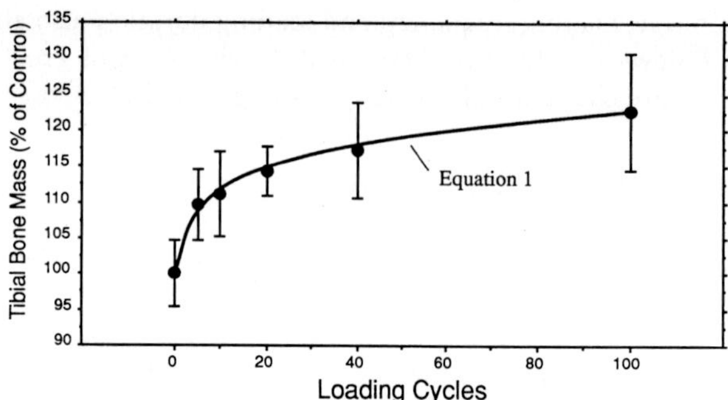

FIG. 3. Umemura et al. [20] trained rats to jump various of numbers of time per day and found that 5 jumps/day were sufficient to increase bone mass, but increasing numbers of jumps gave diminishing returns with respect to bone mass. These data very closely fit the mathematical relationship proposed in Eq. 1

and loading magnitude [13,21]. For each of these previous experiments, bone formation can be presented as a function of strain stimulus calculated using Eq. 1. Equation 1 also closely fits the data of Umemura et al. [20] (Fig. 3).

Feedback Control of Bone Adaptation

Bone adaptation is "error-driven." As stated by Lanyon [22], "The mechanically-adaptive response is dominated not by the numerous cycles of 'normal' strain change engendered during the predominant activity but rather by the far fewer cycles of relatively 'abnormal' strain changes produced during unusual loading situations." This rule reflects adaptation, at a cellular level, that causes bone cells to accommodate to "normal" strain waveforms from routine daily activities like walking or running.

The mathematical function that describes error-driven bone adaptation has the general form

$$\frac{\partial m}{\partial t} = B\{\phi - F\} \qquad (3)$$

where m is bone mass, t is time, ϕ is the local stress/strain state, F is the equilibrium stress/strain state, and B and is a constant [23]. F represents the "normal" loading state to which the bone cells are accustomed. Thus, $\phi - F$ is an error function that drives the system to change bone mass. ϕ can be represented by the daily loading stimulus (S) given in Eq. 1, and F can be characterized as the "normal" loading stimulus ($S_\bullet$). Thus, $S - S_0$ must be the driving force for bone adaptation. Under normal loading patterns, both osteoclast and osteoblast activities are maintained at low levels, but if the error function ($S - S_0$) falls below a lower threshold (i.e., abnormally low loading), osteoclast activity associated with bone remodeling increases. If the error function surpasses an upper threshold, osteoblast activity on bone modeling surfaces is activated, causing sculpting of the shape of long bones or trabeculae. In long bones, which are loaded mostly in bending, the strains along the neutral bending axis are small under normal loading conditions, so we can assume that the bone cells have accommodated to small strains; otherwise we should expect the bone along the neutral axis to resorb away. The strains increase in magnitude as the distance from the neutral bending axis increases, and thus the cells should be accommodated to different strains at each point across the long-bone section. Large deviations from equilibrium, i.e., abnormal loading states, drive adaptation. This may explain why experimental loading regimens that produce bending along an abnormal neutral axis have a dramatic effect on bone formation, even though the strain magnitudes achieved are well within physiological limits [19]. In this scenario, the difference between "abnormal" and "normal" loading stimuli at different points within the bone tissue can be quite large.

New Theory of Mechanical Usage Windows

The formula for daily loading stimulus given in Eq. 1 can be adapted to the concept of mechanical usage windows put forth by Frost. Frost's windows can be defined in terms of peak dynamic strain magnitude, the number of loading cycles, and loading frequency. From our studies of applied loading to the tibiae of rats, we can define the mechanical usage windows as follows.

The error function $(S - S_0)$ must surpass a threshold, the minimum effective strain stimulus (MESS), to activate bone formation on modeling surfaces. This MESS was measured in the rat tibia as 1050 microstrain for a loading regimen of 36 cycles per day at 2 Hz [13]. Thus, from Eq. 1,

$$MESS = 1050 \times 2 \times \log(1 + 36) = 3293$$

This threshold defines the boundary between the physiological and mild overuse windows in terms of peak strain and number of loading cycles (Fig. 4) or in terms of peak strain and loading frequency (Fig. 5). There is no definitive experimental evidence defining a threshold for disuse. Therefore, we guessed that the threshold for bone loss occurs at strains below 200 microstrain for less than 100 cycles per day. This threshold is represented by the dashed line in Figs. 4 and 5. The damage window for the rat tibia was defined by ex vivo fatigue tests conducted in our laborating (Akhter, unpublished data). The stiffness for the rat tibia was monitored while oscillating bending forces were applied to the bone. The levels of peak strain and the number of loading cycles in which detectable losses in the tibial stiffness were observed were defined as the lower boundary of the damage window. The levels of peak strain and the number of loading cycles in which tibial stiffness was reduced by over 30% defined the failure line (Figs. 4 and 5). The mechanical usage windows for the rat tibia loading in bending thus can be defined from experimental data and the theoretical relationship in Eq. 1.

Cellular Mechanotransduction

The mechanisms by which bone adaptation works are poorly understood, but they require some form of cellular mechanotransduction. Mechanotransduction, or the conversion of a biophysical force into a cellular response, is an essential mechanism

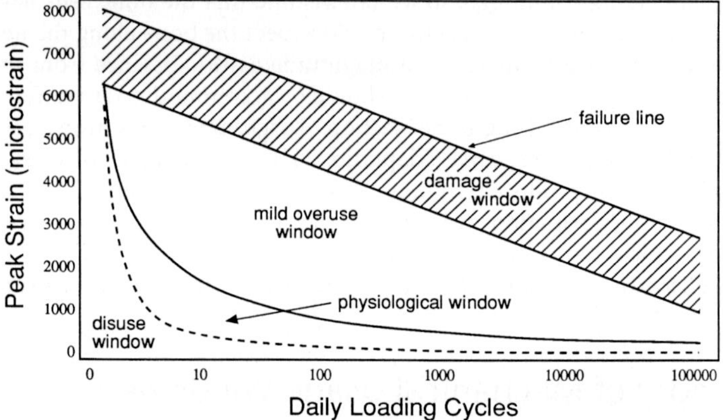

FIG. 4. New model for mechanical usage windows presented in terms of peak strain magnitude and number of loading cycles. The physiological window is bordered by the minimum effective strain stimulus (*solid line*) and the lower threshold (*dashed line*). The MESS was defined based upon data from loading experiments using four-point bending of the rat tibia [13]. These experiments were done using a fixed loading frequency of 2 cycles per second (Hz). The damage window was defined by a series of bending fatigue experiments with rat tibiae. The lower boundary of the damage window represents loading conditions under which detectable damage, measured as loss of stiffness, began to occur in the tibia. The failure line represents the loading conditions under which the stiffness of the tibia was reduced by 30%

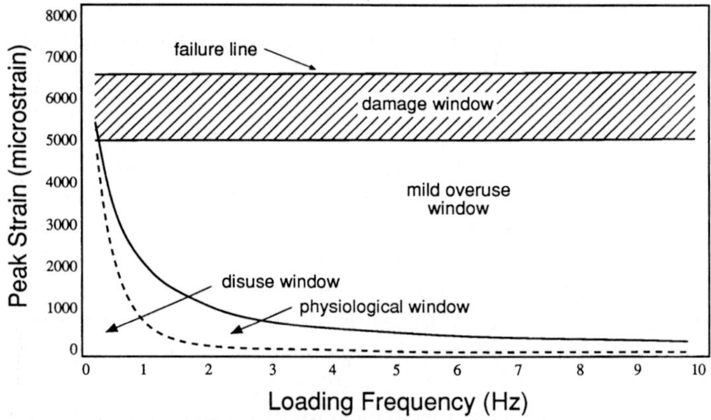

FIG. 5. New model for mechanical usage windows presented in terms of peak strain magnitude and loading frequency. The physiological window is bordered by the minimum effective strain stimulus (*solid line*) and the lower threshold (*dashed line*). The MESS was defined based upon data from our loading experiments using four-point bending of the rat tibia [13]. These experiments were done using a fixed loading frequency of 2 Hz. The damage window was extrapolated from data from a series of bending fatigue experiments using rat tibiae and done at a loading frequency of 2 Hz. It is assumed that loading frequency does not affect the strain level at which damage occurs in the bone

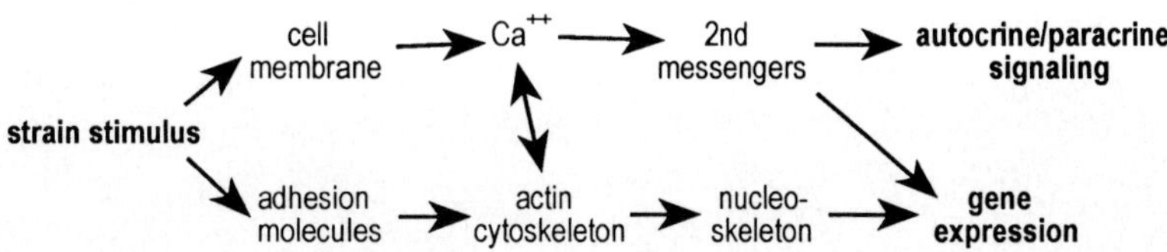

FIG. 6. Mechanochemical pathways for bone adaptation. Mechanical signals (strain stimulus) are detected by mechanoreceptors in the cell membrane or by transmembrane adhesion molecules. Within the cell membrane is a G protein-linked mechanoreceptor that causes increased intracellular calcium (Ca^{++}), through membrane ion channels or from intracellular stores, and second messengers such as prostaglandins and nitric oxide; these messengers can travel outside the cell and initiate both autocrine and paracrine signaling, or remain within the cell and influence gene expression. The adhesion molecules, e.g., integrins or cadherins, are directly linked to the actin cytoskeleton, which is linked to the nucleoskeleton, which in turn is linked to DNA. It is proposed that mechanical signals can cause restructuring of the actin cytoskeleton, affecting the direct mechanical link to the genes, and thus regulate gene expression

for a wide variety of physiologic functions that allow living organisms to respond to their mechanical environment. There is now evidence of several mechanochemical transduction pathways within bone cells (Fig. 6). One involves a mechanotransducer that resides in the cell membrane. This transducer is G protein-linked and also interacts with a stretch-activated cation channel, the inositol triphosphate messenger pathway, and constituitive isoforms of cyclo-oxygenase (COX) and nitric oxide synthase (NOS). The second pathway involves a direct linkage between the transmembrane integrins, the actin cytoskeleton, and the nuclear transcription machinery. The induction of COX is dependent upon this pathway.

In bone cell culture, mechanical loading or fluid shear stress increases intracellular calcium levels and production of prostaglandins and nitric oxide within minutes [24–27]. This stimulation of prostaglandins can be blocked by 70–80% with G protein inhibitors GDPβS and pertussis toxin, indicating that a G protein-associated mechanotransducer attached to the cell membrane may be responsible for prostaglandin production. Constituitive isoforms of COX and NOS are typically bound to the cell membrane and thus would be available for mechanochemical transduction involving G proteins. The movement of extracellular calcium ions across the cell membrane also appears to play a role in mechanotransduction, as does calcium release from intracellular stores [24,28]. One way in which extracellular calcium can pass across the cell membrane is through a stretch-activated cation channel [29]. Increase in intracellular calcium occurs within minutes in osteoblasts exposed to fluid shear stresses, and this response is partially blocked by $GdCl_3$, which blocks the stress-activated calcium channels in the cell membrane [24]. It is not clear yet what interaction the inositol triphosphate pathway, which controls release of intracellular calcium, has with the stretch-activated cation channel or the G protein mechanotransducer, but these systems may be interrelated.

Another pathway by which mechanotransduction occurs is through the integrin-cytoskeleton complex. Integrins are heterodimeric transmembrane proteins that bind to the extracellular matrix (ECM) on the outside of cells and are linked to the actin cytoskeleton via the short cytoplasmic domain of the β subunit on the inside of cells

No flow (f-actin/c-fos)   Flow 1 h (f-actin/c-fos)

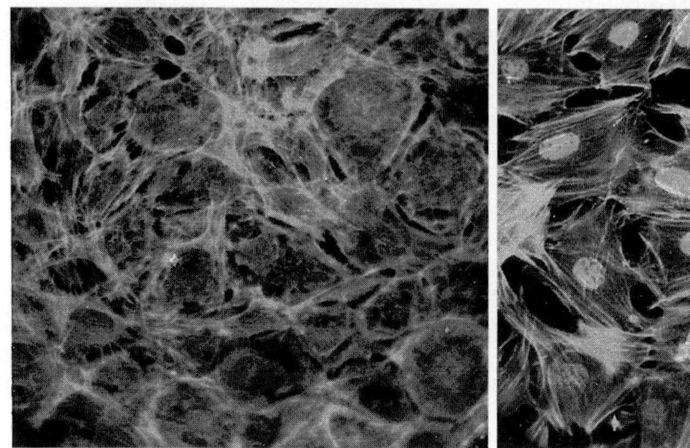

FIG. 7. MC3T3-E1 osteoblasts subjected to fluid shear (12 dynes/cm²) for 60 min undergo dramatic reorganization of the actin cytoskeleton and express the early response gene c-fos. *Left panel*: Control cells not subjected to flow have poorly organized stress fibers labeled with Texas red-phalloidin (*green*), and expression of c-fos is not present. *Right panel*: Cells subjected to fluid flow for 60 min develop prominent stress fibers labeled with Texas red-phalloidin and demonstrate clear nuclear staining of c-fos protein (*red*). Copyright 1998 by Neil X. Chen, used with permission

as specialized sites known as focal adhesions. Several lines of evidence using various cell types, including fibroblasts, epithelial cells, endothelial cells, and neutrophils, as well as osteoblasts, indicate that a key molecule in mediating the linkage of actin filaments to integrin cytoplasmic domains is the protein α-actinin [30–32]. Fluid flow on bone cells induces recruitment of integrins to focal adhesions and causes the actin filaments in the cell to reorganize into large bundles of actin filaments called stress fibers [33] (Fig. 7). Coincident with fluid flow-induced changes in cytoskeletal organization is an increase in expression of c-fos, an early response gene, and cyclooxygenase-2 (COX-2), an enzyme important in bone mechanotransduction [34]. Anchorage of actin filaments at focal adhesions via α-actinin is necessary for both the formation of stress fibers and up-regulation of c-fos and COX-2 expression that is normally induced when osteoblasts are subjected to fluid shear [33].

Osteocytes and bone lining cells make up over 95% of all cells of the osteoblastic lineage that are attached to bone [35]. These cells are interconnected with each other through functional gap junctions [36,37] and are responsive to mechanical loading stimuli in vivo [38,39]. For these reasons, it is commonly assumed that these cells act as sensors of mechanical stimuli, but, since neither bone lining cells nor osteocytes can actively form or resorb bone, they must signal to "effector cells" (osteoblasts or osteoclasts) before a change in bone structure can be initiated. The most likely intermediaries for cell-to-cell communication between sensor cells and effector cells are the prostaglandins and nitric oxide (NO). Mechanical stimuli applied to cell and tissue culture causes production of several prostaglandins and NO [25,40–44]. Blockade of prostaglandin production in vivo, particularly with selective inhibitors of the inducible isoform of cyclooxygenase, eliminates mechanically induced bone formation [34,45]. Inhibitors of NO synthases also suppress mechanically induced bone formation in rats [46,47].

Discussion

It is unlikely that pathways for bone cell regulation will be completely selective for mechanotransduction, but more likely signals from hormones or paracrine factors share these pathways to some extent. Certainly, most of the mechanotransduction pathways identified to this point involve rather ubiquitous messengers such as intracellular calcium, prostaglandins, cyclic AMP, and NO as the downstream targets of mechanical effects. These messenger systems are used by many different cell types in various tissues to initiate responses to hormonal, paracrine, and mechanical signals. The nature of interactions between hormonal and mechanical effects on bone cells is of great interest. A little over 10 years ago, Frost [48] proposed that hormones interact with bone adaptation by altering a series of mechanical loading "thresholds," which determine when bone cells will be activated to remove or add new bone to the skeleton. This theory, called the "mechanostat theory," implies that hormones enhance or inhibit mechanical loading effects at some fundamental level within the bone cell signal transduction machinery. A recent study showed that mechanical loading fails to induce bone formation in thyroparathroidectomized rats, but when these rats are given a dose of parathyroid hormone shortly before mechanical loading, the mechanically induced bone formation response is restored [49]. This result supports the prospectus put forth by Frost that hormones and other systemic factors act by modulating cellular mechanotransduction pathways.

In summary, the mechanisms for bone adaptation are beginning to come into focus. Adaptation involves a mechanosensory apparatus in bone and several mechanochemical pathways. Since efficient bone adaptation improves skeletal performance and reduces the risk of fracture, often a fatal affliction in ancient times, the process of evolution probably preserved and enhanced the ability of bone cells to respond appropriately to mechanical loads. Cellular mechanotransduction may thus be a fundamental process in bone cell biology. Bone adaptation can be predicted, to some extent, by mathematical formulas derived from fundamental rules: bone adaptation is driven by dynamic, rather than static, loading, and extending the loading duration has a diminishing effect on further bone adaptation. These mathematical rules, when combined with Frost's theory of mechanical usage windows, allow prediction of bone adaptation in animal models. Further work is needed to determine whether these rules can also predict bone adaptation in the human skeleton.

References

1. Roux W (1895) Gesammelte Abhandlungen. Vol. 1. Engelmann, Leipzig
2. Wolff J (1892) Das Gesetz der Transformation der Knochen. Hirschwald, Berlin
3. Pauwels F (1980) Biomechanics of the locomotor apparatus. Springer-Verlag, Berlin
4. Thompson D (1961) On growth and form (abridged edition, JT Bonner, ed) Cambridge (originally published in 1917)

5. Frost HM (1964) The laws of bone structure. Charles C Thomas, Springfield, IL
6. Qin Y-X, McLeod KJ, Guilak F, Chiang F-P, Rubin CT (1996) Correlation of bony ingrowth to the distribution of stress and strain parameters surrounding a porous-coated implant. J Orthop Res 14:862–870
7. Pidaparti RMV, Turner CH (1997) Cancellous bone architecture: advantages of nonorthogonal trabecular alignment under multidirectional joint loading. J Biomech 30:979–983
8. Frost HM (1990) Structural adaptations to mechanical usage (SATMU): 1. Redefining Wolff's law: the bone modeling problem. Anat Rec 226:403–413
9. Frost HM (1990) Structural adaptations to mechanical usage (SATMU): 2. Redefining Wolff's law: the bone remodeling problem. Anat Rec 226:414–422
10. Burr DB, Martin RB, Schaffler MB, Radin EL (1985) Bone remodeling in response to in vivo fatigue microdamage. J Biomech 18:189–200
11. Mori S, Burr DB (1993) Increased intracortical remodeling following fatigue damage. Bone 14:103–109
12. Uhthoff HK, Jaworski ZFG (1978) Bone loss in response to long-term immobilisation. J Bone Joint Surg 60-B:420–429
13. Turner CH, Forwood MR, Rho J, Yoshikawa T (1994) Mechanical loading thresholds for lamellar and woven bone formation. J Bone Miner Res 9:87–97
14. Turner CH (1992) Functional determinants of bone structure: beyond Wolff's law of bone transformation. Bone 13:403–409
15. Duncan RL, Turner CH (1995) Mechanotransduction and the functional response of bone to mechanical strain. Calcif Tissue Int 57:344–358
16. Lanyon LE, Rubin CT (1984) Static vs dynamic loads as an influence on bone remodelling. J Biomech 17:897–905
17. Liskova M, Hert J (1971) Reaction of bone to mechanical stimuli. Part 2. Periosteal and endosteal reaction of tibial diaphysis in rabbit to intermittent loading. Folia Morphologica 19:301–317
18. Turner CH, Owan I, Takano Y (1995) Mechanotransduction in bone: role of strain rate. Am J Physiol 269:E438–E442
19. Rubin CT, Lanyon LE (1984) Regulation of bone formation by applied dynamic loads. J Bone Joint Surg 66A:397–402
20. Umemura Y, Ishiko T, Yamauchi T, Kurono M, Mashiko S (1997) Five jumps per day increase bone mass and breaking force in rats. J Bone Miner Res 12:1480–1485
21. Turner CH, Forwood MR, Otter MW (1994) Mechanotransduction in bone: do bone cells act as sensors of fluid flow? FASEB J 8:875–878
22. Lanyon LE (1992) The success and failure of the adaptive response to functional loading-bearing in averting bone fracture. Bone 13:S17–S21
23. Fyhrie DP, Schaffler MB (1995) The adaptation of bone apparent density to applied load. J Biomech 28:135–146
24. Hung CT, Allen FD, Pollack SR, Brighton CT (1996) Intracellular Ca^{2+} stores and extracellular Ca^{2+} are required in the real-time Ca^{2+} response of bone cells experiencing fluid flow. J Biomech 29:1411–1417
25. Johnson DL, McAllister TN, Frangos JA (1996) Fluid flow stimulates rapid and continuous release of nitric oxide in osteoblasts. Am J Physiol 271:E205–E208
26. Jones DB, Bingmann D (1991) How do osteoblasts respond to mechanical stimulation? Cells Materials 1:329–340
27. Reich KM, Frangos JA (1991) Effect of flow on prostaglandin E_2 and inositol triphosphate levels in osteoblasts. Am J Physiol 261:C428–C432
28. Reich KM, McAllister TN, Gudi S, Frangos JA (1997) Activation of G proteins mediates flow-induced prostaglandin E2 production in osteoblasts. Endocrinology 138:1014–1018

29. Duncan RL, Kizer N, Barry EL, Friedman PA, Hruska KA (1996) Antisense oligodeoxynucleotide inhibition of a swelling-activated cation channel in osteoblast-like osteosarcoma cells. Proc Natl Acad Sci USA 93:1864–1869

30. Otey CA, Pavalko FM, Burridge K (1990) An interaction between α-actinin and the β1 integrin subunit in vitro. J Cell Biol 111:721–730

31. Pavalko FM, Burridge K (1991) Disruption of the actin cytoskeleton after micro-injection of proteolytic fragments of alpha-actinin. J Cell Biol 114:481–491

32. Pavalko FM, LaRoche SM (1993) Activation of human neutrophils induces an interaction between the integrin β2 subunit (CD18) and the actin-binding protein α-actinin. J Immunol 151:3795–3807

33. Pavalko, FM, Chen NX, Turner CH, Burr DB, Atkinson S, Hsieh Y-F, Qui J, Duncan RL (1998) Fluid shear-induced mechanical signaling in MC3T3-E1 osteoblasts requires cytoskeleton-integrin interactions. Am J Physiol 275:C1591–C1601

34. Forwood MR (1996) Inducible cyclo-oxygenase (COX-2) mediates the induction of bone formation by mechanical loading in vivo. J Bone Miner Res 11:1688–1693

35. Parfitt AM (1983) The physiologic and clinical significance of bone histomorphometric data. In: Bone histomorphometry (Recker RR, ed) CRC Press, Boca Raton, FL, pp 143–223

36. Donahue HJ, McLeod KJ, Rubin CT, Andersen J, Grine EA, Hertzberg EL, Brink PR (1995) Cell-to-cell communication in osteoblastic networks: cell line-dependent hormonal regulation of gap junction function. J Bone Miner Res 10:881–889

37. Doty SB (1981) Morphological evidence of gap junctions between bone cells. Calcif Tissue Int 33:509–512

38. Inoaka T, Lean JM, Bessho T, Chow JWM, Mackay A, Kokubo T, Chambers TJ (1995) Sequential analysis of gene expression after an osteogenic stimulus: c-fos expression is induced in osteocytes. Biochem Biophys Res Commun 217:264–270

39. Skerry TM, Bitensky L, Chayen J, Lanyon LE (1989) Early strain-related changes in enzyme activity in osteocytes following bone loading in vivo. J Bone Miner Res 4:783–788

40. Klein-Nulend J, van der Plas A, Semeins CM, Ajubi NE, Frangos JA, Nijweide PJ, Burger EH (1995) Sensitivity of osteocytes to biomechanical stress in vitro. FASEB J 9:441–445

41. Klein-Nulend J, Burger EH, Semeins CM, Raisz LG, Pilbream CC (1997) Pulsating fluid flow stimulates prostaglandin release and inducible prostaglandin G/H synthase mRNA expression in primary mice bone cells. J Bone Miner Res 12:45–51

42. Pitsillides AA, Rawlinson SC, Suswillo RF, Bourrin S, Zaman G, Lanyon LE (1995) Mechanical strain-induced NO production by bone cells: a possible role in adaptive bone (re)modeling? FASEB J 9:1614–1622

43. Rawlinson SC, Mohan S, Baylink DJ, Lanyon LE (1993) Exogenous prostacyclin, but not prostaglandin E2, produces similar responses in both G6PD activity and RNA production as mechanical loading, and increases IGF-II release, in adult cancellous bone in culture. Calcif Tissue Int 53:324–329

44. Somjen D, Binderman I, Berger E, Harell A (1980) Bone remodeling induced by physical stress is prostaglandin E_2 mediated. Biochim Biophys Acta 627:91–100

45. Chow JW, Chambers TJ (1994) Indomethacin has distinct early and late actions on bone formation induced by mechanical stimulation. Am J Physiol 267:E287–E292

46. Fox SW, Chambers TJ, Chow JW (1996) Nitric oxide is an early mediator of the increase in bone formation by mechanical stimulation. Am J Physiol 270:E955–E960

47. Turner CH, Takano Y, Owan I, Murrell GAC (1996) Nitric oxide inhibitor L-NAME suppresses mechanically-induced bone formation in rats. Am J Physiol 270:E634–E639

48. Frost HM (1987) Bone "mass" and the "mechanostat": A proposal. Anat Rec 219:1–9

49. Chow JW, Fox S, Jagger CJ, Chambers TJ (1998) A role for parathyroid hormone in the mechanical responsiveness of rat bone. Am J Physiol 274:E146–E154

Biomechanics of Articular Joints: Review of a Decade of Progress of the Niigata Biomechanics Group

Toshiaki Hara[1], Yuji Tanabe[1], and Makoto Sakamoto[2]

Summary. A survey of some of the advances made over the past 10 years in the understanding of joint mechanics by the Niigata biomechanics researchers are presented. We have conducted research on joint mechanics with an awareness that approaches from both experimental and mathematical analysis are important. Topics covered in this chapter include: measurement of joint contact pressure under experimental conditions using a pressure-sensitive conductive rubber sensor which we have developed; and mathematical analysis of joint contact, in particular, using the anisotropic cartilage model that introduces the idea of a specific alignment for collagen fiber.

Key words. Biomechanics, Joint, Contact stress, Mechanical properties

Introduction

The Niigata Biomechanics Group was formed in 1987 by Dr. Tatsuya Tajima, Professor Emeritus of the Department of Orthopaedic Surgery in Niigata University; Dr. Hideaki Takahashi, Professor of the Department; Dr. Yoshio Koga; and Toshiaki Hara, Professor of the Department of Mechanical Engineering. At the time of its formation, the participants exchanged their ideas from their specialty either as orthopaedic surgeons or mechanical engineers. The group conducted its first study under the theme of limb elongation by callotasis on the growth plate [1] initiated by Professor Takahashi, which became a pioneering work, providing the first biomechanical data in Japan. It resulted in numerous subsequent studies such as the development of a measuring system of joint contact pressure, joint dynamics, mechanical characteristic of bone, sports engineering, and other important topics in the research field of biomechanics.

[1] Department of Mechanical Engineering, Niigata University, 8050 Ikarashi 2, Niigata 950-2181, Japan
[2] Department of Mechanical Engineering, Niigata College of Technology, 5-13-7 Kamishin'ei-cho, Niigata 950-2076, Japan

In 1989, T. Hara was invited as visiting professor to the Orthopaedic Surgery Biomechanics Laboratory at the Mayo Clinic led by Professor Edmund Y. S. Chao, who was a close friend of Professors Tajima and Takahashi. This collaboration gave momentum to the study operation with an international focus to the group. In particular, Hara conducted an experimental study together with Professor Chao on the biomechanics of the wrist joint and published some interesting data [2]. In 1992, Yuji Tanabe of the Department of Mechanical Engineering of Niigata University carried out research with Professor W. Bonfield of London University, who is known for his study of the biomaterials, and his research on the mechanical properties of bone [3]. In 1993, Professor Chao moved to the Johns Hopkins University. Makoto Sakamoto, who obtained the first doctorate under Professor Hara, became a visiting scientist at this time, and joined in the research on the indentation test of biological tissue [4] as well as on mathematical models of joints. Orthopedic surgeons, who studied biomechanics with the Niigata group, are conducting research and achieving results, mainly on artificial joints [5], under Professor Ramon B. Gustilo and Dr. Joan E. Bechtold of the University of Minnesota.

This chapter reviews the studies of the Biomechanics group of Niigata, especially those on the mechanical loading of joints.

The effect of loading on bone causes pressure on the articular cartilage attached to the surface of a joint. It is extremely important to analyze the characteristics of joint contact in conjunction with joint mechanics. To ascertain a joint contact mechanism, first the size of the contact area and second the distribution of contact pressure should be determined. There are two approaches for dealing with these questions (1) measurement of the contact area and contact pressure distribution of joints experimentally using cadaver limbs and (2) calculation of the contact stress using mathematical models of joints.

A number of specialists in mechanical engineering have been working on the contact problem, which is known as one of the most difficult problems to solve in the field. Our group has proceeded with the study of the joint contact problem using both the experimental and mathematical models. The following is an outline of our current findings with those models.

Experimental Analysis

It is important when measuring the contact area and pressure distribution that the sensor used in the experiment not destroy the conformity of the joint surface, since the joint surface is generally curved and three-dimensional.

Methods such as dye staining [6] and silicon rubber casting [7] may be used to measure only the contact area. These time-consuming and labor-intensive methods are applied only to determine the contact area. Therefore, further development of these methods is not foreseen in the future.

Pressure-sensitive film (Prescale, Fuji Photo Film, Tokyo, Japan) is widely used to measure the contact pressure distribution of joints. In this method, two-sheet films are inserted between contacting joints, and the amount of pressure is measured by the density of red color, which deepens when the contact pressure is high. The films are used at wrist joints [8], patellofemoral joints [9], tibiofemoral joints [10], and elbow joints [11]. The pressure-sensitive film method has the advantage of being easy to use, but it has the major disadvantage of not being able to measure a continuous change in the pressure distribution.

There are other methods such as using a miniature load cell [12], pressure pin [13], or Buldon tube pressure gauge [14]. These methods require creating complex measuring systems for making holes on the joint surface and setting transducers beneath the surface. Given the complexity of the measuring systems and the structure of transducers used, it is questionable whether they measure the exact contact pressure. To solve these problems, we have developed a pressure-sensitive sensor using conductive rubber.

Pressure-Sensitive Conductive Rubber Sensor

The pressure-sensitive conductive rubber was developed in Japan (CS57-7RSC, Inaba Rubber, Osaka, Japan), and the pressure-sensitive conductive rubber sensor (PSRS) was developed in the Niigata Biomechanics Laboratory. The mechanism of differential electrical conductivity of the PSRS was based on the distributed volume of carbon black particles within the rubber. When external pressure is applied to the PSRS, electrical resistance decreases as structures of carbon black particles come into contact pressure. The rubber, 0.49 mm thick, is sandwiched between a pair of mylar film electrodes (0.07 mm thick), and sealed with plastic film for waterproofing. The entire device is 0.8 mm thick. Hara et al. [2] first reported on the PSRS and its application for the wrist joint, and they described the following advantages of the sensor: 1. On approximate thickness of 0.8 mm, with minimal disruption of the contact interface 2. Its resilience and flexiblity, enabling it to accommodate to an uneven contact surface easily 3. As a variable resistor, it can measure contact pressure successively. The outcome of research measuring contact pressure of an unresurfaced patella in a total knee arthroplasty using PSRS follows.

Contact Pressure of Unresurfaced Patella in Total Knee Arthroplasty

In this study, the PSRS has an active area of 50×96 mm, and a high-resolution grid system of 2560 measuring points as shown in Fig. 1. The active range of pressure is 0–2.5 MPa.

After the knee was stripped of muscle, leaving the quadriceps tendon intact, the PSRS was attached to the patellar articular surface with cyanoacrylate and several accessory sutures. The position of the sensor was confirmed by X-ray. Three-dimensional patellar tracking was measured with two sets of high-resolution CCD cameras (TR3, Sony, Tokyo, Japan) using the direct linear transformation method. Each camera tracked the markers that were strategically placed on the patella and femur, and three-dimensional patellar tracking against the femur was obtained as shown in Fig. 2. Three-dimensional motion between tibia and femur was measured with a 6-DOF electromechanical goniometer (G-II, Niigata Biomech Lab., Japan) attached to both bones with screws. After these preparations were completed, the knee joint was mounted on a specially designed frame. The quadriceps mechanism was loaded at 200 N with a pulley and the following configurations were tested in each

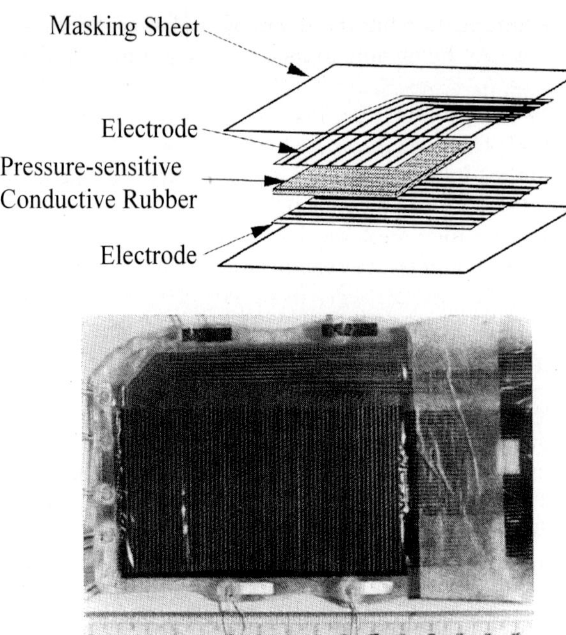

Measuring Area: 96×50 mm
Measuring Points: 2560

Fig. 1. Basic structure of the pressure-sensitive conductive rubber sensor (PSRS). The rubber, 0.49 mm thick, is sandwiched between a pair of mylar film electrodes which are 0.07 mm thick, and sealed with plastic film for waterproofing. The entire device is 0.8 mm thick. In this case, the sensor has an active area of 50 × 96 mm, and a high-resolution grid system of 2560 measuring points. The active range of the pressure is 0–2.5 MPa

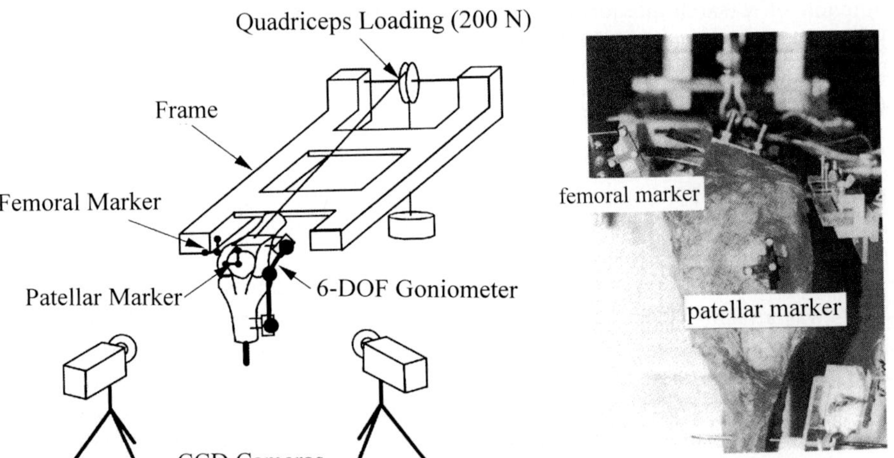

Fig. 2a,b. Set-up of experiment. a Schematic diagram. A cadaveric knee joint is mounted to the frame and the quadriceps tendon is loaded at 200 N. The 6-DOF goniometer is affixed to the lateral side of the knee joint with screw for 3-D motion between tibia and femur. 3-D patellar tracking is measured using two sets of CCD cameras with DLT methods. b Two markers are strategically placed on the patellar and femur to represent the 3-D positions specimen in this order (1) intact knee, (2) bicompartmental knee arthroplasty with tibial and femoral components, leaving the patella unresurfaced (Bi-TKA), and (3) tri-compartmental knee arthroplasty with tibial, femoral, and patellar components (Tri-TKA). The patellar component used in this study was dome-shaped and implanted on the patella using an onset technique. The center of the prosthetic patellar implant was aligned with the central ridge of the original patella. The difference of the patellar thickness before and after patellar resurfacing was within 2 mm. For each experimental configuration the knee flexion was investigated.

Contact pressure distribution on the patella was graphically altered between the intact knee, Bi-TKA, and Tri-TKA. In an intact knee, the contact pattern was a horizontal band. This band of contact moved upward from inferior to superior over the patellar articular surface with the increase of knee flexion. This contact pattern was similar to that which other previous investigators have reported [15]. In Bi-TKA, the unresurfaced patellar contact against the femoral component showed a band-like distribution up to 30° of knee flexion, a round shape from 30° to 90°, and band-like again over 90°. At more than 60° of knee flexion, the unresurfaced patellar contact did not shift with knee flexion but tended to remain around the center of the articular surface. After the patella was resurfaced, the patellar contact showed line contact and shifted inferior to superior over the patellar component with knee flexion (Fig. 3).

The mean contact pressure was conversely highest for Tri-TKA, followed by Bi-TKA, and the intact knee. The mean pressure of Bi-TKA was 76.5% to 197.7% (average 143.1%) of that of intact knee. In Tri-TKA, the mean pressure was 133.1% to 270.1% (average 222.7%) of that of intact knee. The mean pressure was significantly higher in Tri-TKA than in Bi-TKA from 0 to 30° of knee flexion ($P < 0.05$), than in intact knee at

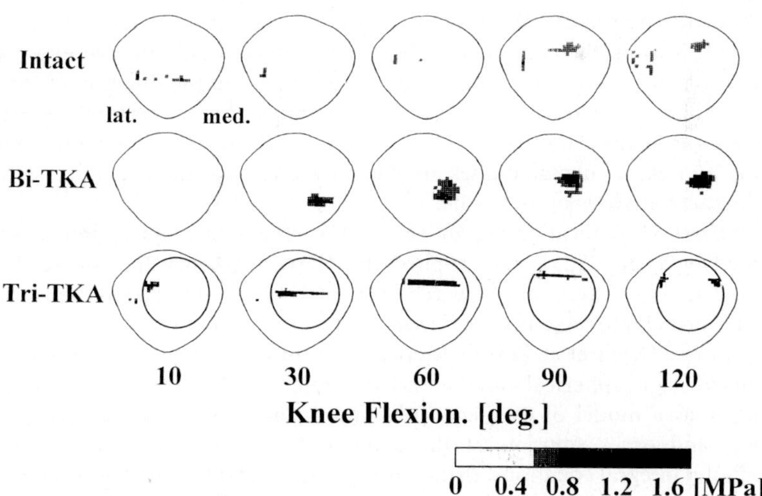

FIG. 3. Typical contact pressure distributions on the patellae in *intact* knee, *Bi-TKA*, and *Tri-TKA* with knee flexion. Intact knee shows bandlike contact, Bi-TKA shows round contact at more than 60° of knee flexion, and Tri-TKA shows line contact

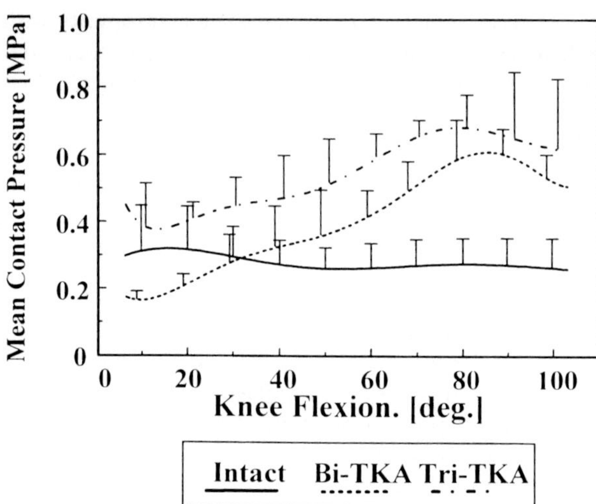

FIG. 4. Mean contact pressure on the patella. The mean pressure is significantly higher in Tri-TKA than in Bi-TKA from 0° to 30° of knee flexion ($P < 0.05$). In Bi-TKA, the mean contact pressure was significantly higher than in intact knee more than 80° of knee flexion ($P < 0.05$)

30° and 50° to 100° of knee flexion ($P < 0.05$). In Bi-TKA, the mean pressure was significantly higher than in intact knee from 80° to 100° of knee flexion ($P < 0.05$) (Fig. 4).

Apart from the patellofemoral joint, PSRS has been applied to the tibiofemoral [16,17], wrist [18], hip [19], and elbow joints [20].

Mathematical Model Analysis

Mathematical models have proved to be an effective means for studying structural elements of the musculoskeltal system. This tool makes it cost-effective to simulate joint activities using the computer rather than perform costly in vivo experimental procedures. Also, for ethical reasons, one may test ideas on the function of the different components of the joints using modeling techniques before performing such tests in vitro and/or in vivo. However, models must be validated experimentally. Therefore, modeling and experimental studies are considered as two interdependent strategies that help and complement each other.

The theoretical determination of articular cartilage stresses in joints was first performed by Hirsch [21], who applied the Hertzian theory for contact between two elastic spheres. Zarek and Edwards [22] used the same Hertzian theory and the associated principal stress field to justify a structure–function relationship for the collagen fibrils. Hayes et al. [23] developed the solution using the Fredholm integral equations for rigid spherical and flat-ended indentation of an elastic layer on a rigid foundation, as a model of cartilage indentation. Sakamoto et al. [4] presented the analytical and exact solution of the same indentation model instead of using the Fredholm integral equations. Using the biphasic model for cartilage [24], Mow and Lai [25] calculated stresses in a cartilage layer subjected to a moving, parabolically distributed normal surface traction. Recently, a rigid-body-spring model (RBSM) was developed. It is simple in theory, and joint contact stress can be calculated within a short time. The accuracy of RBSM was discussed by Li et al. [26].

Eberhardt et al. [27,28] developed a solution for the contact problem of elastic spheres, with either one or two isotropic elastic layers to model cartilage. Sakamoto et al. [29,30] extended the model of Eberhardt et al. as follows.

Mathematical Joint Contact of Anisotropic Cartilage Model

We simulated an axisymmetric articular joint model of which a subchondral bone is a rigid substrate and an articular cartilage is a transversely isotropic layer (z-axis: principal direction of anisotropy) as shown in Fig. 5. Using the assumptions of the Hertzian theory, the boundary conditions on the layer are as follows:

1. A prescribed displacement, according to Hertzian theory, within the contact zone
2. Zero normal stress outside of the contact region
3. Zero shear stress, inside and outside of the contact region
4. Zero displacements across the interface

The formulation results in a pair of integral equations which may be solved using a technique developed by Sakamoto et al. [31]. The problem is reduced to solutions of two sets of unknown coefficients (b_n, c_n) from a system of simultaneous equations as follows:

$$\sum_{n=0}^{\infty}(b_n,c_n)\int_0^{\infty}t(\lambda)J_m^2(\lambda a/2)J_{n+1/2}(\lambda a/2)J_{-n-1/2}(\lambda a/2)d\lambda$$

$$= (\delta_{0m},\delta_{0m}-\delta_{1m}/2),\quad (m=0,1,2,\ldots), \tag{1}$$

where $J_n(x)$ is the Bessel function, δ_{0m} is Kronecker's delta, and

$$t(\lambda) = (k_2\cosh\lambda h_1 \cdot \sinh\lambda h_2 - k_1\sinh\lambda h_1\cosh\lambda h_2/\gamma)$$

$$/\{2+(\gamma k_2+k_1/\gamma)\sinh\lambda h_1 \cdot \sinh\lambda h_2 - (k_1+k_2)\cosh\lambda h_1 \cdot \cosh\lambda h_2\}, \tag{2}$$

$$k_i = (c_{11}\mu_i - c_{44})/(c_{13}+c_{44}),\quad h_i = h/\mu_i^{1/2},\quad (i=1,2), \tag{3}$$

$$\gamma = (\mu_1/\mu_2)^{1/2} \tag{4}$$

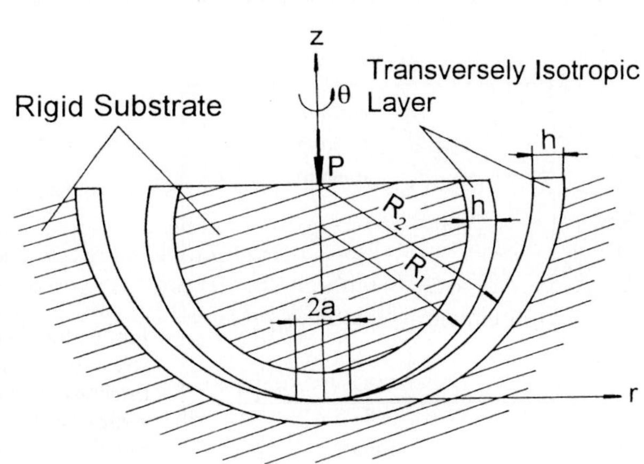

FIG. 5. Geometry of the mathematical joint model which assumes that the subchondral bone is the rigid substrate and the articular cartilage is the transversely isotropic layer. The layered elastic sphere indents the layered elastic cavity. The approach of the sphere with respect to the cavity is along the z-axis

where μ_i, $(i = 1,2)$ are the roots of the following equation:

$$c_{11}c_{44}\mu^2 + \{c_{13}(c_{13} + 2c_{44}) - c_{11}c_{33}\}\mu + c_{33}c_{44} = 0, \tag{5}$$

where $c_{11}, c_{12}, c_{13}, c_{33}$, and c_{44} are five independent elastic constants of the cartilage layer. The normal contact stress $(\sigma_z)_{z=0}$ and the applied load P may be expressed in the following form:

$$(\sigma_z)_{z=0} = -\frac{\kappa}{\pi r(a^2 - r^2)^{1/2}} \sum_{n=0}^{\infty} (b_n - \xi c_n) T_{2n+1}(r/a), \quad (0 \le r \le a), \tag{6}$$

$$P = -2\pi \int_0^a r(\sigma_z)_{z=0} dr = 2\kappa \sum_{n=0}^{\infty} (-1)^n (b_n - \xi c_n)/(2n+1), \tag{7}$$

where $T_n(x)$ represents Tchebycheff polynomials and

$$\kappa = c_{44}\alpha\mu_2^{1/2}(1+k_2)/(1-k_2), \quad \xi = a^2 \Big/ 4R\alpha = \sum_{n=0}^{\infty} b_n \Big/ \sum_{n=0}^{\infty} c_n \tag{8}$$

The material properties of both isotropic and transversely articular cartilage layers, chosen from experimental data available in the literature [32], are given in Table 1. To compare the difference in contact stress in the joint due to a different layer-thickness of articular cartilage, three layer thicknesses, $h = 2\,\text{mm}$, $3\,\text{mm}$, and $4\,\text{mm}$, are chosen to represent a thin, moderate thickness, and thick cartilage, respectively. Figure 6 shows the radial distribution of normal contact stress $(\sigma_z)_{z=0}$ for the transversely isotropic layer as a function of layer thickness h. The maximum normal contact stress increases as the cartilage layer thickness becomes smaller. With increasing thickness, the contact area increases. The distribution of $(\sigma_z)_{z=0}$ for the transversely isotropic layer is shown in Fig. 7 for various sphere radii R_1. It is noted that the decrease in the

TABLE 1. Material properties of the articular cartilage

Layer	E (MPa)	E′ (MPa)	G (MPa)	G′ (MPa)	ν	ν′
Transversely isotropic	50	10	17.9	5.4	0.4	0.2
Isotropic	15	15	5.4	5.4	0.4	0.4

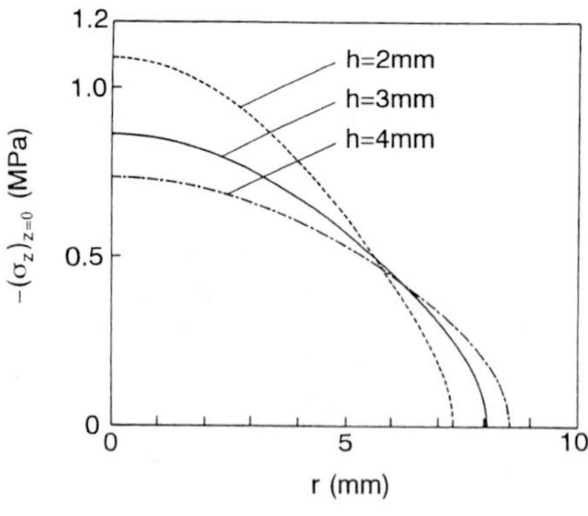

FIG. 6. Radial distribution of normal contact stress $(\sigma_z)_{z=0}$ as a function of cartilage layer thickness h. The applied load P is 100 N, the radius of the sphere R_1 is 30 mm, and the radius of the cavity R_2 is 40 mm

Fig. 7. Radial distribution of normal contact stress $(\sigma_z)_{z=0}$ as a function of radius R_1. The applied load P is 100 N, the layer thickness of cartilage h is 3 mm, and the radius of the cavity R_2 is 40 mm

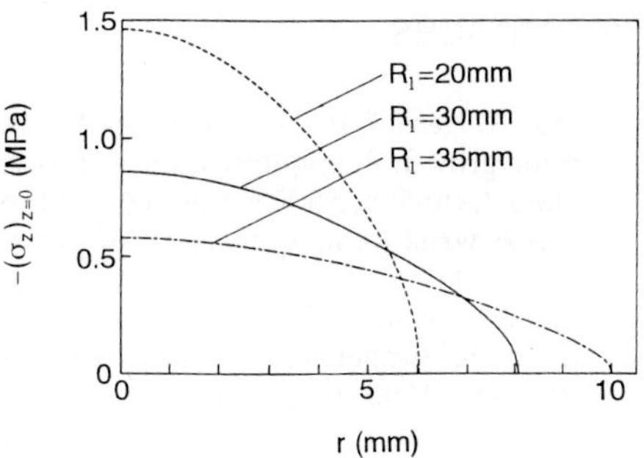

Fig. 8. Radial distribution of normal contact stress $(\sigma_z)_{z=0}$ when (a) the articular cartilage is the transversely isotropic layer (*Trans. Iso.*), and (b) the articular cartilage is the isotropic layer (*Iso.*). The applied load P is 100 N, the layer thickness of cartilage h is 2.5 mm, the radius of the sphere R_1 is 30 mm, and the radius of the cavity R_2 is 40 mm

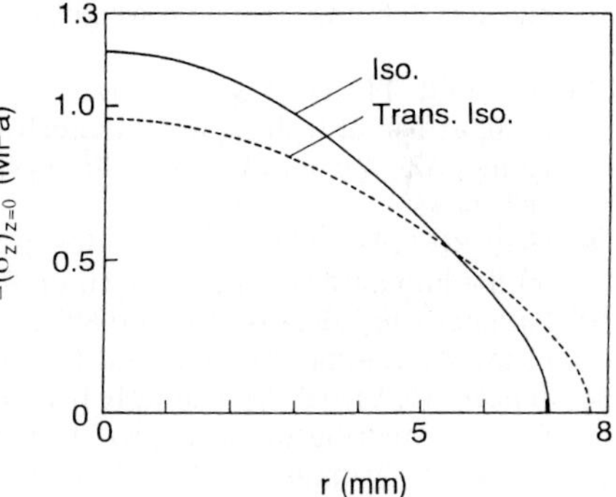

indenting radius results in a decreased contact area and an increase in maximum stress. Figure 8 shows the distribution of $(\sigma_z)_{z=0}$ for both isotropic and transversely isotropic cartilage layers. It is noted that the maximum stress for the transversely isotropic cartilage model is lower than the value for isotropic model. In the transversely isotropic model, tangential stiffness plays an important role in the response of articular cartilage compression behavior, and is thus important for mechanical stress-carrying capacity.

Conclusion

We may conclude that the development of a measuring technique for joint contact stress distribution and a comprehensive three-dimensional anatomical-based mathematical model of joint continue to present a major challenge. Yet it is a subject worthy of continuing study, in agreement with the suggestions for future research directions made by Mow. et al. [33] in their excellent survey of some of the advances made in understanding diarthoidal joint biomechanics.

References

1. Oda R, Hara T, Homma M, Koga Y, Takahashi, HE (1989) Effects of applied stress on bone growth in epiphyseal plate. Tissue Engineering, ASME BMD 14:51–54
2. Hara T, Horii E, An KN, Cooney WP, Linscheid RL, Chao EYS (1992) Force distribution across wrist joint: application of pressure-sensitive conductive rubber. J. Hand Surg, 17:339–347
3. Tanabe Y, Kobayashi K, Sakamoto M, Hara T, Takahashi HE (1994) Identification of the dynamic properties of bone using the split-Hopkinson pressure-bar technique. Biomater Mech Properties, ASTM STP 1173:127–141
4. Sakamoto M, Li G, Hara T, Chao EYS (1996) A new method for theoretical analysis of static indentation test. J Biomech 29:679–685
5. Omori G, Koga Y, Bechtold JE, Gustilo RB, Nakabe N, Sasagawa K, Hara T, Takahashi HE (1997) Contact pressure and three-dimensional tracking of unresurfaced patella in total knee arthroplasty. Knee 4:15–21
6. Black JD, Matejczyk M, Greenwald AS (1981) Reversible cartilage staining technique for defining articular weight-bearing surfaces. Clin Orthop Rel Res 159:265–267
7. Stormont TJ, An KN, Morrey BF, Chao EYS (1985) Elbow joint contact study: Comparison of technique. J Biomech 18:329–336
8. Palmer AK, Werner FW (1984) Biomechanics of the distal radioulnar joint. Clin Orthop 187:26–35
9. Haut RC (1989) Contact pressures in the patellofemoral joint during impact loading on the human flexed knee. J Orthop Res 7:272–280
10. Fukubayashi T, Kurosawa H (1980) The contact area and pressure distribution pattern of the knee. Acta Orthop Scand 51:871–879
11. Tencer AF, Viegas SF, Cantrell J, Chang M, Clegg P, Hicks C, Willamson JB (1988) Pressure distribution in the wrist joint. J Orthop Res 6:509–517
12. Walker PS, Erkman MJ (1975) The role of the menisci in force transmission across the knee. Clin Orthop 109:184–192.
13. Carlson CE, Mann RW, Harris W (1974) A radio telemetry device for monitoring cartilage surface pressure in the human hip. IEEE Trans Biomed Eng 21:257–264
14. Inaba H (1985) A study of the contact pressure of the tibio-femoral joint: A preliminary report. Proc JSOB 7:13–17
15. Huberti HH, Hayes WC (1984) Patellofemoral contact pressure. J Bone Joint Surg [Br] 66:715–724
16. Iwasaki H, Sasagawa K, Hara T, Omori G, Takahashi Y, Koga Y (1992) Experimental study on effect of mechanical axis shift on contact pressure distribution in tibiofemoral joint. Proc JSOB 14:341–344
17. Kimura M, Nakabe N, Hara T, Omori G (1995) Contact pressure measurement in tibiofemoral joint under dynamic loading. J Japanese Soc Clin Biomech Rel Res 16:473–477
18. Nakabe N, Hara T, Hatano Y, Shibata M (1995) Kinematic and kinetic behavior of the radiocarpal joint. J Japanese Soc Clin Biomech Rel Res 16:19–24
19. Genda E, Miura T, Iwasaki H, Sasagawa K, Hara T (1992) An experimental analysis of hip joint contact pressure. Proc JSOB 14:315–318
20. Murata H, Ikuta Y, Horii E, Hara T (1995) Biomechanical studies on the pathogenesis of osteoarthritis in the elbow joint with a new pressure-sensitive conductive rubber sensor. J Japanese Soc Clin Biomech Rel Res 16:5–8
21. Hirsch C (1944) A contribution to the pathogenesis of chondromalacia of the patella. Acta Chir Scand Suppl 83:1–106
22. Zarek JM, Edwards J (1963) The stress-structure relationship in articular cartilage. Med Elect Biol Eng 1:497–507

23. Hayes WC, Keer LM, Herrmann G, Mockros LF (1972) A mathematical analysis for indentation tests of articular cartilage. J Biomech 5:541–551
24. Mow VC, Kuei SC, Lai WM, Armstrong CG (1980) Biphasic creep and stress relaxation of articular cartilage: Theory and experiment. J Biomech Eng 102:73–84
25. Mow VC, Lai WM (1980) Recent developments in synovial joint biomechanics. SIAM Rev 22:275–317
26. Li G, Sakamoto M, Chao EYS (1997) A comparison of different methods in predicting static pressure distribution in articular joints. J Biomech 30:635–638
27. Eberhardt AW, Keer LM, Lewis JL, Vithoontien V (1990) An analytical model of joint contact. J Biomech Eng 112:407–413
28. Eberhardt AW, Lewis JL, Keer LM (1991) Normal contact of elastic spheres with two elastic layers as a model of joint articulation. J Biomech Eng 113:410–417
29. Sakamoto M, Zhu QF, Hara T, Chao EYS (1995) A mathematical model of joint contact. J Jpn Soc Clin Biomech Rel Res 16:193–198
30. Sakamoto M, Hara T (1998) An axisymmetric model for joint static contact stress analysis. In: Middleton J, Jones ML, Pande GN (eds) Computer methods in biomechanics and biomedical engineering 2, Gordon and Breach, 569–576
31. Sakamoto M, Hara T, Shibuya T, Koizumi T (1993) Axisymmetric contact problem for two rigid spheres coated with elastic layers. Trans JSME 59A:963–969
32. Mow VC, Zhu W, Ratcliffe A (1991) Structure and function of articular cartilage and meniscus. In: Mow VC, Hayes WC (eds) Basic orthopaedic biomechanics, Raven, New York, pp 143–198
33. Mow VC, Ateshian GA, Spilker RL (1993) Biomechanics of diarthrodial joints: A review of twenty years of progress. J Biomech Eng 115:460–467

Mechanical Unloading and Bone Marrow Cells

Toshitaka Nakamura, Kenji Sakata, Hiroshi Tsurukami, and Akinori Sakai

Summary. To delineate the influence of mechanical unloading on the osteogenic potential, the effects of mechanical unloading on the trabecular bone formation and the development of osteoblastic cells from bone marrow cells were examined using neurectomized mice. The trabecular osteoclasts and the osteoclastogenic potential of the bone marrow cells were also assessed. In 14 days after sciatic neurectomy, trabecular bone volume in the proximal tibial metaphysis was significantly reduced. The double-labeled surface and bone formation rate (BFR/BS) were significantly reduced. While the numbers of the total bone marrow cells and the nonadherent cells in the neurectomized limbs were not signficantly smaller than that of the sham-operated loaded limbs, the number of the adherent cells in the unloaded limbs was significantly reduced. The number of CFU-f colonies did not differ, but the number of bone nodules developed from bone marrow cells was significantly reduced in the unloaded limbs. The osteoclast-like cell development was increased when the bone marrow cells were incubated with parathyroid hormone. But, the number of CFU-GM colonies did not increase in the unloaded limbs. These data confirmed that the reduction in trabecular bone formation was associated with the reduction in the adherent stromal cells and bone nodule formation of bone marrow cells in the mice tibia after neurectomy. However, in vitro assays including CFU-f and CFU-GM did not identify the changes by unloading. The mechanical unloading affects the development of the bone cells, but may not greatly enhance the capacity for osteoclastogenesis in the bone marrow.

Key words. Neurectomy, Labeled surface, Nodule formation, CFU-f, CFU-GM

Introduction

Skeletal unloading causes a loss of bone in human and animals [1–4], and unloading by immobilization of rat hind limbs is shown to cause a rapid increase in bone resorption and a sustained reduction in bone formation [4]. In histomorphometrical

Department of Orthopedic Surgery, University of Occupational and Environmental Health, 1-1 Iseigaoka, Yahatanishi-Ku, Kitakyushu 807-8555, Japan analyses of trabecular bone surfaces in the tibia, the mineral apposition rate and bone formation rate are reduced [4,5] and the number of trabecular osteoclasts is increased [4–6]. Since bone marrow contains progenitor cells of both osteoblasts [7–9] and osteoclasts [10,11], it is reasonable to presume that unloading would affect the osteogenic and osteoclastogenic capacity of bone marrow cells.

Bone marrow cells contain hematopoietic cells and a heterogeneous non-hematopoietic component including fibroblasts, endothelial cells, reticular cells, adipocytes, and macrophages, which together comprise the marrow stroma [7–9]. The bone marrow culture system reveals mostly nonadherent cells of hematopoietic origin and a smaller adherent cell population, including stromal fibroblastic cells with high alkaline phosphatase (ALP) activity, subsequently leading to mineralized nodule formation [8,9]. These adherent cells are thought to include the precursors of osteoblasts [12–14]. On the other hand, osteoclasts arise from hematopoietic mononuclear cells in the bone marrow [10,11]. While the cell of origin for the osteoclast in bone marrow is still a matter of controversy, the most likely stem cell is contained in a colony-forming unit for granulocytes and macrophages (CFU-GM) [15].

The osteogenic potential of bone marrow cells in the rat femur unloaded by neurectomy is reported to be reduced after surgery [16]. We have recently observed the reduction in the alkalinephosphatase activity of the bone marrow cells and the enhanced formation of osteoclast-like multinucleated cells in the marrow cultures obtained from mice tibia after neurectomy [17]. However, information on the development of the bone-forming cells from bone marrow stroma cells in unloaded bone is insufficient. We present the data on trabecular bone formation of the proximal tibia and the development of osteogenic cells from bone marrow cells after neurectomy in mice.

Materials and Methods

Animals

Forty DDY male mice, 6 weeks of age, were subjected to right sciatic neurectomy and sham surgery was performed on the left side. Right sciatic neurectomy was performed by removing a 0.5 cm section of the nerve in the midthigh, and sham surgery (nerve identification) was performed on the left side under ether anesthesia. At 14 days postoperatively, right and left tibiae were harvested. Twenty animals were used for histomorphometry and an analysis of marrow cells in tibia was carried out in the other 20 animals.

Histomorphometry

Ten samples from the mice with calcein labeling were embedded in methylmethacrylate (MMA) resin. Some other samples ($n = 10$) were embedded in a mixture of MMA, hydroxyglycolmethacrylate, and 2-hydroxyethylacrylate (GMA) [6]. Undecalcified 5-μm-thick frontal sections were obtained with a Reichert-Jung microtome (Model 2050 Supercut) and were measured to determine the percentage of trabecular bone volume and trabecular surface of the proximal metaphyses. Trabecular thickness was then calculated using the equation of the parallel plate model [18]. For the parameters of bone formation and resorption, the percentage of double-labeled surfaces to total trabecular surface and mineral apposition rate were obtained. The ratio of bone formation rate to bone surface (BFR/BS, $\mu m^3/\mu m^2$ per day $\times 10^{-2}$) was calculated. GMA sections were stained for tartrate-resistant acid phosphatase (TRAP). The ratio of trabecular osteoclast number to bone surface was measured on TRAP-stained sections. TRAP-positive cells that formed resorption lacunae at the surface of the trabeculae and contained one or more nuclei were identified as osteoclasts. In the specimens, the metaphyseal cancellous bone area located within 2.0 mm of the growth plate–metaphyseal junction was measured, but the region located within 0.25 mm of the junction was not measured to exclude the spongiosa continuing to the growth plate. The measurements were performed on a CTR monitor with a CCD camera (HCC-1600A, Flovel, Tokyo, Japan) connected to a semiautomatic image analyzing system (Cosmozone 1S, Nikon, Tokyo, Japan).

Bone Marrow Cells

The proximal epiphyseal end and the distal-most third of the cortex were cut away. Marrow cultures were initiated using the method of Maniatopoulos et al. [19]. Bone marrow was flushed out from the proximally cut end, a single-cell suspension was prepared by repeated aspiration, and the whole bone marrow cells were cultured in α-modified Eagle's medium (Flow Lab, Irvine, UK) supplemented with 15% fetal calf serum (Gibco, Grand Island NY USA). The total number of bone marrow cells was calculated using the sample in a hematocytometer. Cells were then grown in 9.6 cm^2-dish. The medium was changed every other day and nonadherent cells in the medium were counted. On day 6 after preparation, adherent cells were trypsinized and counted in a hematocytometer. Bone marrow stroma cells, thus obtained, were disseminated into a 6-well plate (Corning, Corning NY USA) at a concentration of 5×10^5 cells/ml under 2 ml of culture medium for each of CFU-f and CFU-GM and cultured for 10 days. Then the number of colonies was counted. Colonies consisting of more than 50 cells were defined as CFU-f or CFU-GM [20].

Nodule Formation and Osteoclast-Like Multinucleated TRAP-Positive Cell Development

For bone nodule formation, bone marrow cells were seeded at a density of 5×10^4 cells/well in 6-well dishes. Alpha-MEM medium containing 10% FBS, 2.2 mg/ml NaHCO$_3$, 12.5 μg/ml ascorbic acid phosphate, 2.5 mM sodium β-glycerophosphate was exchanged every 2–3 days. At day 14, cells were fixed with 10% neutral formaldehyde on day 21 and stained with alizarin red S (Wako, Tokyo, Japan). Then the number of bone nodules was counted [20]. For producing osteoclast-like cell development, bone marrow cells obtained from the tibia were disseminated into a 24-well plate at a concentration of 7.5×10^6 cells/ml. The culture medium was α-MEM containing 10% FCS, 2.0 g/l NaHCO$_3$, and 10^{-8} mol/l per milliliter of parathyroid hormone (PTH).

These cells were cultured on the plate for 8 days in 5% CO_2 and 95% air in a humidified atmosphere. Half the volume of the culture medium was replaced every other day. Then the culture medium was removed, fixed in 10% formalin for 10 min, and refixed in ethanol-acetone for 1 min. After the culture plate dried, the samples were treated with 5 mg naphthol AS-MX phosphate (Sigma) dissolved in 0.5 ml N,N-dimethylformamide (Wako) containing 50 mmol/l sodium tartrate (Wako) and 30 mg fast red violet LB salt (Sigma) in 50 ml of 0.1 mol/l sodium acetate buffer (pH 5.0) for 15 min at room temperature. Then the number of TRAP-positive multinucleated osteoclast-like cells was counted under a light microscope.

Statistics

Results were expressed as the mean +/− SEM. The differences between unloaded and loaded limbs were compared by Student's *t* test. A *P* value of less than 0.05 was considered significant.

Results

Histomorphometry

The metaphyseal trabecular bone volume in the proximal tibia of unloaded limbs was significantly reduced (Fig. 1). The trabecular thickness values were also significantly reduced. The osteoclast surface values in the unloaded limb did not significantly differ from the values in the loaded limb. Double-labeled surface values for the unloaded limbs were significantly reduced (Fig. 2). The difference in the mineral apposition rate values were not statistically significant. Bone formation rate values in the unloaded limbs were also significantly reduced.

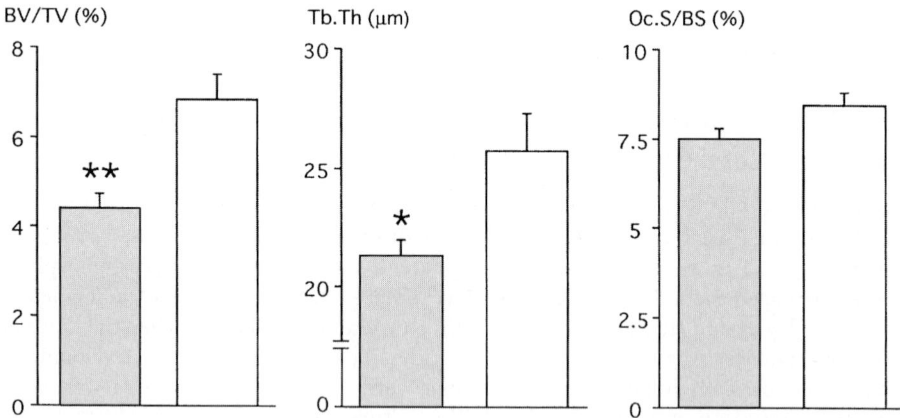

FIG. 1. Bone volume (*BV/TV*), trabecular thickness (*Tb.Th*), and osteoclast surface (*Oc.S/BS*) in the proximal tibia after neurectomy in mice. *P < 0.05 vs sham; **P < 0.01 vers sham. *Shaded bars*, neurectomized limb; *white bars*, sham-operated limb

Bone Marrow Cells

The total number of bone marrow cells in the tibia of the unloaded limbs did not significantly differ from the value in the loaded limbs (Fig. 3). The number of nonadherent bone marrow cells did not differ, but the number of adherent bone marrow cells in the unloaded limbs was significantly smaller than the value in the loaded limbs. The numbers of CFU-f colonies from the bone marrow cells of the tibia did not differ between the unloaded and loaded limbs, nor did the numbers of CFU-GM colonies differ significantly (Fig. 4).

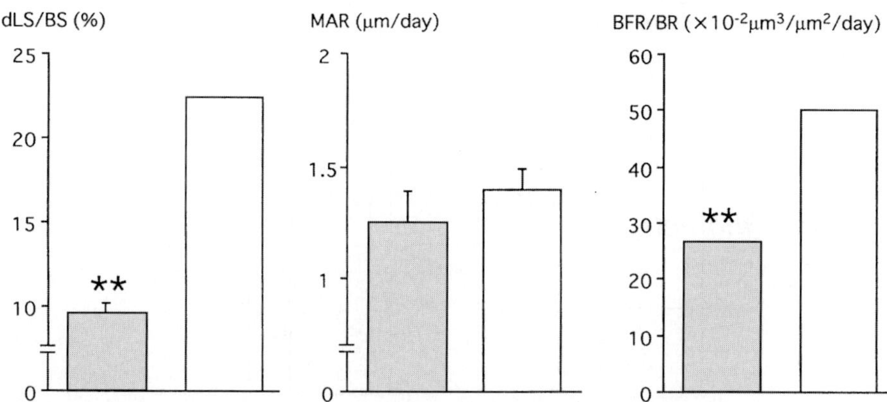

FIG. 2. Double-labeled surface (*dLS/BS*), mineral apposition rate (*MAR*), and bone-formation rate (*BFR/BS*) in the proximal tibia after neurectomy in mice. **$P < 0.01$ vs sham. *Shaded bars*, neurectomized limb; *white bars*, sham-operated limb

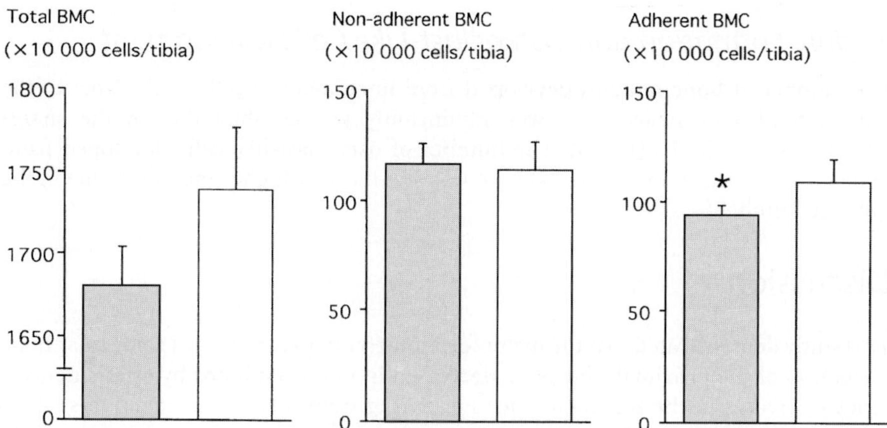

FIG. 3. Number of bone marrow cells (*BMC*) in the proximal tibia after neurectomy in mice. *$P < 0.05$ vs sham. *Shaded bars*, neurectomized limb; *white bars*, sham-operated limb

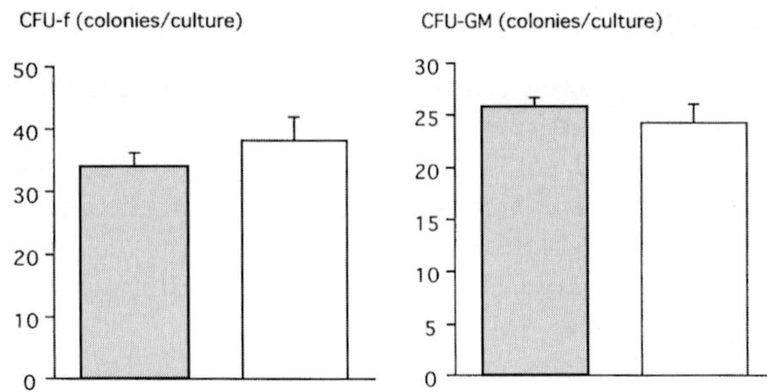

FIG. 4. Numbers of *CFU-f* and *CFU-GM* colonies from bone marrow cells of the tibia after neurectomy in mice. *Shaded bars*, neurectomized limb; *white bars*, sham-operated limb

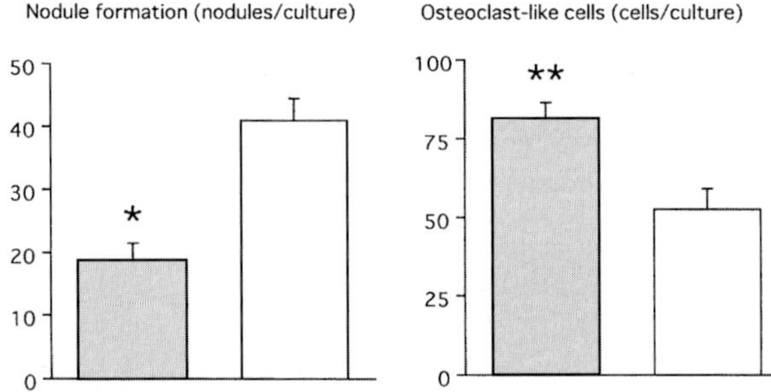

FIG. 5. Numbers of bone nodules and osteoclast-like cells developed from bone marrow cells in the tibia after neurectomy in mice. *$P < 0.01$ vs sham; **$P < 0.01$ vs sham; *Shaded bars*, neurectomized limb; *white bars*, sham-operated limb

Nodule Formation and Osteoclast-Like Cell Development

The number of bone nodules developed from bone marrow cells of the tibia in the limb unloaded by neurectomy was significantly smaller than that in the sham-operated loaded limbs (Fig. 5). The number of osteoclast-like cells developed from bone marrow cells in the unloaded limb was significantly higher than the value in the unloaded limb.

Discussion

This study demonstrated that the histomorphometrical parameters of trabecular bone formation of the proximal tibia were decreased in unloaded limbs by sciatic neurectomy. Decreases in the parameters for measuring trabecular mineralization such as mineralized surface and bone formation rate were associated with a decrease in the osteogenic capacity of bone marrow cells, which was evaluated by nodule formation from bone marrow cells. It was also confirmed that in the 14 days after neurectomy, bone marrow cells of the tibia were characterized by a reduced capacity for adherent stromal cells, consistent with our previous observation [17] and the reported findings in the denervated rat femur [16]. These changes reflect a reduction in the population of nonhematopoietic stromal cells in the bone marrow. Since it has been observed consistently that the fraction of the trabecular bone surface lined by osteoblasts is not changed in the unloaded limbs in rats [21], a decrease in the trabecular bone surface is associated with a concomitant decrease in the total number of trabecular osteoblasts. Thus, the unloading by neurectomy not only reduces the bone mass, but seems to reduce the bone marrow capacity for adherent cells by affecting their development.

The number of CFU-f colonies of equal density that developed from the cells obtained from a mixed population of stem and progenitor cells did not change by unloading after neurectomy. However, bone nodule formation from the cells was significantly reduced in the neurectomized limbs. These data strongly indicate that while the proliferative activity of CFU-f colonies was not reduced, the fraction of osteogenic cells in the colonies was down-regulated by unloading. The population of CFU-f cells does not consist only of an osteogenic component but also contains stromal fibroblast providing a microenvironment supportive of hematopoiesis [8]. Therefore, the maintained values of CFU-f colonies, obtained by seeding bone marrow cells at equal density, would be due to an increase in the fraction of nonosteogenic stromal fibroblasts both contributing to the expansion of bone marrow tissues and filling the space formerly occupied by the trabecular bone after neurectomy. Thus, it may be expected that mechanical stimulation regulates the fractional components of osteogenic and nonosteogenic cell populations that develop from CFU-f cells.

The production of osteoclast-like cells by PTH from bone marrow cells was enhanced by unloading. Since the number of trabecular osteoclasts measured in the same experiment did not increase, the increased osteoclastogenesis from bone marrow cells induced by unloading may occur early, before the increase in bone resorption in the unloaded limbs after neurectomy. In our study, however, the number of CFU-GM colonies which developed from bone marrow cells did not signifi cantly differ between the unloaded and loaded limbs. Thus, it is reasonable to expect that the PTH-dependent component of the final steps in the differentiation of cells committed to the osteoclast pathway was increased by unloading. It has been well confirmed that osteogenic cells have a role of facilitating osteoclast development from bone marrow cells in a co-culture system [23]. Therefore, unloading may be related to the terminal differentiation of osteoclasts from osteoclastogenic cells.

The results of in vivo studies have suggested consistently a role for PTH in the development of osteopenia in unloaded limbs after neurectomy. For example, removal of the parathyroid gland alleviated the osteopenia by unloading in dogs [24]. Administration of the PTH antagonist WR-2721 lessens the increase in osteoclast number after hind limb neurectomy in rats [25]. Calcium deficiency, obviously associated with increased PTH secretion, augments bone resorption after hind limb neurectomy in rats [26]. These reported data and our observation strongly suggest that PTH plays a role in the increase of bone resorption in immobilized bone. However, while the increase in the osteoclast number was observed in the neurectomy model, it was not observed in the rat bone of the unloading model by tail suspension which does not impose surgical stress on the animals and allows the free movement of the limbs [27]. We did not observe any difference in CFU-GM numbers for bones in the unloaded and loaded limbs. Thus, it is assumed that the unloading itself may not greatly increase the osteoclastogenic potential in the bone marrow cells.

In conclusion, our study has confirmed that a reduction in trabecular bone formation is associated with a reduction in the number of adherent stromal cells and the capacity for nodule formation from bone marrow cells in mice tibia after neurectomy. However, in vitro assays including CFU-f and CFU-GM were not able to identify the reduction in osteogenic potential or the increase in producing osteoclastogenic potential of the bone marrow. Thus, mechanical unloading affects the development of the osteogenic cells, but may not greatly enhance the capacity for producing osteoclastogenic cells in the bone marrow. Further studies are necessary before the exact role of loading on the development of bone cells in the bone marrow can be defined conclusively.

References

1. Globus RK, Bikle DD, Morey-Holton E (1986) The temporal response of bone to unloading. Endocrinology 118:733–742
2. Morey ER, Baylink DJ (1978) Inhibition of bone formation during space flight. Science 201:1138–1141
3. Rabin R, Gordon SL, Lymn RW, Todd PW, Frey MA, Sulzman FM (1993) Effects of spaceflight on the musculoskeletal system: NIH and NASA future directions. FASEB J 7:396–398
4. Weinreb M, Rodan GA, Thompson DD (1989) Osteopenia in the immobilized rat hind limb is associated with increased bone resorption and decreased bone formation. Bone 10:187–194
5. Shaker JL, Fallon MD, Goldfarb S, Farber J, Attie MF (1989) WR-2721 reduced bone loss after hindlimb tenotomy in rats. J Bone Miner Res 4:885–890
6. Murakami H, Nakamura T, Tsurukami H, Abe M, Barbier A, Suzuki K (1994) Effects of tiludronate on bone mass, structure, and turnover at the epiphyseal, primary, and secondary spongiosa in the proximal tibia of growing rats after sciatic neurectomy. J Bone Miner Res 9:1355–1364
7. Beresford, JN (1989) Osteogenic stem cells, and the stromal system of bone and marrow. Clin Orthop 240:270–280
8. Friedenstein AJ, Chailkhyan RK, Gerasimov UV (1987) Bone marrow osteogenic stem cells: In vitro cultivation and transplantation in diffusion chambers. Cell Tissue Kinet 20:263–272
9. Owen M, Cave J, Joyner CJ (1987) Clonal analysis in vitro of osteogenic differentiation of marrow CFUf. J Cell Sci 87:731–738
10. Roodman GD, Ibbotson KJ, MacDonald BR, Kuel TJ, Mundy GR (1985) 1,25(OH)$_2$ vitamin D$_3$ causes formation of multinucleated cells with osteoclast characteristics in culture of primate marrow. Proc Natl Acad Sci USA 82:8213–8217
11. Suda T, Takahashi N, Martin J (1992) Modulation of osteoclast differentiation. Endocrine Rev 13:55–80
12. Leboy PS, Beresford JN, Devlin C, Owen M (1991) Dexamethasone induction of osteoblast mRNA in rat bone marrow stromal cell cultures. J Cell Physiol 146:370–378
13. Malaval L, Modrowski D, Gupta AK, Aubin JE (1994) Cellular expression of bone-related protein during in vitro osteogenesis in rat bone marrow stromal cell cultures. J Cell Physiol 158:555–572

14. Rickard DJ, Sullivan TA, Shenker BJ, Leboy PS, Kazhdan I (1994) Induction of rapid osteoblast differentiation in rat bone marrow stromal cell cultures by dexamethasone and BMP-2. Dev Biol 161:218–228

15. Mundy GR (1993) Bone resorbing cells. Favus MJ Ed. Primer on the metabolic bone diseases and disorders of mineral metabolism, 2nd edn. Raven New York, pp 25–32

16. Keila S, Pitaru S, Grosskopf A, Weinreb A (1994) Bone marrow from mechanically unloaded rat bone expresses reduced osteogenic capacity in vitro. J Bone Miner Res 9:321–327

17. Sakai A, Nakamura T, Tsurukami H, Okazaki R, Nishida S, Tanaka Y, Norimura T, Suzuki K (1996) Bone marrow capacity for bone cells and trabecular bone turnover in immobilized tibia after neurectomy in mice. Bone 18:479–486

18. Parfitt AM, Mathews CHE, Villanueva AR, Kleerekoper M, Frame B, Rao DS (1983) Relationship between surface, volume and thickness of iliac trabecular bone in aging and osteoporosis: Implications for the microanatomic and cellular mechanisms of bone loss. J Clin Invest 72:1396–1409

19. Maniatopoulos C, Sodek J, Melcher AH (1988) Bone formation in vitro by stromal cells obtained from bone marrow of young rats. Cell Tissue Res 254:317–330

20. Worton RG, McCulloch EA, Till JE (1969) Physical separation of hemopoietic stem cells from cells forming colonies in culture. J Cell Physiol 74:171–182

21. Weinreb M, Rodan GA, Thompson DD (1991) Depression of osteoblastic activity in immobilized limbs of suckling rats. J Bone Miner Res 6:725–731

22. Rickard DJ, Kazhdan I, Leboy PS (1994) Importance of 1,25-dihydroxyvitamin D_3 and the nonadherent cells of marrow for osteoblast differentiation from rat marrow stromal cells. Bone 16:671–678

23. Suda T, Takahashi N, Martin J (1992) Modulation of osteclast differentiation. Endocrine Rev 13:66–80

24. Burkhart JM, Jowsey J (1967) Parathyroid and thyroid hormones in the development of immobilization osteopenia. Endocrinology 81:1053–1062

25. Shaker JL, Fallon MD, Goldfarb S, Farber J, Attie MF (1989) WR-2721 reduces bone loss after hindlimb tenotomy in rats. J Bone Miner Res 4:885–890

26. Weinreb M, Rodan GA, Thompson DD (1991) Immobilization-related bone loss in the rat is increased by calcium deficiency. Calcif Tissue Int 48:93–100

27. Halloran BP, Bikle DD, Wronski TJ, Globus RK, Levens MJ, Morely-Holton E (1986) The role of 1,25-dihydryxyvitamin D in the inhibition of bone formation induced by skeletal unloading. Endocrinology 116:948–954

Changes in Bone Tissue of Tail-Suspended Rats

Yoshiaki Kodama[1], Konosuke Nakayama[2], Hiroaki Fuse[3],
Takahide Kurokawa[1], Toshitaka Nakamura[4], and
Toshio Matsumoto[5]

Summary. Skeletal unloading by space flight or loss of weight bearing causes a marked loss of bone. Tail-suspended rats are suitable models to analyze changes in bone tissue that occur during unloading. To clarify how the changes in bone formation and resorption affect bone tissue after skeletal unloading, we have investigated the effects of unloading on bone mineral density (BMD), bone strength, and hte histology of hindlimb bones using tail-suspended rats. After 14 days of tail-suspension, the BMD and the strength of the femur markedly decreased compared to those of the control rats at both the metaphysis and the diaphysis. Histological analysis showed that the trabecular bone volume of the proximal tibia was decreased with a reduction in bone formation in tail-suspended rats, and that hindlimb elevation caused a reduced cortical bone thickness of the femoral diaphysis with a decrease in periosteal mineral apposition rate only at the periosteal side. Administration of a potent antiresorptive agent, pamidronate, restored BMD, bone strength, and the histology of the femoral metaphysis in tail-suspended rats, but could not recover those of the diaphysis. These data suggest that the deficit in BMD and bone strength in trabecular bone of tail-suspended rats are associated with enhanced bone resorption as well as reduced bone formation, and that the reduced bone volume and strength in cortical bone results from mainly suppressed periosteal bone formation.

Key words. Mechanical unloading, Bone formation, Periosteum, Bone mineral density, Bisphosphonate

[1] Department of Orthopedic Surgery, University of Tokyo School of Medicine, 7-3-1 Hongo, Bunkyo-ku, Tokyo 113-0033, Japan
[2] Fourth Department of Internal Medicine, University of Tokyo School of Medicine, 3-28-6 Mejirodai, Bunkyo-ku, Tokyo 112-0015, Japan
[3] Teikoku Hormone Manufacturing Co., 1604 Simosakunobe, Takatsu-ku, Kawasaki, Kanagawa 213-0033, Japan
[4] Department of Orthopedic Surgery, University of Occupational and Environmental Health, 1-1 Iseigaoka, Yahatanishi-ku, Kitakyushu, Fukuoka 807-0804, Japan
[5] First Department of Internal Medicine, University of Tokushima School of Medicine, 3-18-15 Kuramoto-cho, Tokushima, Tokushima 770-0042, Japan
Corresponding author: Y. Kodama

Introduction

Mechanical stress plays an essential role in the maintenance of bone mass, bone shape, and bone strength. Skeletal unloading by space flight or loss of weight bearing causes a marked reduction in bone mass and strength [1,2].

In 1978, Morey and Baylink reported that space flight decreased bone formation at the periosteum, whereas bone resorption remained unchanged. They also found that the suppressed bone formation was restored under normal gravity after space flight [1]. Since then, impaired bone formation or osteoblastic function have been shown using various animal models simulating skeletal unloading, such as immobilization by tenotomy [3] or sciatic neurectomy [4], or tail-suspension [5]. Although the reduction in bone mass has been reported to be mainly due to an inhibition of bone formation [1,4,6], a transient increase in bone resorption is observed in immobilized rat hindlimbs [3]. In addition, inhibition of bone resorption by bisphosphonates prevents bone loss caused by mechanical unloading after sciatic neurectomy [7] or tail-suspension [8,9], which suggests that impaired bone resorption is associated with unloading-induced bone loss.

To clarify how the impaired bone formation and resorption alterations occur during skeletal unloading and how these changes affect bone mass and strength, we have examined the effects of hindlimb elevation on BMD, bone strength, and histology using tail-suspended rats.

Tail-Suspended Rat Model

Skeletal unloading by tail suspension, first developed as a model simulating space flight by Bikle et al. [10], shows a remarkable bone loss in hindlimbs of growing rats within 2 weeks compared to their control rats. Tail-suspended rats, whose tails are kept elevated to unload hindlimbs, are suitable models for the study of local effects of bone loss by unloading, because they can freely take food and water and because it does not affect any systemic factors.

The decreased bone formation is thought to be a main cause of the bone loss. In this model of growing rats, bone formation exceeds bone resorption and the effect of enhanced bone resorption on bone loss is far less than that of bone formation [5,11]. Cytokines, such as insulin-like growth factors (IGFs) and transforming growth factor-beta (TGF-β), may in part mediate this process [11,12].

Several agents have been shown to successfully prevent the trabecular bone loss induced by tail-suspension in vivo. Stimulation of bone formation by administration of TGF-β_2 [13] or intermittent treatment with parathyroid hormone [14] preserves the trabecular bone volume in tail-suspended rats. Inhibition of bone resorption by bisphosphonates almost completely prevents bone loss caused by hindlimb elevation [8,9].

To better understand the cellular and molecular mechanism in this unloaded model, or to precisely evaluate the effects of these agents on prevention of the bone loss, it is necessary to know the precise mechanism of how bone turnover changes at different sites of unloaded bones during tail-suspension.

Fig. 1. Effect of tail-suspension on the bone mineral density (BMD) of different regions of the femur in control and tail-suspended rats. After 7 (*upper panel*) or 14 (*lower panel*) days of tail-suspension, the femora were dissected. The femoral BMD was measured by dual energy X-ray absorptiometry. BMD of the femur was determined in 20 equally divided regions with equal longitudinal length. *Closed circles*, control group; *open circles*, tail-suspended group. Region 1 is the distal end of the femur, and region 20 is the proximal end of the femur

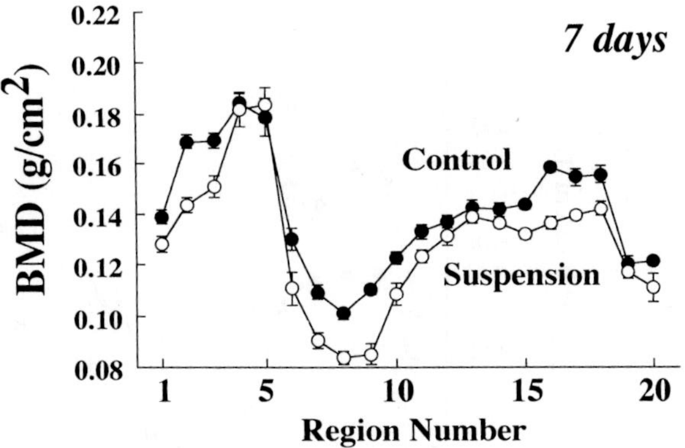

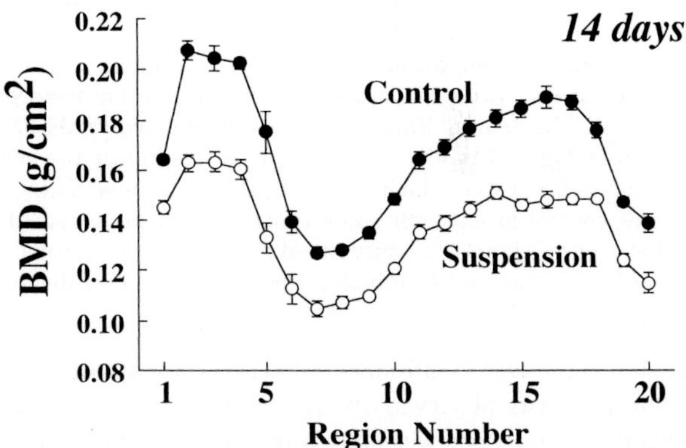

Bone Mineral Density

As bone turnover differs between trabecular and cortical bone, we examined the changes in BMD of different regions of the femur with different composition of trabecular and cortical bone during tail-suspension.

Four-week-old male Sprague-Dawley rats were randomly assigned to control or tail-suspension groups. To suspend the tail, a strip of elastic tape was applied spirally to the whole tail. The end of the tape was fixed to the overhead bar to maintain the hindlimbs suspended above the floor of the cage [15]. At 7 or 14 days after hindlimb elevation, rats were sacrificed and the femora were dissected. Femoral BMD was measured by dual energy X-ray absorptiometry (DXA) using QDR-1000 plus (Hologic, Waltham, MA, USA) with ultra-high-resolution mode (line spacing 0.0254 cm, point resolution 0.0127 cm). Then femoral BMD was analyzed at longitudinally divided 20 equal regions of the femur.

As shown in Fig. 1, tail-suspension for 7 days resulted in a lower BMD in regions 5–8, which represents distal metaphysis rich in trabecular bone, compared to control rats, whereas BMD of regions 9–12, which represents diaphysis rich in cortical bone, was not different between these rats. After 14 days of tail-suspension, BMD of each

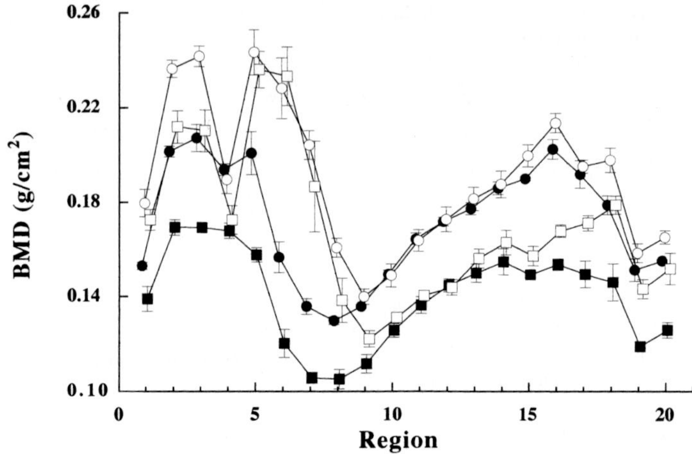

FIG. 2. Effect of pamidronate on the BMD of different regions of the femur in control and tail-suspended rats. After 14 days of tail-suspension, the femora from 4 rats in each group were dissected. The femoral BMD was measured and analyzed in 20 equally divided regions as mentioned in Fig. 1. Pamidronate (1 mg/ml saline/kg) or the vehicle was given to rats intraperitoneally twice a week during tail-suspension. *Closed circles*, control group with vehicle; *open circles*, control group with pamidronate treatment; *closed squares*, tail-suspended group with vehicle; *open squares*, tail-suspended group with pamidronate treatment. Region 1 is the distal end of the femur, and region 20 is the proximal end of the femur

region was lower in tail-suspended rats than in nonsuspended rats (Fig. 1). Thus, rapid bone loss was observed in trabecular bone in the initial phase of unloading and sustained bone loss was shown in cortical bone in the latter phase.

To clarify whether the impaired bone resorption plays any role in the reduction of bone volume in tail-suspended rats, we examined the effect of the inhibition of bone resorption by a potent bisphosphonate, pamidronate. Pamidronate (1 mg/kg) in 1 mg/ml normal saline was injected to rats intraperitoneally twice a week during the 2 weeks of tail-suspension.

As shown in Fig. 2, 14 days of tail-suspension caused a marked reduction in the BMD at all regions of the femur compared to control rats. At the distal metaphysis composed of mainly trabecular bone, treatment with pamidronate markedly increased the BMD in both control and tail-suspended rats to a similar level. In contrast, pamidronate had almost no effect on the BMD of the diaphysis, composed of mainly cortical bone in either control or tail-suspended rats. These results suggest that a transient surge of bone resorption is associated with the trabecular bone loss, but not with the loss of cortical bone induced by skeletal unloading.

Bone Strength

Physical strength of femoral diaphysis is maintained mostly by volume and structure of bone. As there is a remarkable difference in changes in BMD between femoral diaphysis and metaphysis during tail-suspension (Figs. 1,2), we evaluated effects of unloading on bone strength at both femoral midshaft and femoral neck.

TABLE 1. Effect of pamidronate on the physical strength of the femoral midshaft and neck in control and tail-suspended rats

	Pamidronate	Breaking force	
		Femoral midshaft (newtons)	Femoral neck (newtons)
Before suspension		$19.3 \pm 0.7^{*,**}$	$28.3 \pm 2.7^{*}$
Control	−	55.7 ± 4.0	82.3 ± 11.7
	+	$56.9 \pm 1.5^{**}$	$91.6 \pm 8.7^{**}$
Suspension	−	$36.9 \pm 3.4^{*}$	$40.4 \pm 4.7^{*}$
	+	$34.5 \pm 0.6^{*}$	$74.1 \pm 5.8^{**}$

The femur was obtained before and after 14 days of tail-suspension. Pamidronate (1 mg/ml saline/kg) or the vehicle was given to rats intraperitoneally twice a week.

* Significantly different from control group without pamidronate ($P < 0.05$).

** Significantly different from tail-suspended group without pamidronate ($P < 0.05$).

Mechanical strength of the midshaft of the femur was measured by the 3-point bending test, and the mechanical strength of the femoral neck was evaluated by a compression bending test using a load torsion tester (Tensilon SS207-EP; Baldwin, Tokyo, Japan) as reported previously [15].

As shown in Table 1, the breaking force of the femoral midshaft was markedly reduced in tail-suspended rats, a reduction that was not prevented by administration of pamidronate. The breaking force of the femoral neck was also lower in tail-suspended rats than in control rats; however, administration of pamidronate prevented most of the reduction in femoral neck strength. These changes in bone strength were closely associated with the changes in BMD of the femur. In parallel with the increase in the BMD of the femoral neck, the reduction in physical strength of the femoral neck was prevented by pamidronate in tail-suspended rats. In contrast, the lack of effect of pamidronate on the BMD of cortical bone was associated with the failure in preventing reduction in physical strength of the femoral diaphysis (Fig. 1). Apseloff et al. reported that treatment of tail-suspended rats with aminohydroxybutane bisphosphonate prevented the reduction in BMD of the whole femur but could not prevent the reduction in bone strength measured by three-point bending of the femoral diaphysis [9]. As the physical strength of femoral diaphysis is determined in part by bone volume, there is a possibility that inhibition of bone resorption by bisphosphonate increased only trabecular bone volume in the metaphysis and failed to recover cortical bone volume.

These results demonstrate that bisphosphonates can maintain the volume and strength of trabecular bone but cannot preserve those of cortical bone caused by a reduction in periosteal bone formation due to mechanical unloading.

Histological Analysis

Previous reports demonstrated that tail-suspension reduced trabecular bone volume in the proximal tibia compared to control rats with the decrease in histomorphometric parameters of bone formation [5]. The loss of trabecular bone volume and structure might lead to the decrease in bone strength in metaphysis. It has been confirmed

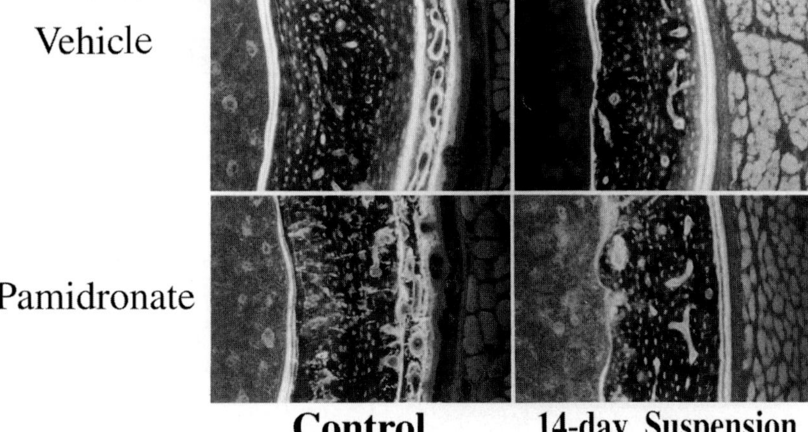

FIG. 3. Cross sections of the femoral diaphysis from control and tail-suspended rats. After 14 days of tail-suspension, the femora were dissected with surrounding soft tissues attached to keep periosteum intact. Pamidronate (1 mg/ml saline/kg) or the vehicle was given to rats intraperitoneally twice a week during tail-suspension. Calcein double-labeling was performed 7 and 3 days prior to death. Undecalcified 25-μm thick ground sections with Villanueva staining were prepared from the mid-portion of the femora. ×30. From [15], with permission

histologically that inhibition of bone resorption by alendronate increases trabecular bone volume by suppressing bone turnover using this model [8].

Although histological analysis reveals that reduced periosteal bone formation is thought to play a key role in cortical bone loss induced by space flight [1,16], the interface between the periosteum and cortical bone has not been analyzed histologically. To examine the periosteal change, we dissected the femur with surrounding soft tissues attached after 14 days of tail-suspension. All the rats were subcutaneously injected with 20 mg/kg calcein 7 and 3 days prior to death. Ground 25-μm thick cross sections at the mid-portion of the femur were obtained by Jung Ultrafrase and Jung Polycute (Leica, Heidelberg, Germany). Histomorphometric measurement was performed using a bone histomorphometry system (System Supply, Nagano, Japan).

Figure 3 shows calcein double-labeling of cross sections of the femoral diaphysis with Villanueva staining. After 14 days of tail-suspension, the thickness of cortical bone was reduced in tail-suspended rats compared to control rats. The distance between the calcein-labeled lines, which represents bone formation, was markedly decreased with a reduction in osteoid formation at the periosteal side. Tail-suspension also caused a change in the thickness of the periosteum adjacent to the surface of cortical bone and the number of cell layers in periosteum, which suggests that the suppressed function of periosteal osteoblastic cells might account for the impaired periosteal bone formation. Pamidronate treatment did not affect the cortical bone thickness, distance between labeled lines, the thickness of periosteum, or the number of periosteal cell layers in either control or tail-suspended rats. These histological observations were confirmed by histomorphometric measurements. As shown in Table 2, mineral apposition rate (MAR) at the periosteal side was much lower in

TABLE 2. Effect of pamidronate on histomorphometric parameters of cross sections of the femoral diaphysis in control and 14-day tail-suspended rats

	Pamidronate	Cortical bone area (mm^2)	Endosteal area (mm^2)	Periosteal MAR (mm/day)	Endosteal MAR (mm/day)
Before suspension		1.65 ± 0.02 *,**	3.10 ± 0.03	N.D.	N.D.
Control	−	3.66 ± 0.14	3.05 ± 0.13	11.93 ± 0.61	1.51 ± 0.38
	+	3.73 ± 0.12**	3.19 ± 0.14	12.74 ± 0.92**	1.23 ± 0.41
Suspension	−	2.68 ± 0.06*	3.13 ± 0.25	6.16 ± 1.07*	1.30 ± 0.43
	+	2.76 ± 0.14*	3.09 ± 0.12	4.78 ± 1.02*	1.37 ± 0.37

The rats were treated and the samples were obtained as in Table 1.

MAR, mineral apposition rate.

* Significantly different from control group without pamidronate ($P < 0.05$).

** Significantly different from tail-suspended group without pamidronate ($P < 0.05$).

tail-suspended rats compared to that in the controls, whereas MAR at the endosteal side was not significantly altered by tail-suspension. As a result, tail-suspension decreased the cortical bone area without affecting the medullary area. Pamidronate did not affect either periosteal or endosteal MAR, and failed to restore the cortical bone area. These data suggest that the deficit in the BMD and breaking force in tail-suspended rats results from the reduced thickness of cortical bone, and that the reduction in cortical area is caused chiefly by suppressed bone formation at the periosteum. Therefore, agents or physical exercises that can stimulate periosteal bone formation are required to restore normal bone strength and bone mass.

Conclusion

Skeletal unloading by tail-suspension results in lower BMD and bone strength in both trabecular and cortical bone compared to the control rats. Rapid bone loss in trabecular bone in the early phase of skeletal unloading is caused by a transient increase in bone resorption, whereas gradual bone loss in the latter phase is due to a sustained decrease in bone formation in cortical bone. The reduction in cortical bone mass results mainly from impaired periosteal bone formation. Inhibition of bone resorption by treatment with pamidronate almost completely reversed the reduced bone mass and breaking force in trabecular bone. However, pamidronate had little effect on the decrease in bone mass and breaking force induced by a sustained decrease in bone formation in cortical bone. To preserve cortical bone mass and strength, stimulation of periosteal bone formation might be required.

References

1. Morey ER, Baylink DJ (1978) Inhibition of bone formation during space flight. Science 201:1138–1141
2. Rabin R, Gordon SL, Lymn RW, Todd PW, Frey MA, Sulzman FM (1993) Effects of spaceflight on the musculoskeletal system: NIH and NASA future directions. FASEB J 7:396–398

3. Weinreb M, Rodan GA, Thompson DD (1989) Osteopenia in the immobilized rat hind limb is associated with increased bone resorption and decreased bone formation. Bone 10:187–194

4. Keila S, Pitaru S, Grosskopf A, Weinreb M (1994) Bone marrow from mechanically unloaded rat bones expresses reduced osteogenic capacity in vitro. J Bone Miner Res 9:321–327

5. Globus RK, Bikle DD, Morey-Holton E (1986) The temporal response of bone to unloading. Endocrinology 118:733–742

6. Machwate M, Zerath E, Holy X, Hott M, Modrowski D, Malouvier A, Marie PJ (1993) Skeletal unloading in rat decreases proliferation of rat bone and marrow-derived osteoblastic cells. Am J Physiol 264:E790–E799

7. Murakami H, Nakamura T, Tsurukami H, Abe M, Barbier A, Suzuki K (1994) Effects of tiludronate on bone mass, structure, and turnover at the epiphyseal, primary, and secondary spongiosa in the proximal tibia of growing rats after sciatic neurectomy. J Bone Miner Res 9:1355–1364

8. Bikle DD, Morey-Holton ER, Doty SB, Currier PA, Tanner SJ, Halloran BP (1994) Alendronate increases skeletal mass of growing rats during unloading by inhibiting resorption of calcified cartilage. J Bone Miner Res 9:1777–1787

9. Apseloff G, Girten B, Weisbrode SE, Walker M, Stern LS, Krecic ME, Gerber N (1993) Effects of aminohydroxybutane bisphosphonate on bone growth when administered after hind-limb bone loss in tail-suspended rats. J Pharmacol Exp Ther 267:515–521

10. Globus RK, Bikle DD, Morey-Holton E (1984) Effects of simulated weightlessness on bone mineral metabolism. Endocrinology 114:2264–2270

11. Machwate M, Zerath E, Holy X, Pastoureau P, Marie PJ (1994) Insulin-like growth factor-I increases trabecular bone formation and osteoblastic cell proliferation in unloaded rats. Endocrinology 134:1031–1038

12. Zhang R, Supowit SC, Klein GL, Lu Z, Christensen MD, Lozano R, Simmons DJ (1995) Rat tail suspension reduces messenger RNA level for growth factors and osteopontin and decreases the osteoblastic differentiation of bone marrow stromal cells. J Bone Miner Res 10:415–423

13. Machwate M, Zerath E, Holy X, Hott M, Godet D, Lomri A, Marie PJ (1995) Systemic administration of transforming growth factor-beta$_2$ prevents the impaired bone formation and osteopenia induced by unloading in rats. J Clin Invest 96:1245–1253

14. Halloran BP, Bikle DD, Harris J, Tanner S, Curren T, Morey-Holton E (1997) Regional responsiveness of the tibia to intermittent administration of parathyroid hormone as affected by skeletal unloading. J Bone Miner Res 12:1068–1074

15. Kodama Y, Nakayama K, Fuse H, Fukumoto S, Kawahara H, Takahashi H, Kurokawa T, Sekiguchi C, Nakamura T, Matsumoto T (1997) Inhibition of bone resorption by pamidronate cannot restore normal gain in cortical bone mass and strength in tail-suspended rapidly growing rats. J Bone Miner Res 12:1058–1067

16. Westerlind KC, Turner RT (1995) The skeletal effects of spaceflight in growing rats: tissue-specific alterations in mRNA levels for TGF-beta. J Bone Miner Res 10:843–848

Bending Load and Bone Formation Response

Hiroshi Hagino, Toru Okano, Makoto Enokida, Hideaki Kishimoto, and Kichizo Yamamoto

Summary. We report here the results of experiments using a 4-point bending device, and review earlier research into the relationship between bending stresses applied to the bone and bone response using this device. Twenty-four 6-month-old female Wistar rats (retired breeder) were randomly assigned to three experimental groups (n = 8/group) to which the following loads were applied: Group A, 25 N; Group B, 30 N; Group C, 35 N. A load was applied on the right tibia by 4-point bending. The tibia was loaded for 36 cycles at 2 Hz 3 days a week, for a total of 9 days with loading. In vivo strain on the lateral periosteal surface was 999, 1320, and 1726 μstrain in Group A, B, and C, respectively. On the lateral periosteal surface, bone formation significantly increased with the magnitude of force. Approximately 800 μstrain was the threshold value for lateral periosteal bone formation, and woven bone formation was observed on tibiae subjected to loads greater than 1500 μstrain.

Key words. Mechanical loading, Bending stress, Bone formation, Bone modeling

Introduction

To tolerate load and maintain morphological integrity, the bone transmits information about applied forces to osteoblasts and osteoclasts, resulting in formation of new bone tissue. This bone formation is considered to be controlled by factors that include the magnitude and frequency of applied forces.

Rubin and Lanyon [1] performed an osteotomy on the ulna of a turkey and inserted pins directly into the bone to apply bending stress. Then they evaluated the relationship between the strain that developed on the bone surface and bone formation. As a result, they were able to observe apparent bone formation when approximately 2000 μstrain bending stress was applied to the ulna 36 times a day. Strain on the bone can be accurately predicted in this experiment in which the bone is directly stressed. However, surgical invasion is inevitable in such experiments and may influence the region of observation [2]. Therefore, a 4-point bending device has been developed as

Department of Orthopedic Surgery, Faculty of Medicine, Tottori University, 36-1 Nishi-cho, Yonago, Tottori 683-8504, Japan an experimental system which can facilitate application of non-invasive bending stress to the bone as well as predicting the magnitude of the strain on the bone [3–7].

In the present study, we report the results of experiments using a 4-point bending device, and generally describe the previously obtained information regarding the relationship between bending stresses applied to the bone and bone formation.

Materials and Methods

Animals

Twenty-four 6-month-old female Wistar rats (retired breeder; bodyweight: 260–315 g, Shimizu Laboratory Supply, Kyoto, Japan) were used. This experiment was approved by the Committee on Laboratory Animals, Faculty of Medicine, Tottori University. During the experimental period, tap water and commercially available food (CE-2 [CLEA Japan, Tokyo, Japan] calcium content: 1.18 g/100 g phosphorus content: 1.09 g/100 g vitamin D_3 content: 250 IU/100 g) were available ad libitum. The lighting duration in the breeding room was 12 h (7:00 a.m. to 7.00 p.m.). Room temperature was 24°C. After 7 days acclimatization, the rats were randomly assigned to three experimental groups (n = 8/group) to which the following loads were applied: Group A, 25 N; Group B, 30 N; Group C, 35 N. Mean body weight did not differ among groups. Between loading sessions, all rats were allowed normal cage activity.

In Vivo External Mechanical Loading

In Vivo Mechanical Loading Was Initiated. Loads were applied using a 4-point bending device (developed and assembled at Creighton University, Omaha, NE, USA). Each rat was anesthetized with ether and its right lower leg was placed between pads in the device (Fig. 1). The load on the right tibia was applied by 4-point bending. The tibia was loaded for 36 cycles at 2 Hz 3 days a week, for a total of 9 days with loading. The applied force for each group was changed by adjusting the point at which the spring was attached to the wheel fixed to a step motor.

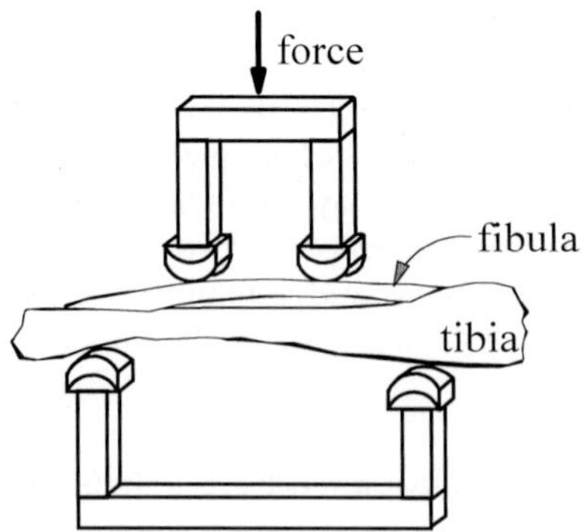

FIG. 1. Four-point bending. Each rat was anesthetized with ether and its right lower leg was placed between pads in the device. Load was applied to the right tibia by 4-point bending. The inner pads are 11 mm apart, and the outer pads are 23 mm apart

The applied force during loading was monitored by a strain gauge attached to the lever arm. Before the experiment, a load cell with a strain gauge was inserted and the force was applied to check the relationship between strain data from the lever arm and the actual force applied at the site between the pads. This load cell had previously been calibrated by applying forces from 0 to 70 N using a mechanical testing machine, and strain data were recorded for each force value. Using the data, the relationship between strain data from the lever arm and the actual force applied at the site between the pads was examined and a positive linear regression was observed. The actual applied load during in vivo 4-point bending was calculated from this regression formula.

Bone Histology

The rats received intraperitoneal calcein injections (6 mg/kg body weight) on experimental days 12 and 19. The rats were killed on day 21.

The region of maximal bending was located in the central diaphysis, 3–13 mm proximal to the tibio–fibula junction (TFJ). Cross sections were prepared from that region and two sections were obtained at 4 mm and 4.5 mm proximal to the TFJ, ground to 60 µm, and mounted on glass slides.

Calculation of In Vivo Strain

In vivo strain was calculated using the moment of inertia of each central diaphyseal cross section. The outline of the cortical bone on each slide was traced and the moment of inertia and section modulus for each cross section were calculated using bone histomorphometry software (System Supply, Nagano, Japan).

Peak compressive strain on the lateral surface was calculated using the beam bending theory as follows: $Ec = MC / EI$ where Ec = peak compressive strain on the lateral surface, M = bending moment (N-m), E = longitudinal Young's modulus (estimated as $29 \times 10^9 \, N/m^2$ here), I = moment of inertia, and C = the distance from the centroid to the lateral surface). In vivo, peak strain (Ep) was predicted from Ec using the following formula:

$Ep = 0.828Ec - 127.16$ [4]

Histomorphometry

We used a camera lucida projecting onto a graphics pad interfaced to a personal computer (PC-9801, NEC, Tokyo, Japan), equipped with bone histomorphometry software.

For both the periosteum and endosteum, we measured single-labeled surface (sLS, %), double-labeled surface (dLS, %), and woven bone surface (WoS, %) (defined as surface with overlying woven bone). WoS was not included in sLS or dLS. Formation surface (FS) was defined as dLS+WoS+(sLS/2). Mineral apposition rate (MAR, µm/day) and surface-based bone formation rate (BFR, µm/day) were calculated. BFR was calculated using the following formula:

$$BFR = MAR \cdot FS$$

Histomorphometric data were collected from the periosteal and the endocortical surfaces of the tibia. The tibial periosteal surface was subdivided into lateral and medial surfaces. The FS value on the left was subtracted from that of the right tibia and the difference was used for the correlation analysis.

Statistical Analysis

Values were compared between right and left using Student's paired t-test. Analysis of variance (ANOVA) was used for comparison among multiple groups. A multiple comparison test was performed using Scheffe's test. $P < 0.05$ was regarded as significant. SPSS software (version 7.5J, SPSS, Chicago IL, USA) was used.

Results

Applied Force and In Vivo Strain

The applied force, averaged for all rats and all days, was 23.8 ± 0.8 N in Group A, 29.9 ± 0.4 N in Group B, and 34.8 ± 0.3 N in Group C. In vivo strain on the lateral periosteal surface was 999.3 ± 192.2 µstrain, 1320.4 ± 196.0 µstrain, and 1726.0 ± 308.7 µstrain in Groups A, B, and C, respectively. Those values showed significant differences between groups ($P < 0.01$). Variation in the strain within each group resulted from variation in the moment of inertia in each rat tibia.

Periosteal Surface

At the lateral surface, FS was increased in Group B and Group C compared with that on the left side (Figs. 2, 3). There was a significant difference between Group A and Group C. FS and strain on the lateral periosteal surface showed a significant positive linear correlation ($P < 0.01$) (Fig. 4), and about 800 µstrain was the threshold for FS increase. As dLS of the left tibia was observed only in Group C, there was a significant difference in MAR only for Group C (Fig. 5). BFR increased with the applied load and periosteal strain; however, this tendency was not significant (Fig. 4). Woven bone was observed at the periosteal surface of the right tibia in Group B and C. Although woven bone formed in rats receiving periosteal strain over 1500 µstrain, there was no correlation between WoS and strain.

At the medial surface, FS increased with the applied force and the magnitude of strain on the periosteal surface, showing significant differences between right and left tibia and groups (Fig. 3). MAR of the right tibia was calculated in 3, 5, and 8 rats in Groups A, B, and C, respectively, and that of the left tibia was calculated in only 2 rats from Groups B and C (Fig. 5). MAR on the medial surface of the right tibia for Groups B and C was about half of that on the lateral surface. There was no difference in BFR at the medial surface among groups.

Endocortical Surface

FS increased with the applied force and there was a significant difference between right and left in Group C (Table 1). MAR was calculated in 2, 4, and 7 rats in Group A, B, and C, respectively, showing no significant difference among groups nor between right and left. There was no woven bone formed at the endocortical surface in any animal.

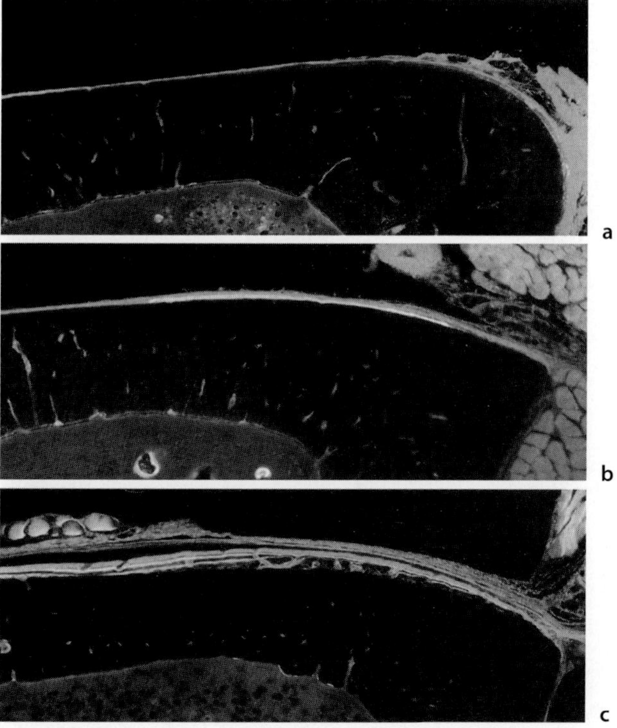

Fig. 2a–c. Increased bone formation. **a** Group A (25 N); **b** Group B (30 N); **c** Group C (35 N)

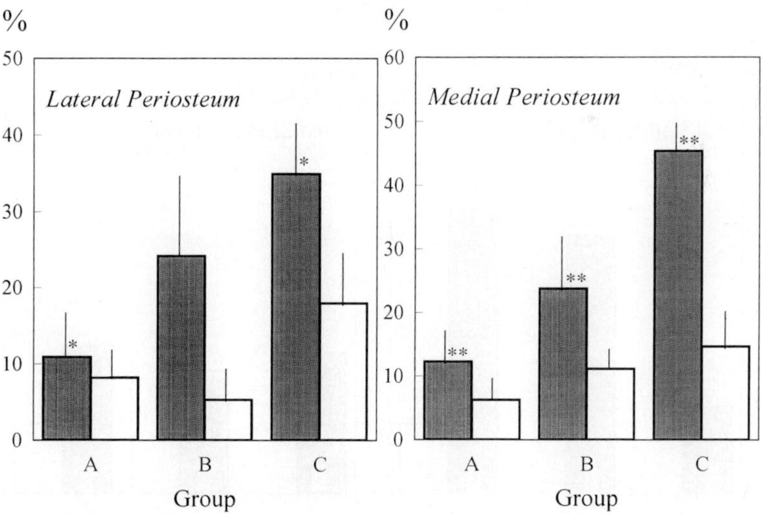

Fig. 3. Formation surface. The difference between right and left was significant in Groups B and C at the lateral surface and in all groups at the medial surface ($P < 0.05$). There was a significant difference between Group A and Group C at the lateral surface and among all groups at the medial surface (*$P < 0.05$, **$P < 0.01$). Data are mean ± SEM. *Shaded bars*, right tibia; *open bars*, left tibia

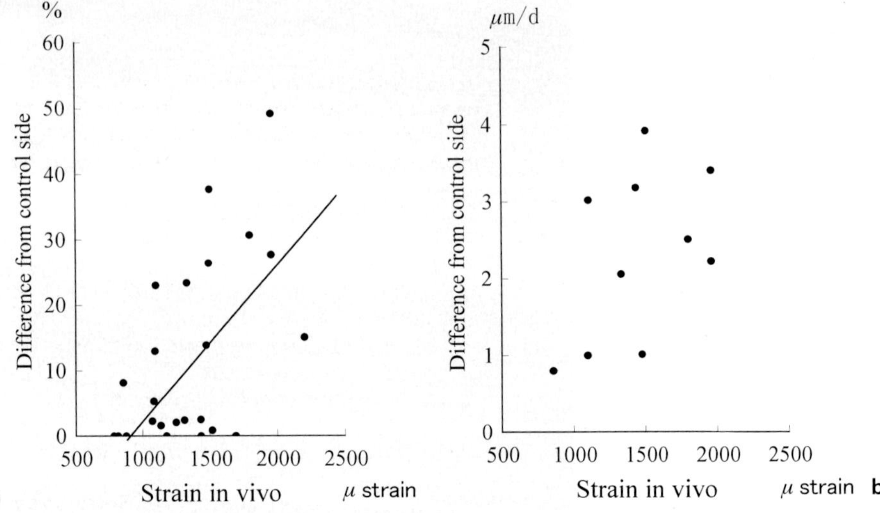

FIG. 4a,b. Formation surface and bone formation rate and strain in vivo. **a** Periosteal formation surface (FS) **b** Bone formation rate (BFR). FS and strain on lateral periosteal surface showed a significant positive linear correlation ($P < 0.01$). BFR increased with the periosteal strain, but the increase was not significant

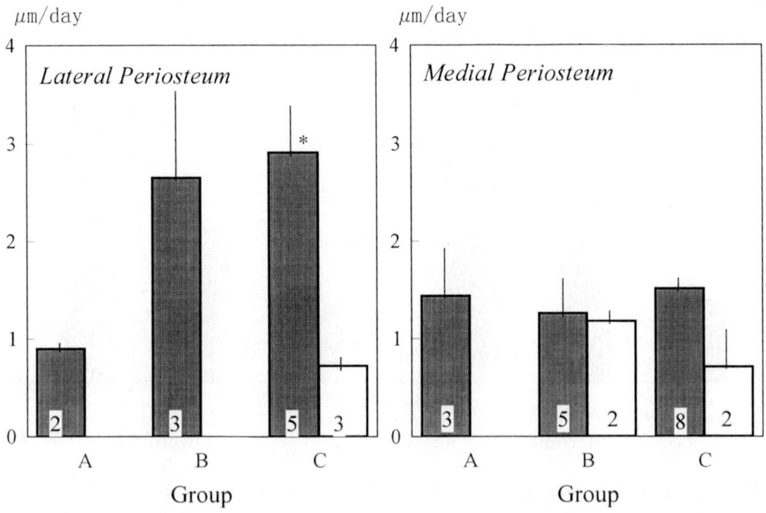

FIG. 5. Mineral apposition rate (MAR). There was a significant difference in MAR only for Group C at the lateral surface (*$P < 0.05$ Rt. vs. Lt.). Data are mean ± SEM. *Shaded bars*, right tibia; *open bars*, left tibia

TABLE 1. Endocortical response

		Group A (25N)	Group B (30N)	Group C (35N)
FS (%)	right	(8) 5.27 ± 2.89	(8) 12.64 ± 15.13	(8) 21.19 ± 9.78]*
	left	(8) 4.89 ± 2.56^a	(8) 4.04 ± 3.44	(8) 3.95 ± 1.99**
MAR	right	(2) 1.60 ± 0.34	(4) 1.61 ± 0.33	(7) 2.55 ± 0.90
(μm/day)	left	(3) 0.55 ± 0.96	(2) 1.85 ± 0.29	(1) 1.12
BFR	right	(2) 0.09 ± 0.05	(4) 0.37 ± 0.28	(7) 0.62 ± 0.31
(μm/day)	left	(3) 0.04 ± 0.06	(2) 0.13 ± 0.08	(1) 0.07

Data are mean ± SD.

FS, formation surface; MAR, mineral apposition rate; BFR, bone formation rate.

Evaluated number of rats are provided in parentheses.

* Significant difference between right and left in Group C ($P < 0.01$).

** Significant difference between Group A and C ($P < 0.05$).

Discussion

In the present study, bending stresses (25–35 N, 2 HZ, 36 cycles) were applied to the tibiae of rats 3 times a week over a 3-week period. As a result, on the lateral periosteal surface, bone formation significantly increased with the magnitude of force. Approximately 800 μstrain was the threshold value for lateral periosteal formation, and woven bone formation was observed on tibiae greater than 1500 μstrain, suggesting a certain relationship between the magnitude of the strain on the periosteal surface and bone formation in rats.

When loads were applied to the bone, the responds of the bone depended on the magnitude of the strain developed. Frost organized the relationship between these mechanical stresses and bone responses into the mechanostat theory, in which strain that induces these threshold values is called the minimum effective strain (MES) [8–9]. There are two different MESs that can either reduce bone remodeling or activate bone modeling. When the strain developed after the force applied to the bone exceeds the first threshold value, bone remodeling is reduced; when the strain exceeds the second threshold value, bone modeling is activated.

Rats used in this study were in the process of growth, that is, animals undergoing bone modeling. Therefore, this experimental system clarified the relationship between the magnitude of strain on the bone and threshold values of the strain that can activate bone modeling. The results suggested that periosteal strain measuring about 800 μstrain was the threshold value for activation of bone remodeling, which corresponded well with the results of previous reports [3].

It was also established that formation is controlled not only by the magnitude of strain, but also by the strain rate. Results obtained from the experiment using a 4-point bending device in four groups classified by strains ranging from 0 to 39 000 μstrain/s demonstrated that the bone formation rate increased with the magnitude of strain rate [10]. In this experiment, there was no increase in bone formation even when 54 N force was continuously applied to the bone (in this case, the strain rate was 0). Therefore, it was suggested that the threshold value of bone formation was more potently influenced by changes in strain rather than by the magnitude of strain.

The effects of duration and frequency of stress on bone formation were examined using a 4-point bending device [3,11]. As a result, it was demonstrated that the long-term stress application was not necessary, and bone formation was increased by stresses applied cyclically 4 times a day for 12 days or 36 times in one day.

Frequency and duration of exercise loading on bone required to increase bone mass remain to be clarified from the clinical point of view. However, based on the information previously obtained using a 4-point bending device, variable loads that induce sufficient strain on the bone are considered effective for increasing bone mass [12]. In addition, relatively short-term loading is sufficient to increase bone mass. Since long-term continuous loading induces stresses on the bone, probably resulting in micro-damage or stress fracture [13], repeated exercise loading at regular intervals is recommended to increase bone mass.

References

1. Rubin CT, Lanyon LE (1984) Regulation of bone formation by applied dynamic loads. J Bone Joint Surg 66A:397–402
2. Frost HM (1983) The regional acceleratory phenomenon: A review. Henry Ford Hosp Med J 31:3–9
3. Turner CH, Akhter MP, Raab DM, Kimmel DB, Recker RR (1991) A noninvasive, in vivo model for studying strain adaptive bone modeling. Bone 12:73–79
4. Akhter MP, Raab DM, Turner CH, Kimmel DB, Recker RR (1992) Characterization of in vivo strain in the rat tibia during external application of a four-point bending load. J Biomechanics 25:1241–1246
5. Raab-Cullen DM, Akhter MP, Kimmel DB, Recker RR (1994) Bone response to alternate-day mechanical loading of the rat tibia. J Bone Miner Res 9:203–211
6. Raab-Cullen DM, Thiede MA, Petersen DN, Kimmel DB, Recker RR (1994) Mechanical loading stimulates rapid changes in periosteal gene expression. Calcif Tissue Int 55:473–478
7. Hagino H, Raab MD, Kimmel DB, Akhter MP, Recker RR (1993) Effect of ovariectomy on bone response to in vivo external loading. J Bone Miner Res 8:347–357
8. Frost HM (1988) Vital biomechanics: Proposed general concepts for skeletal adaptations to mechanical usage. Calcif Tissue Int 42:145–156
9. Frost HM (1992) The role of changes in mechanical usage set points in the pathogenesis of osteoporosis. J Bone Miner Res 7:253–261
10. Turner CH, Owan I, Takano Y (1995) Mechanotransduction in bone: role of strain rate. Am J Physiol 269:E438–E442
11. Forwood MR, Turner CH (1994) The response of rat tibiae to incremental bouts of mechanical loading: A quantum concept for bone formation. Bone 15:603–609
12. Lanyon LE (1992) The success and failure of the adaptive response to functional load-bearing in averting bone fracture. Bone 13:S17–21
13. Martin RB, Burr DB (1989) Structure, function, and adaptation of compact bone. Raven, New York

Adaptive Bone Remodeling Under Mechanical Stimuli

KAZUO TAKAKUDA

Summary. Bone responds to its mechanical environment and changes its form accordingly. However, no adaptive bone remodeling has been reproduced in animal models. Hence we have used experimental animals at various stages of growth and examined bone response to bending loads to investigate the mechanism of adaptive bone remodeling. In this study, we used rats 8 to 34 weeks old, applied non-invasive 3-point bending loads to their tibia, and labeled the newly formed bones with fluorescent dyes. After the animals were killed, successive undecalcified sections were made and observed with a confocal laser scanning microscope. On the basis of the preliminary experiments, the bone growth modified by mechanical stimuli is discussed.

Key words. Bone remodeling, Adaptation, Mechanical stress, Animal experiments

Introduction

Bone may be regarded as a "smart" structure which responds to its mechanical environment and changes its form accordingly. The most remarkable example is observed when a tubular bone such as a femur that has set in an abnormal form after fracture returns to its normal form. In this case, a very sophisticated coupling of bone formation and bone resorption must take place, i.e., the bone formation at the compressive side of the periosteal surface and at the tensile side of the endocortical surface, and the bone resorption at the tensile side of the periosteal surface and at the compressive side of the endocortical surface. The mechanism that enables cells to create such "smart" remodeling has yet to be elucidated. Many researchers have been attracted to this phenomenon. However, no clear findings have been made because adaptive bone remodeling has not been reproduced in animal models.

To investigate the mechanism of adaptive bone remodeling, we have to use experimental animals at various stages at growth and examine bone response to bending loads. Hence in this study we used rats 8–34 weeks old, applied a non-invasive 3-point

Institute for Medical and Dental Engineering, Tokyo Medical and Dental University, Kanda-Surugadai 2-3-10, Chiyoda-ku, Tokyo 101-0062, Japan bending load to their tibia, and labeled the newly formed bones with fluorescent dyes. After the animals were killed, successive undecalcified sections were made and observed with a confocal laser scanning microscope. On the basis of the preliminary experiments, the significance of the bone growth modified by the mechanical stimuli was discussed.

Design of Experiment

Adaptive Remodeling of Bone

An example of typical adaptive remodeling is shown in Fig. 1 [1]. The figure demonstrates the malunion of a tubular bone after fracture and its return to its original shape as a consequence of remodeling. Such examples are commonly experienced in clinical cases, and frequently quoted in literature.

If we examine the relation between bone remodeling and the mechanical conditions of the bone, we may note that the bone is resorbed on the tensile surface and that bone is formed on the compressive surface. This led Bassett [2] to propose his hypothetical rule for bone remodeling.

Basset's Rule of Remodeling. Bone formation takes place on the surface of compressive stress and bone resorption takes place on the surface of tensile stress.

Although this rule looks very reasonable, if we further examine bone remodeling from a biomechanical point of view, we will find that the rule has a serious flaw. The long bone has a tubular shape, hence we have to consider bone formation and resorption on the endocortical surface as well as the periosteal surface. Unfortunately, Bassett's rule is based on the bone response only on the periosteal surface. If we try to predict the change in shape of the bone in the case shown in Fig. 1, assuming that it has a circular cross section and follows Basett's rule, we would have the shape shown in Fig. 2. This bone cannot regain its original shape after remodeling.

To achieve bone remodeling that enables the bone to regain its correct shape, bone formation must take place on the periosteal surface of the compressive side and on the endocortical surface of tensile side. Furthermore, this bone formation must be accompanied by bone resorption that takes place on the periosteal

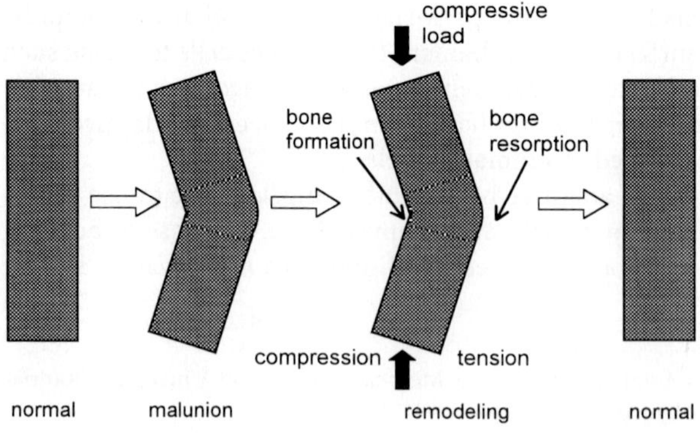

FIG. 1. Schema of the adaptive bone remodeling frequently shown in the literature (lateral view). Adapted from [1]

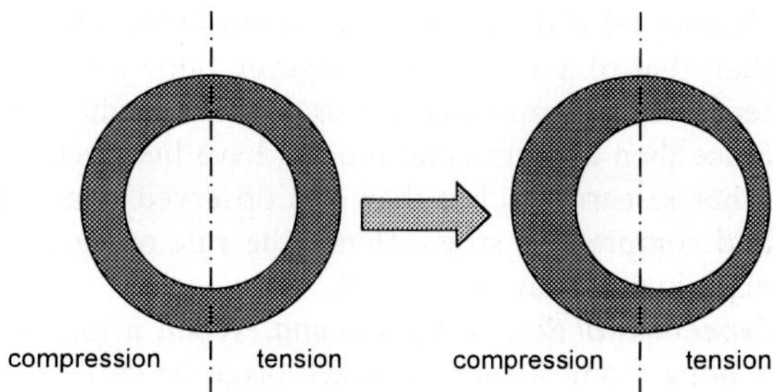

Fig. 2. Unrealistic bone remodeling predicted by Bassett's rule (cross-sectional view)

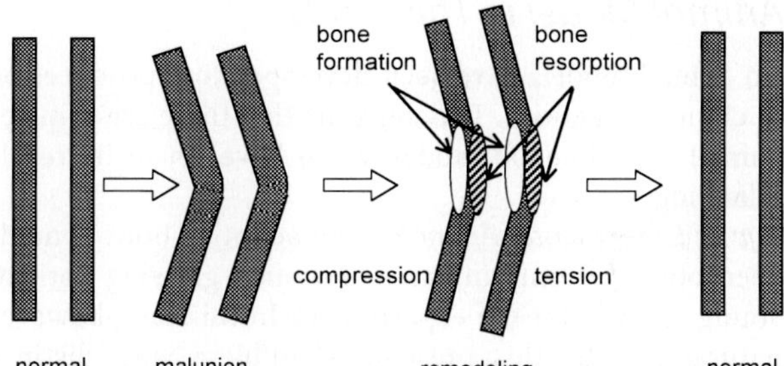

Fig. 3. Schema of adaptive bone remodeling rationale from the biomechanical viewpoint

surface of the tensile side and on the endocortical surface of the compressive side. Figure 3 illustrates this specific coupling of the bone formation and the bone resorption.

It is totally unrealistic to consider that the bone cells on the periosteal and endocortical surfaces receive the mechanical stresses directly as signals for the remodeling. If we assumed that to be true, then we would have to conclude that when the periosteal cells form bone as a response to some mechanical signal, the endocortical cells must then resorb bone inresponse to the same stimulus, and vice versa. Hence the cells would not receive the stress itself as the signal but would receive the other physical quantity. With that argument in mind, Curry [3] suggested a more rational remodeling rule using a concept of strain gradient.

Curry's Rule of Remodeling. Bone formation takes place on the surface where the strain becomes more tensile with depth, and bone resorption takes place on the surface where the strain becomes less tensile with depth.

This rule can simulate nicely the remodeling as shown in Fig. 3, although it is only a hypothesis based on clinical experience. To elucidate the true nature of the phenomena in bones, we had to investigate experimentally with the use of animal models.

Animal Model for the Study of Bone Remodeling

The first attempt to investigate the response of bones to the controlled mechanical stimuli was conducted by Hert [4,5]. He applied a dynamic or a static bending load to a tibia of a rabbit over several months and observed the shape change of the bone.

He found that the effect of a dynamic load on bone remodeling is far more significant than that of a static load. However, bone formation was observed on both sides of tensile and compressive stress, thus contradicting both Bassett's and Currey's rules. Since then experimental models have been refined by Lanyon and Rubin [6,7] and other researchers, but they also observed bone formations on both sides of tensile and compressive stress. Hence the rule of bone remodeling based on these animal experiments may be restated.

Experimental Rule of Remodeling. When a load of sufficient strength is applied to a bone, bone formation takes place on both surfaces of tensile and compressive stress.

Animal Model in This Study

No animal models have been developed to reproduces bone remodeling as observed in clinical situations. This suggests that there are some problems associated with the animal experimental model which have yet to be resolved. These may include the following:

Age of Experimental Animals. The adaptive bone remodeling mentioned earlier has been observed only in cases of young, growing patients. Hence we should choose young animals for the experiments. In this case, however, since bones are formed as natural growth, this presents a problem with distinguishing experimental bone formation from natural bone formation.

Invasion. Invasion of bone has a great influence on bone formation. It is very important to reduce the number of invasions in experiments to as few as possible.

Anesthesia. Since repeated loads must be applied to a bone during an experiment, repeated anesthesia is necessary. But repeated anesthesia affects the condition of the animals significantly. An anesthetic with minimal side effects must be used and its dose kept as low as possible.

Evaluation of the Results. Although woven bone formation was observed in some previous experiments, woven bones are a reaction against strong stimuli and frequently appear in bone fractures. Whether a woven bone formation is a physiological reaction or not remains controversial. Lamellar bone formation must be distinguished from woven bone formations and must be discussed separately.

For the reasons just stated, we have developed a new experimental model, in which a young rat was used and non-invasive 3-point bending was loaded on its tibia.

Materials and Methods

Experimental Animals

Male SD rats of 8 to 34 weeks old were used. They were divided into three groups: a young group (ca. 10 weeks old), a young adult group (ca. 20 weeks old) and an adult group (ca. 30 weeks old). Because most significant adaptive bone remodelings were observed in growing children and not in adults, the age of the experimental animals would have a significant effect in bone remodeling.

Fig. 4. Three-point bending of a rat's tibia

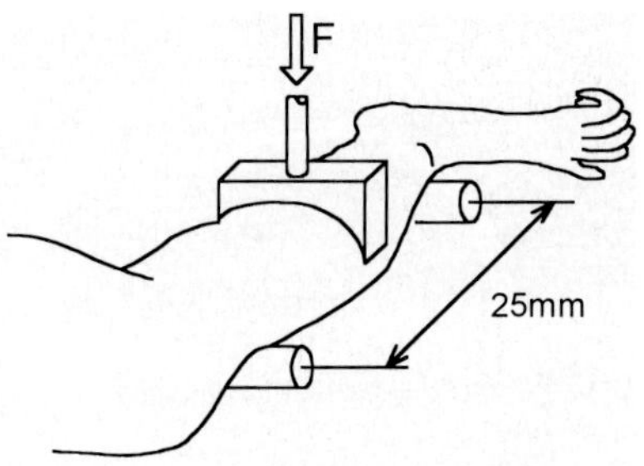

Experimental Apparatus

An apparatus for the application of a 3-point bending load to a rat's tibia was constructed. The schema for the loading is shown in Fig. 4. An air actuator was used in the apparatus for the loading device.

Strain Measurement

The strains induced on the rat's tibia were measured by strain gauges.

Experimental Conditions

The magnitude of force for the 3-point bending was set at 2 kgf, 4 kgf, or 6 kgf. The frequency was 1 Hz and the duration of the stimuli was 5 min per day. The total experimental period was 2 weeks with mechanical stimuli twice a week.

Light Microscopy

The newly formed bone tissue was labeled five times during the experiment with an injection of calcein, alizarin complexeon, calcein again, xylenol orange, and finally calcein. After the animals were killed, successive non-decalcified transverse sections, approximately 0.7 mm thick, were made and examined with confocal laser scanning microscope, which enabled us to visualize the three-dimensional aspect of the bone formation at 1 mm resolution in the longitudinal axis of the tibia.

Results

Strains Induced on Bones

The strains induced by the application of 3-point bending at the medial periosteal surface just opposite to the loading point were 120 to 140 microstrains for 1 kgf loading.

Bone Formation

The natural bone growth observed in the absence of artificial mechanical stimuli was lamellar bone formation on the periosteal or endocortical surfaces (Fig. 5). The bone formation was location specific.

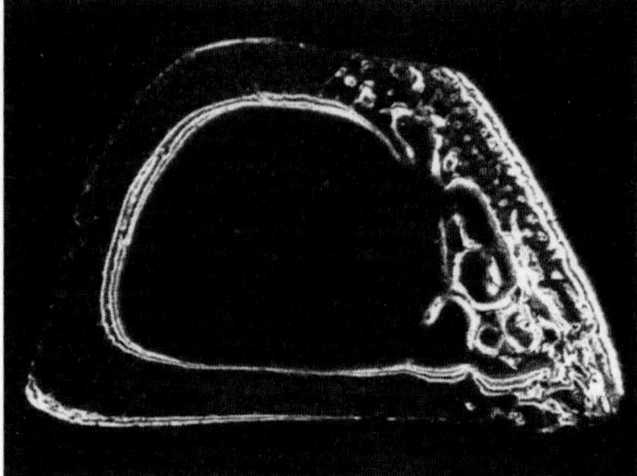

Fig. 5. Lamellar bone formation, 10 mm proximal to the tibiofibular junction (0 kgf, 2 weeks)

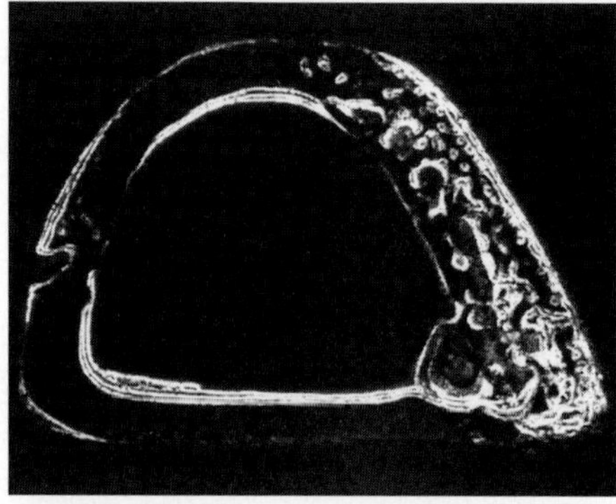

Fig. 6. Lamellar bone formation, 10 mm proximal to the tibiofibular junction (2 kgf, 2 weeks)

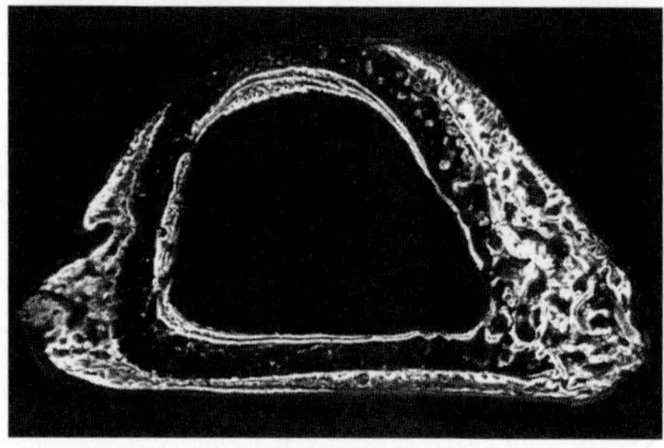

Fig. 7. Lamellar and woven bone formation, 10 mm proximal to the tibiofibular junction (4 kgf, 2 weeks)

The bone formation observed following weak mechanical stimuli (2 kgf loading) was enhanced lamellar bone formation (Fig. 6). The location of the bone formation was mostly similar to those of natural bone growth in the absence of artificial stimuli.

Under the strong mechanical stimuli (4 kgf loading), explosive woven bone formation as well as lamellar bone formation was observed (Fig. 7). Woven bone formation was located on posterior, lateral, and antero-medial sides of the distal periosteal surface of the tibia, which were different locations from those of the lamellar bone formation of natural growth and were locations near the neutral axis of the bending. No woven bone formation was observed on the endocortical surfaces. Conversely, lamellar bone formation was observed on the lateral (compressive stress) side of the periosteal surface and at the medial (tensile stress) side of the endocortical surfaces.

Discussion

By the applying artificial bending loads to bones, significant bone formation was induced. Weak stimuli (2 kgf) enhanced lamellar bone formation, in which the locations of the bone formation was not altered from those of natural bone growth without any artificial mechanical stimuli. This means that the weak stimuli simply enhance the normal bone growth, but do not induce the adaptive bone remodeling. Strong mechanical stimuli (4 kgf) induced woven bone formation, in which bone was formed on the anterior and posterior side of the periosteal surfaces. These locations were close to the neutral axis of the cross-section of the bones under bending load, where no significant bending strains were induced. Hence the woven bone formation resulting from strong mechanical stimuli cannot be the adaptive response of bones. On the other hand, lamellar bone formation resulting from strong mechanical stimuli was observed on the compressive side of the periosteal surfaces and the tensile side of the endocortical surfaces. As was discussed in the previous section, this very peculiar pattern of bone formation may be regarded as adaptive bone remodeling.

In natural bone growth of young animals with normal activity, osteoblasts at particular locations of a bone are activated and deposit new bone whereas cells at other locations are inactive. The weak stimuli in this experiment did not alter the location of the bone formation whereas the strong stimuli did. This may suggest that the weak stimuli could stimulate the activated cells but could not activate the quiescent cells. Strong stimuli seemed necessary to activate the latter. In this case, the induction of lamellar bones by the strong stimuli at locations different from normal bone growth may be the adaptive response of bone.

In this experiment, woven bones were formed in response to strong mechanical stimuli. The woven bone formation is frequently observed in cases of bone fractures. Although woven bone forms quite rapidly, it is replaced by lamellar bone after the succeeding internal remodeling. The reason why woven bone was formed in this experiment is not clear; however, it may be a non-physiological bone response induced by the application of 3-point bending that induced increased intramedullar pressure and/or in-plane bending of cortical bones.

An interesting observation is that the normal bone growth ceased at some locations of the bone subjected to strong stimuli. Because the bone experienced the stresses generated by the normal activity as well as the artificial bending load, it means that the effects of the mechanical stimuli are not so simple. The mechanical stimuli do not simply enhance the bone formation but control the whole shape of the bone as a functional organ.

The bone formation reported in this paper is open to further investigation as to whether it is truly adaptive or not. In any case, the adaptive response of bones under mechanical stimuli seems to be an extremely complicated phenomenon, and intense efforts are required to elucidate it.

References

1. Albert B, Bray D, Lewis J, Raff M, Roberts K, Watson JD (1994) Molecular biology of the cell. 3rd edn. Garland, New York, p 1186
2. Bassett CAL (1971) Biophysical principles affecting bone structure. In: Bourne GH (ed) The biochemistry and physiology of bone, vol.3. Academic, New York, pp 1–76
3. Currey J (1984) The mechanical adaptation of bones. Princeton University Press, Princeton, p 252
4. Hert J, Liskova M, Landgrot B (1969) Influence of the long-term continuous bending on the bone. Folia Morphologica 17:389–399
5. Liskova M, Hert J (1971) Reaction of bone to mechanical stimuli. Part 2. Periosteal and endoosteal reaction of the tibial diaphysis in rabbit to intermittent loading. Folia Morphologica 19:301–317
6. Rubin CT, Lanyon LE (1984) Regulation of bone formation by applied dynamic loads. J Bone Joint Surgery 66A:397–402
7. Brown TD, Douglas RP, Gray ML, Brand RA, Rubin CT (1990) Toward an identification of mechanical parameters initiating periosteal remodeling: a combined experimental and analytical approach. J Biomech 23:893–905

Bone Microdamage and Its Repair: Pathophysiology of Bone Fatigue

Satoshi Mori

Summary. Physiological repetitive loadings of daily activities generate microdamage in the skeleton. Microdamage accumulates with aging. It has been demonstrated with a 3-point bending model of dog's forelimb that microdamage is repaired directly by bone remodeling. Microdamage accumulates in bone, when there is an imbalance between generation and repair of microdamage. Aging bone fragility as well as pathological fracture is caused not only by bone loss but also by the accumulation of microdamage in bone.

Key words. Microdamage, Bone fatigue, Remodeling, Repair, Aging

Introduction

Mechanical loading is an important stimulus for maintaining bone architecture and strength. But repetitive loading imposed during normal daily activities causes skeletal fatigue [1]. Fatigue is defined in engineering as the progressive loss of strength and stiffness that occurs prior to failure in materials subjected to repetitive loadings which are much lower than static breaking strength. These mechanical changes can be attributed to various levels of material damage, from molecular debonding [2] up to macroscopic failure (fracture). At the microscopic level, initiation and propagation of microcracks are observed according to the cycles of the loads before failure, which is in association with the decline of material properties [3]. Every material under repetitive mechanical loading must face deterioration of its mechanical integrity by fatigue. In engineering, the point at which a material exhibits fatigue gives important information for determining a safe, economical, and functional design [4–6]. In living organisms, including bone, mechanical integrity is maintained by repairing microdamage. But if the accumulation of microdamage is more rapid than biological repair, failure such as stress fractures, familiar to joggers or soldiers, occurs. In orthopedics, the mechanism of some pathological fractures like the collapse of the femoral head in avascular necrosis, asymptomatic vertebral compression fractures, or insufficiency

Department of Orthopedic Surgery, Kagawa Medical University, 1750-1 Ikenobe, Miki-cho, Kita-gun, Kagawa 701-0793, Japan fractures of the pelvis can be explained by an accumulation of microdamage. Where production and repair of microdamage is balanced, fatigue may not become apparent as a clinical problem. However once they are imbalanced, serious bone fragility occurs after a number of loadings. There is little information about bone fatigue in the human skeleton and its pathophysiological aspects. Microdamage distribution in the human skeleton and the repairing system of microdamage will be reviewed in this chapter.

Staining Microdamage

Microdamage in the human skeleton was first demonstrated in ribs using bulk stain methods by Frost [7] (1960), and this was supported by Burr and Stafford [8] (1992). Because processing of bone specimens also causes artifactual cracks, specimens are first soaked en bloc in 1.0% basic fuchsin in graded ethanol to stain in vivo cracks before processing. In vivo microdamage has a sharp, deep-stained edge and may have a stained halo around the crack. The artifactual crack is light or non-stained. There is the possibility for underestimating the exrent of the microdamage number with this method, because not all of the in vivo microdamage may be stained.

Microdamage in Human Cortical Bone

Thirteen left 9th ribs from female cadavers aged 60–93 years old were bulk-stained for 2 months and cut as 250 μm thick sections at 12 cm distal from the tubercle and ground to 150 μm [9] (Fig. 1). While the percentage of cortical area did not differ between younger (<80 years old, 42.1 ± 2.98 [SED]%) and older subjects (≥ 80 years old, 40.0 ± 3.17%), microcrack density (Cr.N/cortical area) was higher in older than younger (<80 years old, 0.12 ± 0.03/mm^2, >80 years old, 0.28 ± 0.04/mm^2, $P < 0.01$). Microcrack density showed a positive correlation with age ($r^2 = 0.58$, $P < 0.05$).

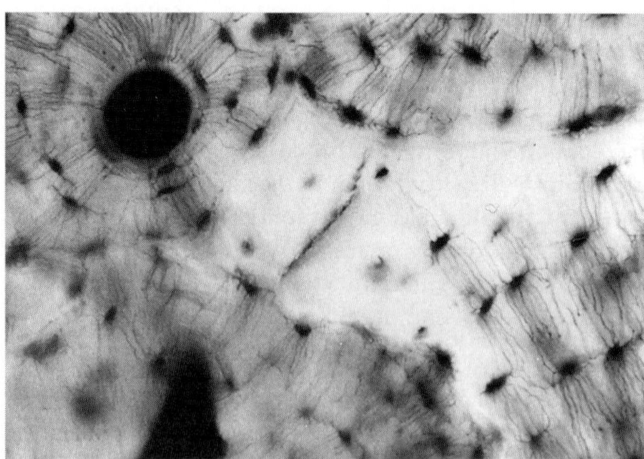

Fig. 1. Microdamage in human rib cortex, stained with bulk stain technique. Microdamage exists in the interstitial osteon where osteocytes and their dendrites are poorly stained (coarse osteocyte network). This suggests that microdamage preferentially appears on aged packets in bone (×62.5)

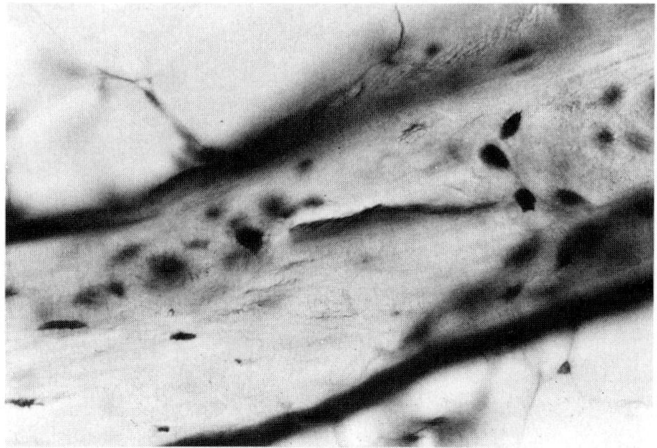

FIG. 2. Microdamage in principal compressive trabeculae in human femoral head, stained with bulk stain technique. Microdamage exists in aged packet with poorly stained osteocytes (×62.5)

These findings suggest that (1) the increased microdamage generation and/or reduced microcrack repair occurs in elderly subjects, and (2) the fragility of the bone can be caused by microdamage accumulation even without reduction of bone mass. Other studies [10] also showed that microcrack number increased with age and is greater in women than men. Norman (1997) [11] reported that 62.4% of microcracks run between the surrounding interstitial bone and the cement line, suggesting that microdamage preferentially appears in aged pieces of bone and is trapped at cement lines.

Microdamage in Human Trabecular Bone

Twenty-eight non-osteoarthrotic femoral heads, 9 from younger adults (<70 years old), 12 from older adults ($\geq$ 70 years old) and seven from femoral-neck-fractured adults (56–90 years old) were stained en bloc with 1% basic fuchsin, embedded in MMA, cut and ground to 150 µm thick [12] (Fig. 2). Microdamage density was evaluated in the principal compressive trabecular area. The percent of trabecular area was significantly lower in older adults (16.8 + 7.6%; $P < 0.05$) or fractured (16.6 + 4.4%; $P = 0.05$) than in younger subjects (24.7 + 6.3%), and microcrack density in older subjects with and without fractures was more than double that in young subjects ($P < 0.01, P < 0.05$). While there was little change in microcrack density before the age of 70, it rapidly increased after 70. Some individuals over 70 had a crack density (Cr.Dn) four- to five-fold greater than the average. The relationship of (Cr.Dn) and trabecular area (Tb.Ar) fit well into a quadratic model, $Cr.Dn = 1.504 - 0.109 \times Tb.Ar + 0.002 \times TbAr^2$ ($P < 0.01$), suggesting that microcracks accumulate more rapidly as the bone volume available to bear loads decreases.

Trabecular Microfractures

Both microcrack and trabecular microfracture are the results of trabecular bone fatigue, but their manifestations are quite different. While microcracks are the fatigue damage itself, microfracture is the trabecular fracture callus. If the fracture healing

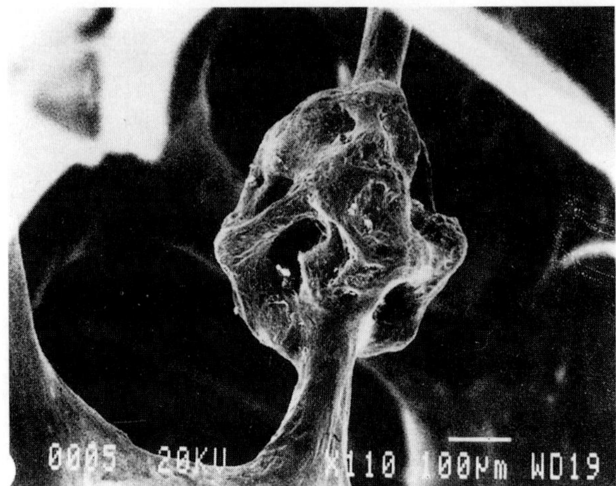

Fig. 3. Trabecular microfracture in human vertebral body under scanning electron microscopy. Massive callus formation appears at the fracture site. (From (13), with permission)

process does not work on the fracture site (non-union), trabecular microfractures cannot be observed. Instead, trabecular disconnection occurs. Microcallus in vertebral trabeculae, clearly demonstrated by Mosekilde (1990) using scanning electron microscopy (Fig. 3) [13], was seen more frequently in elderly individuals. Wicks (1982) [14] and Vernon-Roberts [15] also found that the number of trabecular microfractures exponentially increases with age in normal femoral heads and vertebral bodies.

Histological examination of the human skeleton has revealed that microdamage accumulates in normal skeleton under physiological conditions with age.

Repair of Microdamage

There are two repair potentials in living bone. One is pathological repair working under non-physiological conditions such as fractures. Trabecular microfracture is repaired by the processes in which endochondral ossification, woven bone production, callus formation, and remodeling occur in stages. The other repair potential works under physiological conditions. The fact that repetitive loading within a physiological range produces substantial microdamage [6] suggests that physiological repair is an important metabolic mechanism for maintaining the integrity of bone. Although it has not been proved directly, lamellar bone remodeling is considered to repair microdamage in physiological conditions. Tschantz and Rutishauser [16] first demonstrated the correlation between damage and remodeling with their dog ulnar overload model of resecting a portion of the radius.

A repetitive 3-point bending load model of dog's forelimb was established by Martin and Burr [17], and Mori and Burr [18] demonstrated that remodeling occurs preferentially in fatigue damaged regions. This suggests a direct cause-and-effect relationship between the generation of microdamage in bone and its repair. In the experiment the dog's left radius was loaded first in 3-point bending at 2 Hz, 10 000 cycles with a peak strain on the tensile surface of the radius of 2500 microstrain to generate fatigue microdamage. Eight days later the right radius was loaded in the same

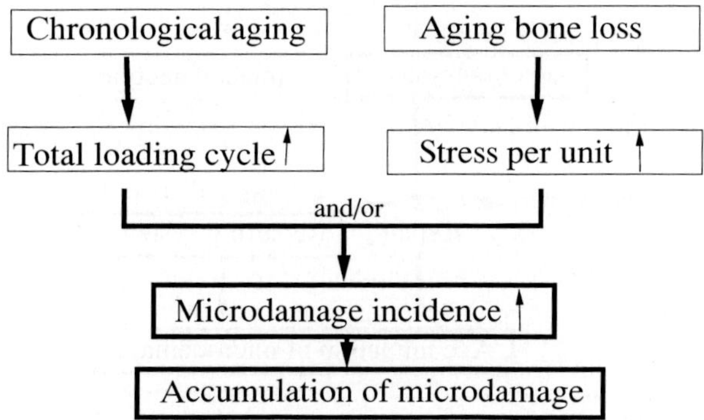

Fig. 4. Possible mechanisms of increasing microdamage incidence

manner to allow the time for the initiation of new remodeling in left radius. Histological examination with a bulk stain technique revealed no difference in micro-crack density between the first and second loaded radius, but a significant increase in resorption number and microcracks associated with resorption space in the first loaded radius compared to the second. These results strongly suggest that remodeling directly repairs microdamage.

Detection of Microdamage

Before remodeling is initiated at the site of microdamage, it must be detected by a biological system. It is has been suggested that osteocytes network with the communication works as a mechanoreceptor of microdamage for the following two reasons [19]: (1) the osteocyte is the first cell in contact with microdamage when it generates and grows, and (2) osteocytes can detect microdamage consistently anywhere in the bone matrix, because they form a large cell communication network in bone with their dendrites. We have found that osteocyte density decreases after 70 years, especially in interstitial packets, which is consistent with the fact that microcrack density is higher in elderly subjects.

Mechanism of Microdamage Accumulation

The extent of microdamage in bone is determined by the balance between generation and repair of microdamage. Microdamage accumulates in bone, when an imbalance exists, either increasing generation or decreasing repair of microdamage (Fig. 4). Increasing microdamage generation is induced either by increasing cycles of loading or by increasing stress: (1) chronological aging which leads to more cycles of loading, and (2) aging bone loss which induces less cross-sectional area and relatively more stress per unit of bone, causing an increase in microdamage generation in bone. A decrease in microdamage repair is induced either by a reduced repair function (remodeling) or by a decrease in detection of microdamage (Fig. 5). Reduced bone

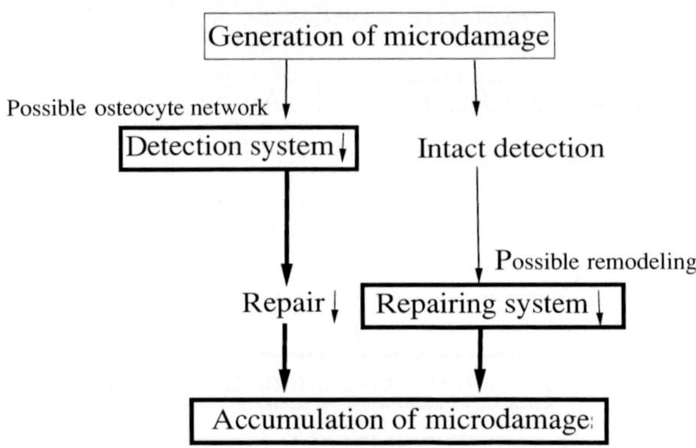

FIG. 5. Possible mechanisms of increasing microdamage repair

turnover or bone resorption as well as a coarse osteocyte network will slow down or shut off removal of microdamage in bone. Under normal bone metabolism, fatigue accumulation can be prevented, if given enough time for repair of microdamage. Disorders of bone resorptive function or remodeling cause skeletal fragility after cycles of loading such as in irradiation or steroid treatment, Cushing's syndrome, Paget's disease, or "marble bone" disease. Special attention must be paid to bisphosphonate treatment in continuous mode, because this treatment may inhibit bone remodeling in the repair of microdamage [20].

It should be also pointed out that bone volume and bone resorptive function are directly or indirectly associated with bone fatigue pathophysiology. Our data have shown that trabecular microdamage accumulates after the age of 70 years. There is a time lag between postmenopausal bone loss and the occurrence of senile fracture. Bone mineral density rapidly decreases during the 10–15 years following the onset of menopause at about the age of 50. The incidence of femoral neck fracture rapidly increases concurrently with microdamage accumulation. This suggests that fragility of aging bone is caused not only by bone loss but also by bone fatigue and therefore is a component of bone fragility that is independent of bone mass [21].

References

1. Suresh S (1991) Fatigue of materials. Cambridge University Press, New York
2. Reifsnider KL, Shulte K, Duke JC (1983) Long-term fatigue behavior of composite materials. In: O'Brien TK (ed) Long-term behavior of composites (ASTM ATP813). American Society for Testing and Materials, Philadelphia
3. Boiler and pressure vessel code (1973) American Society of Mechanical Engineering
4. Airplane damage tolerance requirements (1974) (MIL-A-83444) Air Force Aeronautical Systems Division
5. Federal aviation regulation airworthiness standards (1978) (FAR25.571) Federal Aviation Administration
6. Burr DB, Martin RB, Schaffler MB, Radin EL (1985) Bone remodeling in response to in-vivo fatigue microdamage. J Biomech 18:189–200
7. Frost HM (1960) Presence of microscopic cracks in vivo in bone. Henry Ford Hosp Med Bull 8:27–35

8. Burr DB, Stafford T (1990) Validity of bulk-staining technique to separate artifactual from in vivo bone microdamage. Clin Orthop Relat Res 260:305–308
9. Isa S, Mori S, Ibaraki K (1993) Distribution of microcracks in human ribs. Presented at 13th annual meeting of Japanese Society of Bone Histomorphometry
10. Schaffler MB, Choi K, Migrom C (1995) Aging and matrix microdamage accumulation in human compact bone. Bone 17(6):521–525
11. Norman TL, Wang Z (1997) Microdamage of human cortical bone: Incidence and morphology in long bones. Bone 20(4):375–379
12. Mori S, Harruff R, Ambrosius W, Burr DB (1997) Trabecular bone volume and microdamage accumulation in the femoral heads of women with and without femoral neck fractures. Bone 21(6):521–526
13. Mosekilde L (1990) Consequence of remodeling process for vertebral trabecular bone structure: a scanning electron microscopy study (uncoupling of unloaded structures). Bone Miner 10:13–35
14. Wicks M, Garrett R, Vernon-Roberts B, Fazzalari N (1982) Absence of metabolic bone disease in the proximal femur in patients with fracture of the femoral neck. J Bone Joint Surg 64(B):319–322
15. Vernon-Roberts B, Pirie CJ (1973) Healing trabecular microfractures in the bodies of lumbar vertebrae. Ann Rheum Dis 32:406–421
16. Tschantz P, Rutishauser E (1967) La surcharge mécanique de l'os vivant. Les déformations plastiques initiales et l' hypertrophie d' adaptation. Ann Anat Pathol 12:223–248
17. Martin RB, Burr DB (1982) A hypothetical mechanism for the stimulation of osteonal remodeling by fatigue damage. J Biomech 15:137–139
18. Mori S, Burr DB (1993) Increased intracortical remodeling following fatigue damage. Bone 14:203–109
19. Frost HM (1981) Bone remodeling and skeletal modeling errors. CC Thomas, Springfield, IL
20. Burr DB (1993) Remodeling and repair of fatigue damage. Calcif Tissue Int 53:S74–81
21. Burr DB, Forwood M, Fyhrie D, Martin B, Schaffler MB, Turner C (1997) Bone microdamage and skeletal fragility in osteoporotic and stress fractures. J Bone Miner Res 12(1):6–15

Part 3
Joint Destruction and Its Regulation in Rheumatoid Arthritis

The Immune System Under the Regulation of the Autonomic Nervous System

Toru Abo[1] and Soichiro Yamamura[2]

Summary. Multicellular organisms developed an autonomic nervous system to make it possible for a single cell to cooperate with others when they act for a single purpose. Many cells in living beings, therefore, have surface adrenergic or cholinergic receptors which accept stimuli from the autonomic nervous system. Leukocytes which constitute the immune system are no exception to this rule. Two major components of leukocytes, namely, granulocytes and lymphocytes, have adrenergic receptors and cholinergic receptors, respectively. In this regard, granulocytes are activated in number and function by sympathetic nerve stimulation, whereas for lymphocytes this is done by parasympathetic nerve stimulation. This new concept is extremely important in our understanding of the close relationship among physical conditions (e.g., stress), immune functions, and inflammation (e.g., tissue damage).

Key words. Immune system, Autonomic nervous system, Lymphocytes, Granulocytes, Nonsteroidal anti-inflammatory drugs

Introduction

We know empirically that severe stressors sometimes induce mucosal damage such as gastric ulcer and ulcerative colitis while obesity and shortage of exercise inversely induce certain allergic diseases such as allergic rhinitis and hay fever. However, mechanisms connecting physical conditions with host defense systems (including the immune system) are largely unknown. In a series of recent studies, we have demonstrated that granulocytes and lymphocytes carry adrenergic receptors and cholinergic receptors on the surface, respectively. In other words, two major components of leukocytes are regulated by the autonomic nervous system, similar to the way other cells in the body are.

If we introduce the above-mentioned concept into our host defense systems, the mechanisms involved in many diseases can be clarified. Two arrays of such

[1] Departments of Immunology and [2] Department of Orthopedics, Niigata University School of Medicine, 1 Asahimachi-dori, Niigata 951-8510, Japan

mechanisms include 1) severe stressors → sympathetic nerve stimulation → activation of granulocytes (e.g., release of free and oxygen radicals) → tissue damage; and 2) obesity and shortage of exercise → parasympathetic nerve dominance → activation of lymphocytes (e.g., elevation of prostaglandin synthesis) → excessive allergic reactions. In this chapter, we have reviewed our recent evidence for the regulation of host defense systems by the autonomic nervous system.

Expression of Adrenergic and Cholinergic Receptors on Leukocytes

Macrophages are the most basic leukocytes of the host defense system in multicellular organisms [1]. It has been found that these macrophages have both adrenergic and cholinergic receptors on the surface [2]. When macrophages are activated by adrenergic stimulation, their chemotactic function seems to be activated. On the other hand, when they are activated by cholinergic stimulation, their phagocytic function and the excretion of cytoplasmic granules seems to be activated. During phylogenic development, ancient macrophages gave rise to granulocytes and lymphocytes for greater efficiency of host defense systems (Fig. 1). Granulocytes increased the phagocytic function of ancient macrophages whereas lymphocytes inhibited this phagocytic function and inversely developed a recognition system (i.e., immune system) by modulating adhesion molecules of ancient macrophages (Fig. 1). At this point of evolution, granulocytes mainly took over adrenergic receptors and lymphocytes the cholinergic receptors, although this variation was not an all-or-nothing phenomenon. In other words, granulocytes still carry to some extent cholinergic receptors and lymphocytes some adrenergic receptors.

Several papers have reported the existence of adrenergic receptors on granulocytes [3–5]. However, the authors of these papers have emphasized only the suppressive in vitro effects of the excretion of cytoplasmic granules on granulocytes by sympathetic

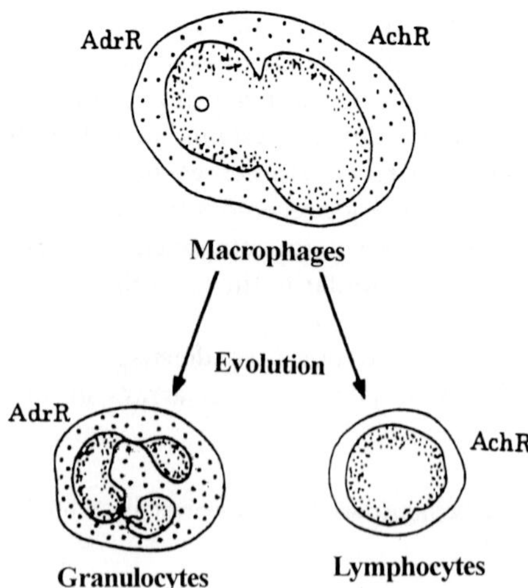

Fig. 1. Evolution of leukocytes and their expression of adrenergic and cholinergic receptors. Ancient macrophages gave rise to granulocytes and lymphocytes in phylogenic development. Macrophages carry both adrenergic (*AdrR*) and cholinergic receptors (*AchR*). However, during evolution, granulocytes acquired mainly the AdrR, lymphocytes mainly the AchR

nerve stimulation. We recently demonstrated in vivo that sympathetic nerve stimulation activated granulocytes in number and function [6,7]. Although the existence of cholinergic receptors on lymphocytes is controversial, our recent study showed that lymphocytes, especially T and B cells, have surface cholinergic receptors [8]. Primitive lymphocytes such as NK cells have both adrenergic and cholinergic receptors on the surface. In this situation, the number of NK cells is increased by sympathetic nerve stimulation while their function (i.e., NK activity) is increased by parasympathetic nerve stimulation (Abo and Yamamura, 1998, unpublished).

Physiological Variation of Leukocytes

The autonomic nervous system is known to vary according to physiological rhythms. One such rhythm is the circadian rhythm, in which the sympathetic nerves are dominant in the daytime while the parasympathetic nerves are dominant at night [2]. Reflecting this situation, leukocyte components also show a circadian rhythm (Fig. 2).

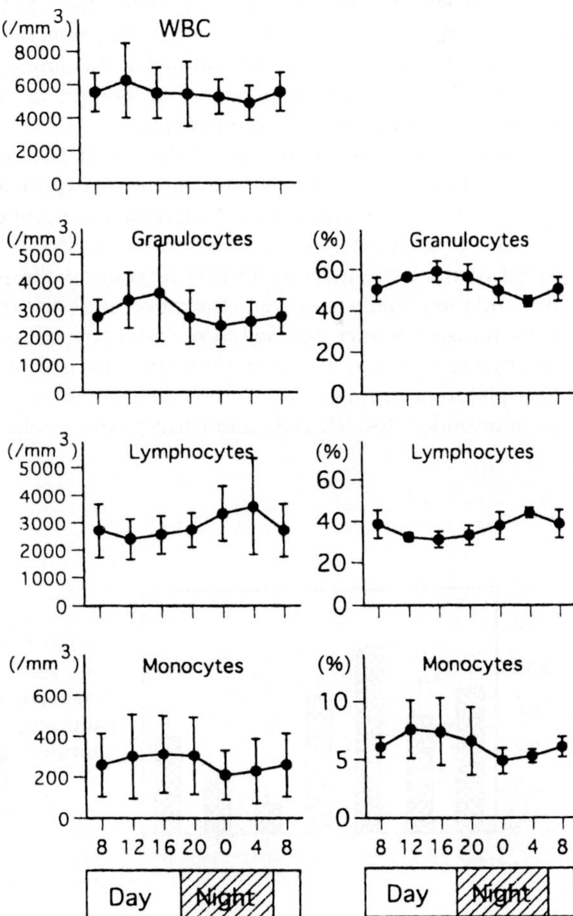

FIG. 2. Circadian rhythm of leukocytes. The numbers and proportions of granulocytes and monocytes show daytime rhythm, and the number and proportion of lymphocytes show night rhythm (n = 8)

Although the total number of leukocytes (i.e., white blood cells [WBC]) is relatively stable during the day, the numbers and relative proportions of granulocytes, lymphocytes, and monocytes (i.e., blood macrophages) vary, showing a clear circadian rhythm. The numbers and proportions of both granulocytes and macrophages increase in the daytime and decrease at night (i.e., daytime rhythm). In sharp contrast, the number and proportion of lymphocytes decrease in the daytime and increase at night (i.e., night rhythm). These variations arise from the fact that granulocytes and monocytes have mainly adrenergic receptors while lymphocytes have predominantly cholinergic receptors on the surface.

Expression of Adrenergic Receptors on Primitive Lymphocytes

Recent advances in immunology have shown that lymphocytes consist of many subsets, including T cells, B cells, NK cells, and extrathymic T cells (NKT cells) in mice [9–11] and in humans [12,13]. To determine how these lymphocyte subsets express β-adrenergic receptors in humans, a specific binding of ^{125}I-cyanopindolol to purified subsets were examined (Fig. 3). For a direct comparison, monocytes (M Φ) and granulocytes (Gra) were examined in parallel. It was found that NK cells and extrathymic T cells (CD56$^+$ NKT cells) expressed β-adrenergic receptors at a high level, similar to the cases of monocytes and granulocytes.

We have demonstrated that the behavior of NK cells and extrathymic T cells is similar to that of granulocytes when mice are exposed to restraint stress [6,14]. That is, severe stressors simultaneously increase the numbers of NK cells, extrathymic T cells, and granulocytes. More precisely, acute stressors induce granulocytes which resided in the bone marrow, to first migrate to the periphery (e.g., the blood and liver) and then finally to move to the mucosal tissues (e.g., gastric mucosa). When the gastric mucosa in mice exposed to restraint stress is examined at 24h, many NK and extrathymic T cells as well as granulocytes are isolated from the corresponding site. These phenomena might result from their common expression of adrenergic receptors in granulocytes, NK cells, and extrathymic T cells.

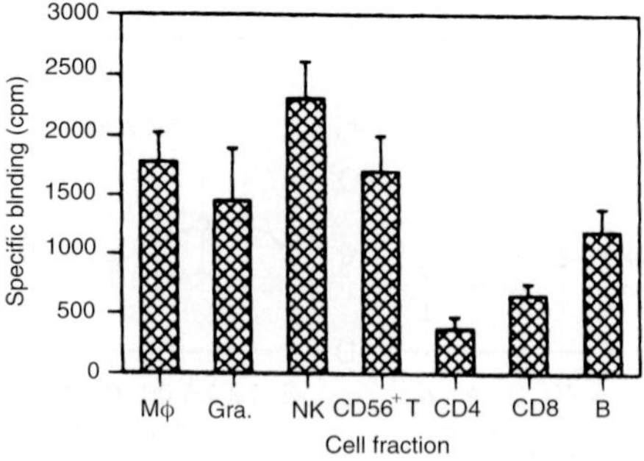

FIG. 3. Expression of β-adrenergic receptors on various subsets of leukocytes. ^{125}I-cyanopindolol was used to identify β-adrenergic receptors on the surface of purified leukocyte subsets. Macrophages (M Φ), granulocytes (Gra), NK cells, and extrathymic T cells (CD56$^+$T) expressed a high level of adrenergic receptors (AdrR), whereas T cells (CD4$^+$ and CD8$^+$) and B cells expressed a relatively low level of AdrR

Why Leukocytes have Adrenergic or Cholinergic Receptors

We have demonstrated that primitive lymphocytes such as NK and extrathymic T cells are primarily present in the digestive tract (i.e., endodermal epithelia) (Fig. 4). Since the gills (which gave rise to the thymus) and liver (a fetal hematopoietic organ) were also developed from the same endodermal epithelia [1], almost all lymphoid organs originated from the digestive tract. The digestive tract function is regulated by the parasympathetic nervous system (e.g., movement of the intestine and secretion of the enzymes). In the normal course of the digestive tract function, it is easy to speculate that many foreign antigens such as viral particles and digested foreign peptides may invade the host. In this regard, lymphocytes should function in collaboration with the digestive tract in response to the parasympathetic nervous system. As a result, it is critical for lymphocytes to carry predominantly cholinergic receptors on the surface.

When living beings are stimulated by the sympathetic nervous system and are active in their external environment they might be invaded by many different bacteria via their feet and other body sites. The phagocytic function of granulocytes (especially neutrophils) is therefore extremely important to the host for protecting it from bacterial infection. As a result, granulocytes carry adrenergic receptors on the surface.

Age-Associated Change in the Numbers of Granulocytes and Lymphocytes

From fetal to adult stages of development, the numbers of granulocytes and lymphocytes vary, showing a unique pattern (Fig. 5). It is well known that the numbers of total white blood cells and granulocytes (mainly neutrophils) are extremely high in

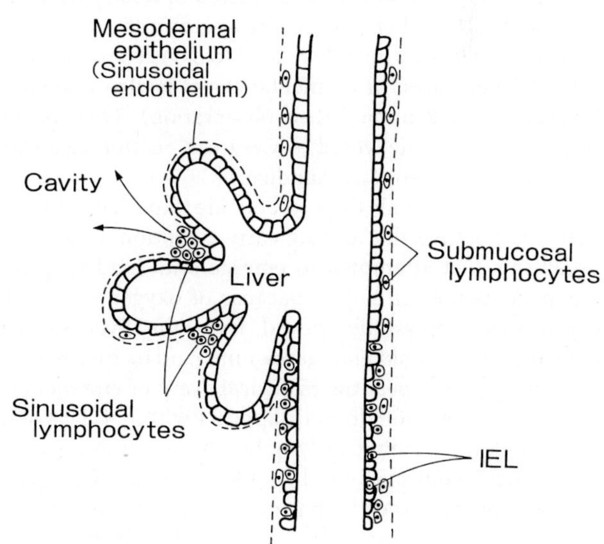

Fig. 4. Extrathymic development of lymphocytes in the digestive tract. The intraepithelial site in the intestine originally developed NK cells and extrathymic T cells from ancient macrophages. Since the sinusoidal site in the liver originated primarily from the intraepithelial site in the intestine, this site also has many NK and extrathymic T cells. *IEL*, intraepithelial lymphocytes

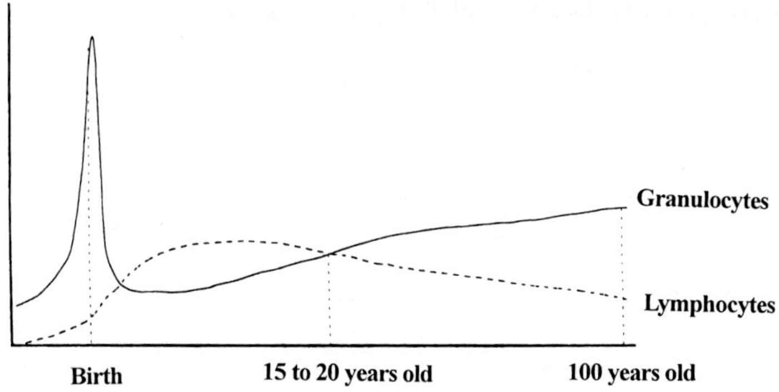

FIG. 5. Age-related change in the numbers of granulocytes and lymphocytes. Neonatal granulocytosis is seen at birth because of the commencement of pulmonary respiration. Thereafter, the predominance of lymphocytes continues into childhood. Around 15 to 20 years of age, the number of granulocytes exceeds the number of lymphocytes, and this tendency gradually predominates

neonates (i.e., neonatal granulocytosis). However, the physiological significance of this phenomenon had remained unclear. We have demonstrated that neonatal granulocytosis is induced by the commencement of pulmonary respiration [15]. A high level of oxygen induces sympathetic nerve activation in the newborn and then granulocytes which have surface adrenergic receptors are activated in number and function. These activated granulocytes severely damage hepatocytes and hematopoietic cells in the liver of neonates. As a result, the well-known phenomena neonatal jaundice and transient hepatitis (neonatal fatty liver) are seen in the newborn [15].

In a subsequent study, the detection of a fatty liver in chickens after the initiation of respiration and before hatching also prompted us to speculate that neonatal granulocytosis is more intimately related to oxygen stress at birth than to the stress of delivery, although physical or mental stress is also known to induce granulocytosis (T. Kawamura, 1998 unpublished observation). This speculation seems to be valid, as neonates that are delivered by Cesarean Section also show granulocytosis after birth and experience neonatal jaundice.

We suggest that all these events are experienced by living beings with lungs and that it is possible that during early evolution a similar phenomenon confronted all organisms that attempted to emerge onto land [15]. It is likely that many of these attempts resulted in failure because of oxygen stress. Only when the hematopoietic organ was successfully moved from the liver to the bone marrow (i.e., adult hematopoiesis) could emergence onto land be successful. At birth, neonates of animals with lungs may repeat the historical event of emergence onto land.

Neonatal granulocytosis disappears within 4 days after birth in humans. Then, in childhood, the number of lymphocytes is always greater than that of granulocytes. This pattern continues until an adolescent is 15–20 years old. In adults, the number of granulocytes exceeds that of lymphocytes and becomes more remarkable with aging. We know empirically that many allergic diseases such as atopic dermatitis and

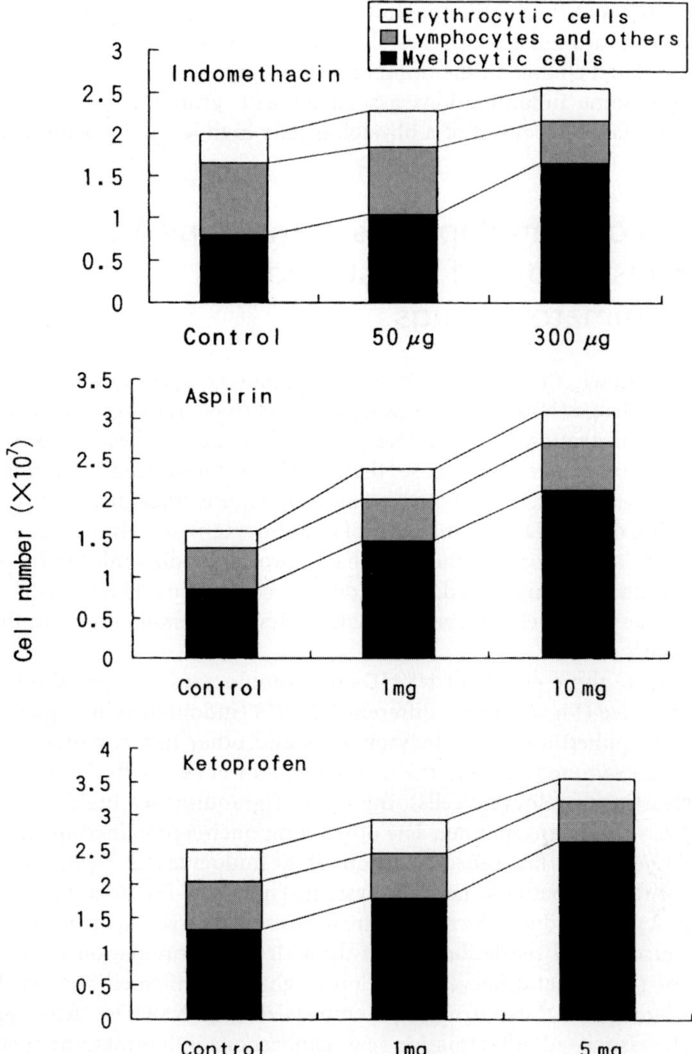

FIG. 6. Selective increase in the proportion of myelomonocytic cells in the bone marrow of mice treated with NSAIDs. Three different types of NSAIDs were injected into mice intraperitoneally and the distributions of various types of cells were compared. Irrespective of type, NSAIDs induced an increase in the proportion and absolute number of myelomonocytic cells (Mac-1[+] or Gr-1[+] cells) in a dose-dependent manner. The proportions of erythroid cells, lymphoid cells, and myelomonocytic cells were identified by the corresponding mAb against each antigen; namely, TER119, a mixture of CD3 and B220, and a mixture of Mac-1 and Gr-1, respectively

asthma are frequent in childhood. However, these allergic diseases naturally disappear with aging (around 15–20 years old). This phenomenon might be explained by this age-associated change in the number of leukocytes.

In old age, some inflammations associated with granulocytes (e.g., pulmonary infections) are fatal as a result of a physiologically high level of granulocytes in aged persons.

Induction of Granulopoiesis in the Bone Marrow by Administrations of Nonsteroidal Anti-inflammatory Drugs

It is widely known that a high dose or continuous doses of nonsteroidal anti-inflammatory drugs (NSAIDs) induce mucosal or tissue damage, irrespective of the routes of administration [7]. Since NSAIDs inhibit the synthesis of prostaglandins via the inhibition of cyclooxygenase, the prostaglandin–related inflammations (i.e., catarrhal, phlegmonous, and allergic inflammation) are efficiently suppressed by the administration of NSAIDs. The majority of lymphocyte-related immune responses are this type of inflammation. On the other hand, prostaglandins inhibit the production of catecholamines. In this regard, a high dose or continuous doses of NSAIDs induce many signs of sympathetic nerve stimulation. Severe granulocytosis in the blood is one such sign.

To investigate these effects of NSAIDs on granulocytes, a single dose of NSAIDs was given to mice (Fig. 6). Three different NSAIDs (indomethacin, aspirin, and ketoprofen) were applied and granulocytopoiesis and other hematopoiesis in the bone marrow were examined. Among the components of erythrocytes, lymphocytes, and granulocytes (i.e., myelocytic cells), the level of granulocytes highly increased in a NSAIDs dose-dependent manner. The other components remained unchanged.

As explained thus far, the generation of granulocytes is regulated under the influence of the sympathetic nervous system. Therefore, the present results suggest that granulocytosis induced by the administration of NSAIDs is intimately associated with the mucosal and tissue damage of these drugs. A circulation failure as one of the signs of sympathetic nerve activation might be confirmed with such mucosal or tissue damage of these drugs. We emphasize that NSAIDs rather grow worse granulocyte-associated inflammation (e.g., gangrenous inflammation). It is extremely important to understand this concept when treating inflammatory diseases.

Acknowledgments. The authors wish to thank Mrs. Masako Watanabe for preparation of the manuscript.

References

1. Abo T, Watanabe H, Sato K, Iiai T, Moroda T, Takeda K, Seki K (1995) Extrathymic T cells stand at an intermediate phylogenetic position between natural killer cells and thymus-derived T cells. Nat Immun 14:173–187
2. Suzuki S, Toyabe S, Moroda T, Tada T, Tsukahara A, Iiai T, Minagawa M, Maruyama S, Hatakeyama K, Endo K, Abo T (1997) Circadian rhythm of leukocytes and lympho-

cyte subsets and its possible correlation with the function of autonomic nervous system. Clin Exp Immunol 110:500–508

3. Panosian JO, Marinetti GV (1983) α_2-Adrenergic receptors in human polymorphonuclear leukocyte membranes. Biochem Pharmacol 32:2243–2247

4. Wiedemann RA, Kohse KP, Wisser H (1988) Alterations of β-adrenoceptors on human leukocyte subsets induced by dynamic exercise: effect of prednisone. Clin Exp Pharmacol Physiol 15:43–53

5. Landmann RMA, Müller FB, Perini CH, Wesp M, Erne P, Büher FR (1984) Changes of immunoregulatory cells induced by psychological and physical stress: relationship to plasma catecholamines. Clin Exp Immunol 58:127–135

6. Tsukahara A, Tada T, Suzuki S, Iiai T, Moroda T, Maruyama S, Minagawa M, Musha N, Shimizu T, Hatakeyama K, Abo T (1997) Adrenergic stimulation simultaneously induces the expansion of granulocytes and extrathymic T cells in mice. Biomed Res 18:237–246

7. Yamamura S, Arai K, Toyabe S, Takahashi EH, Abo T (1996) Simultaneous activation of granulocytes and extrathymic T cells in number and function by excessive administration of nonsteroidal anti-inflammatory drugs. Cell Immunol 173:303–311

8. Toyabe S, Iiai T, Fukuda M, Kawamura T, Suzuki S, Uchiyama M, Abo T (1997) Identification of nicotinic acetylcholine receptors on lymphocytes in periphery as well as thymus in mice. Immunology 72:201–205

9. Sato K, Ohtsuka K, Hasegawa K, Yamagiwa S, Watanabe H, Iwanaga T, Takahashi-Iwanaga H, Asakura H, Abo T (1995) Evidence for extrathymic generation of intermediate TCR cells in the liver revealed in thymectomized, irradiated mice subjected to bone marrow transplantation. J Exp Med 182:759–767

10. Watanabe H, Miyaji C, Kawachi Y, Iiai T, Ohtsuka K, Iwanaga T, Takahashi-Iwanaga H, Abo T (1995) Relationships between intermediate TCR cells and NK1.1[+]T cells in various immune organs. NK1.1[+]T cells are present within a population of intermediate TCR cells. J Immunol 155:2972–2983

11. Osman Y, Watanabe T, Kawachi Y, Sato K, Ohtsuka K, Watanabe H, Hashimoto S, Moriyama Y, Shibata A, Abo T (1995) Intermediate TCR cells with self-reactive clones are effector cells which induce syngeneic graft-versus-host disease in mice. Cell Immunol 166:172–186

12. Takii Y, Hashimoto S, Iiai T, Watanabe H, Hatakeyama K, Abo T (1994) Increase in the proportion of granulated CD56[+]T cells in patients with malignancy. Clin Exp Immunol 97:522–527

13. Okada T, Iiai T, Kawachi Y, Moroda T, Takii Y, Hatakeyama K, Abo T (1995) Origin of CD57[+]T cells which increase at tumour sites in patients with colorectal cancer. Clin Exp Immunol 102:159–166

14. Moroda T, Iiai T, Tsukahara A, Fukuda M, Suzuki S, Tada T, Hatakeyama K, Abo T (1997) Association of granulocytes with ulcer formation in the stomach of rodents exposed to restraint stress. Biomed Res 18:423–437

15. Kawamura T, Toyabe S, Moroda T, Iiai T, Takahashi-Iwanaga H, Fukuda M, Watanabe H, Sekikawa H, Seki S, Abo T (1997) Neonatal granulocytosis is a postpartum event which is seen in the liver as well as in the blood. Hepatology 16:1567–1572

Effects of Stem Loosening on Periprosthetic Bone Remodeling After Cementless Hip Replacement

Takashi Nishii[1], Masao Tanaka[2], Nobuhiko Sugano[1], Shinichi Tamura[3], Kenji Ohzono[1], and Takahiro Ochi[1]

Summary. We studied the influence of stem stability on periprosthetic bone remodeling around a cementless femoral component in bone densitometric examinations and determined if the specified bone remodeling patterns according to stem stability can be explained by mechanical environment. Using dual-energy X-ray absorptiometry (DEXA), we examined bone mineral density (BMD) distribution of the proximal femur in 48 hips with a press-fitted collared stem and 45 hips without a stem. Those hips operated on included 34 and 14 hips with stable and loose stems, respectively, as shown on plain radiographs. For mechanical assessment, we analyzed three-dimensional finite element (FE) models of the proximal femur with a stable stem, with an unstable stem, and without a stem. The DEXA evaluations revealed significant differences of BMD distribution with regard to stem stability. A remarkable increase in BMD in the proximal medial region was a salient feature of femora with loose stems. The biomechanical analysis with the FE model for the unstable stem showed an elevation of equivalent stresses in the proximal medial cortical bone. The stress distribution of the stable and unstable FE models was correlated well with BMD distribution of the stable and loosening groups, respectively. The present study suggests that stability of the stem influences bone remodeling enough to be evident in the evaluation of BMD distribution, and that the analyses of periprosthetic BMD distribution offer the possibility for estimating the stability of the stem per se, based on biomechanical environment.

Key words. Bone remodeling, Hip replacement, Finite element analysis, Dual-energy X-ray absorptiometry

[1] Department of Orthopaedic Surgery, Osaka University Medical School, 2-2 Yamadaoka, Suita, Osaka 565-0871, Japan
[2] Department of Mechanical Engineering, Faculty of Engineering Science, Osaka University, 1-1 Machikaneyama, Toyonaka, Osaka 560-0043, Japan
[3] Division of Functional Diagnostic Imaging, Biomedical Research Center, Osaka University Medical School, 2-2 Yamadaoka, Suita, Osaka 565-0871, Japan

Introduction

Following the insertion of a cementless femoral component, periprosthetic femoral bone is involved in adaptive bone remodeling in terms of bone mineral density (BMD) change and bone contour deformation so as to adapt to the new mechanical environment of the stem bone configuration. Clinically, bone atrophy in the proximal-medial femur is a typical manifestation of bone remodeling after total hip arthroplasty (THA) [1,2]. The femoral component shares part of the mechanical load, which would be transferred through the proximal aspect of the femoral bone without a femoral component, and the reduction of stress and strain in the proximal part of the femoral bone will eventually constitute a remodeling stimulus for the reduction of bone mass and BMD [3–5].

A number of investigators have studied the factors influencing bone remodeling and have striven for optimal femoral components which subsequently induce favorable bone remodeling (preservation of bone stock in the proximal part of the femur). As a result, large diameter, stiff material, and full porous coating of the femoral component are considered to exert an unfavorable influence on bone remodeling [1,6–8]. Other than the factors associated with the femoral component itself, the stability of the femoral component was also assumed to substantially influence the proximal biomechanical environment.

Engh et al. [1] considered proximal bone loss on a radiograph as one of the radiographic signs of stable fixation with bone ingrowth. Based on this concept, it can be hypothesized conversely that the loss of stability of the femoral component may change the environment of mechanical loading around the proximal femur and result in a different bone remodeling pattern relative to the stable femoral component. From a similar point of view, some authors expect that the evaluation of periprosthetic BMD may predict aseptic loosening of the femoral component before radiographic or clinical signs of the loosening are evident [9]. Hence, we measured BMD around a cementless hip prosthesis using dual-energy X-ray absorptiometry (DEXA) in patients with stable and loose stems, and evaluated the remodeling patterns with respect to the stability of the femoral component. In addition, to clarify whether those specific bone remodeling patterns are based on the change of periprosthetic mechanical environment corresponding to implant stability, we performed a computational biomechanical evaluation using a finite element (FE) analysis.

Materials and Methods

Bone Remodeling Evaluation Using DEXA

Forty-eight hips of 42 patients who had an uncemented hip replacement with a press-fitted Omnifit collared femoral stem (Osteonics, Allendale, NJ, USA) with a normalized smooth surface were the subject of this study. A DEXA examination was performed at a time interval of 38 to 101 months (average, 63 months) following the operation using a DPX-L (Lunar, Madison, WI, USA). There were 17 men and 25 women, with an average age of 49 years (range, 25–63 years), in the group. They had been operated on because of osteoarthrosis of the hip in 25 cases and osteonecrosis of the femoral head in 23 cases. With the use of the Omnifit collared femoral stem, 24 hips had undergone a bipolar hip replacement and the remaining 24 had undergone a total hip arthroplasty, according to the degree of disease involvement in the acetabular constitution.

All of the patients were evaluated clinically and radiographically at 6-month intervals after the operation. Radiographically, vertical subsidence of the femoral component was measured on anteroposterior radiographs by taking the vertical distance from the proximal tip of the greater trochanter to the superolateral corner of the component. Stem loosening was defined as a progressive subsidence of more than 4mm or a progressive angular shift of more than 5° [10]. If those changes stopped before the end of the first year after operation, the component was not judged as loosening. As a result, a progressive angular shift of the stem was found in nine hips and progressive subsidence was seen in eight hips at the final follow-up examination. Consequently, 14 hips were judged as unstable due to stem loosening and the stems of the other 34 hips were considered to be stable.

There was no statistical difference with regard to the gender ratio, disease ratio for operation, use of steroid (Fisher's exact test), age, and time interval since operation (Mann-Whitney test) between the two groups. The large stems of more than No. 8 size were used in 56% of patients of the stable group and in 71% of patients of the loosening group.

To evaluate the relevance of the existence of the femoral component on BMD distribution, a DEXA examination was also performed on 45 proximal femora without an implant in 42 patients as a control group. These hips included 20 normal hips, 20 early osteoarthritic hips, and five cases of osteonecrosis of the femoral head without collapse. There were 13 men and 29 women in the group, with an average age of 52 years old (range, 24–75 years). None of the hips in the control group had notable limitation of motion that might prohibit complete positioning of the leg and precise measurement of BMD at the DEXA examination, or involvement of arthritic change at the femoral neck portion.

The periprosthetic BMD was measured by DEXA from the anteroposterior view. Thirteen periprosthetic regions were defined according to the length of the inserted stem (Fig. 1). To evaluate the precision of the DEXA measurements, 10 patients received three consecutive scans following dismounting and remounting on the table during each scan. The average precision at each zone was as follows. Zone 1: 5.3%, Zone 2: 4.9%, Zone 3: 3.9%, Zone 4: 4.5%, Zone 5: 3.6%, and Zone 6: 2.8% on the lateral side; Zone 1: 6.4%, Zone 2: 5.9%, Zone 3: 4.6%, Zone 4: 3.5%, Zone 5: 2.2%, and Zone 6: 4.8% on the medial side; Zone 7: 2.1%. Although the precision of proximal area measurements (Zone 1 and Zone 2 laterally and medially) was relatively high as compared to the other zones, the range of precision was comparable to precision reported by other authors [7].

When comparing the periprosthetic BMD distribution among the three groups including the stable, loosening, and control groups, bone density ratio (BDR) was calculated by dividing the BMD value at each zone with that at the most distal zone (Zone 7) and multiplying by 100 for the percent expression. Although large variations of absolute BMD value exist between individual patients, we consider that this relative index can reduce the effect of the variation in a comparative study. One-way analysis of variance (ANOVA) and the Scheffe F-test were used to examine the differences of BDRs at the 12 zones excluding Zone 7.

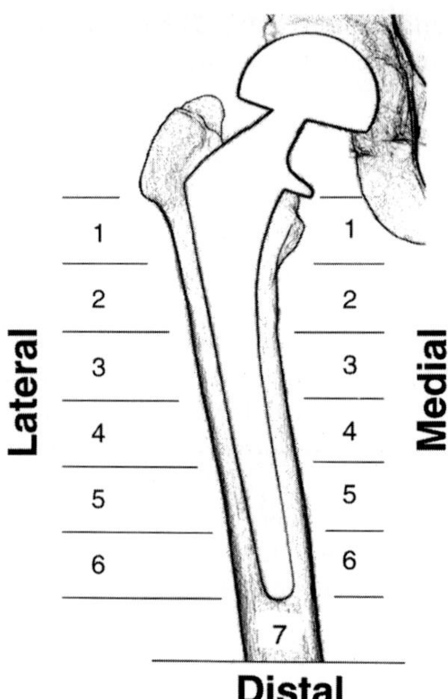

Fig. 1. The location of the 13 regions of interest (Zone 1 to Zone 6 laterally and medially, and Zone 7), defined according to the length of the inserted stem in dual-energy X-ray absorptiometry (DEXA) examinations

Biomechanical Analysis Using a Finite Element Analysis

Three-dimensional FE models of the proximal femur with an implant were developed using CT images of a 31 year-old woman with unilaterally involved osteonecrosis of the femoral head. Eventually, she underwent a bipolar hip replacement with a press-fitted Omnifit Number 7 implant on her left side due to collapse of the femoral head. The right proximal femur was normal in geometrical shape according to radiographic examination and of normal BMD shown by DEXA.

Before the operation, both hips were scanned in consecutive slices of 3 mm, which were 20 mm apart over the femoral head and 140 mm apart below the lesser trochanter. The CT image data was transferred to a Sun SPARC station (Sun Microsystems, Mountain View, CA, USA), and a three-dimensional solid model of the right proximal femur was generated after detection of cancellous, cortical, and sub-chondral bone areas on each CT image with the use of Laplacian-of-Gaussian filtering with thresholding as the contour extraction algorithm [11]. The surgical simulation of implantation of the Omnifit Number 7 solid model into the femoral bone model was performed using the Application Visualization System (AVS) (Advanced Visual Systems, Waltham, MA, USA), a three-dimensional visualization software, on the Sun workstation. During the simulation the AVS enabled the whole view of the femoral and stem models to be visualized simultaneously from anterior and lateral directions as well as multiple cutting planes perpendicular to the femoral axis which contained the transverse stem image superimposed on the transverse femoral bone image. The direction and the distance of insertion of the stem model was determined with the use of the anterior-posterior and medio-lateral radiographs of the femur after the operation. The femoral model with the stem was converted to a basic three-

Fig. 2. **a** Three-dimensional finite element model of the femur with the femoral component. The applied loads were the 2727 N compressive load (components: 1194 N in medial to lateral direction, 732 N in anterior to posterior direction, 2340 N in proximal to distal direction) on the proximal end of the stem, and the 2073 N tensile load (components: 1074 N in lateral to medial direction, 666 N in posterior to anterior direction, 1644 N in distal to proximal direction) on the greater trochanter, assuming a body weight of 600 N [19,20]. These forces represent the case during the single stance phase of normal gait. All nodes on the distal end of the femur were rigidly constrained in all directions. **b** Cross section in the midst of the model. A thin layer of elements (*black layer*) was modeled around the stem elements (two inner elements, arranged radially around the center of the section), and the mechanical property of the elements in the thin layer was altered according to the stability of the stem (cancellous bone or fibrous tissue). Between the thin layer and the stem, nonlinear interface with no friction was modeled to allow tensile separation and local slip

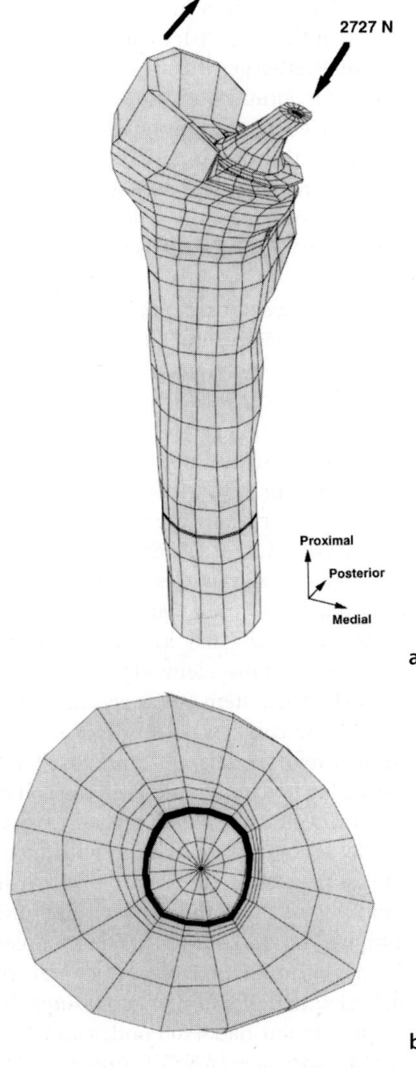

dimensional FE model using linear, eight-noded brick and six-noded wedge elements (Fig. 2a). The elastic moduli were assumed as 110 GPa for elements of the stem, 17 GPa for those of the cortical bone, and 1 GPa for those of the cancellous bone, based on data available in the literature [12,13]. A Poisson ratio of 0.3 was assumed for all elements.

After generation of the basic FE model, we added nonlinear interface elements around the entire stem surface under the collar, to represent the condition at the interface of the press-fitted Omnifit stem surface [3,5]. These interface elements transmit only the compressive stress component and allow tensile separation and local slide to occur with no friction. We then provided thin elements in a width of 0.4 mm along the radial direction just outside of the interface elements from the calcar portion to the stem tip (Fig. 2b), to account for stem stability.

Van Rietbergen et al. [5] reported, using an animal experimental model and a computer simulation model, that bone remodeling around press-fitted stems was reproduced in the computer simulation more satisfactorily when using a FE model in which the proximal fibrous gap was accounted for, compared to a model with direct bone and stem contact at all interfaces. Therefore, we assigned the mechanical property of cancellous bone to the distal half of the thin elements and the mechanical property of fibrous tissue to the proximal half of the thin elements, for the stable model.

Clinically, extensive radiolucent lines were often found around the surface of a loose stem on radiographs, and a thick fibrous membrane was commonly observed at the stem-bone interface at revision surgeries of failed cementless femoral stems [10,14]. Hence, we assigned the mechanical property of fibrous tissue to all thin elements in the case of an unstable stem. The mechanical property of fibrous tissue was represented by a piece-wise linear expression of five stages in a stress–strain relationship. This nonlinear property provides a very low initial stiffness, but progressively increasing stiffness with large strains when compressed. By calculation based on the equation of Weinans et al. [13], the elastic modulus of the element was 13 MPa when the strain was less than 0.2, 29 MPa when the strain was between 0.2 and 0.4, 816 MPa when the strain was between 0.4 and 0.6, 3776 MPa when the strain was between 0.6 and 0.8, and 101 097 MPa otherwise. A high Poisson ratio of 0.49 was assigned to those elements.

Initially the stem collar was assumed to be separated from the calcar. For the stable model, the collar was assumed not to make contact with the calcar. For the unstable model, two models were prepared to study the effect of collar/calcar contact: one assuming no contact between the collar and calcar, the other assuming a collar contact transmitting only compressive stress component.

The model of intact femur without a stem (control model) was also generated using the same meshes as the model with a stable stem under the calcar portion. The elastic modulus of the elements for subchondral bone encapsulating the femoral head was assigned as 1.3 GPa [15]. The completed FE models with both stable and unstable stems without collar contact contained 3631 nodes and 3703 elements. The unstable model with collar contact contained 3631 nodes and 3751 elements. The model of the normal femur had 4400 nodes and 4380 elements. The FE models were analyzed with ANSYS software (ANSYS, Houston, PA, USA).

The results of the FE analyses were compared between the four models including the control model, the stable model, the unstable model without collar contact, and the unstable model with collar contact, in terms of von Mises equivalent stress and strain energy density in the elements around the mid-frontal plane of the cortical bone. For the stable and unstable models, the equivalent stresses at the whole stem surface and relative displacements between the stem and the bone or fibrous layer along the interface were evaluated. Distribution patterns of those mechanical parameters for the stable and the unstable models were correlated with BMD distribution patterns for the stable and the loosening groups in the DEXA analysis.

Results

Bone Remodeling Analysis Using DEXA

In the control group, average BDR on the lateral and medial sides decreased gradually as the zones moved proximally, and in the most proximal zone (Zone 1) average BDRs were approximately 54% laterally, and 60% medially (Fig. 3). In comparison with the control group, the stable group showed significantly higher BDRs at the distal-lateral zones (lateral Zone 5 and 6), and significantly lower BDRs at the proximal-medial zones (medial Zone 2 and 3) ($P < 0.01$, ANOVA, and Scheffe F-test). The loosening group, on average, presented a similar bone density distribution as the stable group. However, at the medial Zone 1, the average BDR showed a remarkable difference. Although the average BDR at the medial Zone 1 was lower in the stable group than the control group, the loosening group showed a significantly higher BDR,

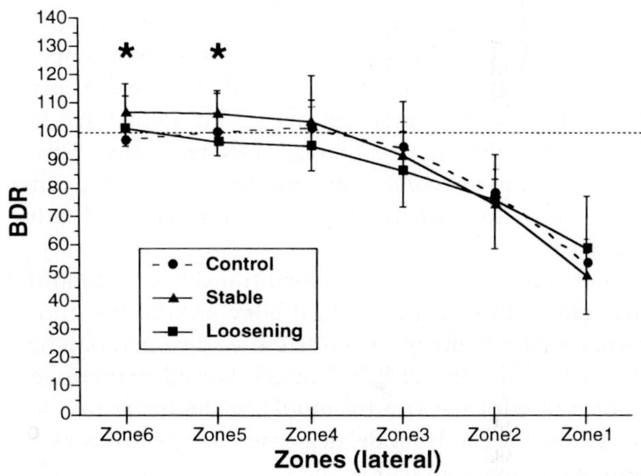

FIG. 3. **a** Bone density ratio (*BDR*) of the lateral zones. One-way analysis of variance (ANOVA) and the Scheffe *F*-test showed a significant difference at lateral Zone 5 and Zone 6 between the control and stable group (*P* < 0.01). **b** BDR of the medial zones. Both operated-on groups showed significant lower values at medial Zone 3 and Zone 2 as compared to the control group, however, at the most proximal zone the unstable group represented a significantly higher value compared to the other two groups (*P* < 0.01)

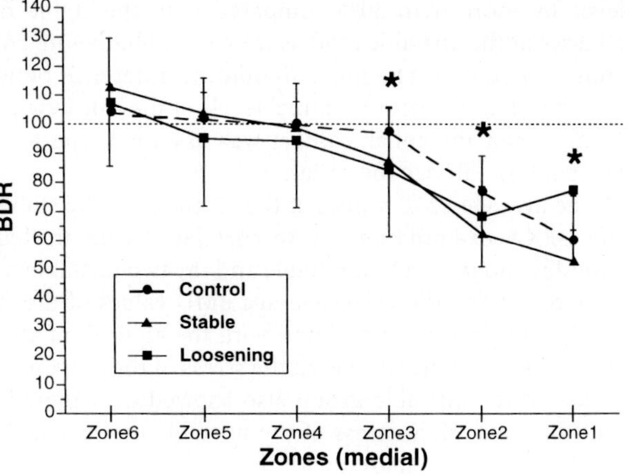

conversely, in comparison with the control group as well as the stable group ($P < 0.01$, ANOVA, and Scheffe F-test).

Biomechanical Analysis with FE Models

The equivalent stress distribution at the surface of the stem is shown for the stable and the unstable models in Fig. 4. In the stable model high stresses were mostly observed in the distal two-thirds of the stem surface (Fig. 4a). The unstable model without collar contact revealed a rather uniform stress distribution at the entire stem surface as compared to the stable model (Fig. 4b). When collar contact was assumed in the unstable model, the stresses in the distal two-thirds of the stem surface decreased more, and significantly high stresses were generated at the lower surface of the collar (Fig. 4c). These stress distribution modes at the stem surface indicated that loss of stability shifted the prime load transmission area upward even if collar contact was not assumed, and the collar contact led to concentration of the load transmission at the collar-calcar interface.

When subsidence of the stem relative to the bone or the fibrous layer was represented by positive values, all the models resulted in positive displacements on the medial side in combination with negative displacements on the lateral side, due to the bending moment by the hip-joint force (Fig. 5). The displacements in the two unstable models increased by more than 50% relative to the stable model. These findings are consistent with the radiographic criteria of stem loosening, which define loosening when progressive migration of more than a determined value occurred.

Subsequent to the changed load transmission condition at the stembone interface, equivalent stress in the cortical bone around the mid-frontal plane showed a great variance among the three models after the operation and the control models (Fig. 6). On the lateral side, the stable model showed an increase of stresses by more than 30% compared with the control model in the distal half levels. On the medial side, the stresses of the stable model decreased progressively as the area moved proximally and resulted in less than half of the stresses of the control model. On the other hand, the two unstable models revealed an increase of the stresses in the proximal one-third level, by more than 30% compared with the stable model. These increases in the stresses of the unstable models were found both with collar contact and without collar contact assumed. The most significant difference between the two unstable models was found in the most proximal levels of the calcar, where the stresses increased drastically when the collar contact was assumed, due to the concentration of the load transmission under the collar.

The average BMD values at the 12 zones of the stable and the loosening groups in the DEXA examinations were correlated with the equivalent stress at the corresponding bone area of the stable and the two unstable models in the FE analysis, using Pearson's correlation. The average BMD values of the stable group showed a strongly significant positive correlation with the equivalent stress of the stable model (0.892, $P < 0.0001$), as compared with the stress of the two unstable models. The average BMD values of the unstable group also showed a strongly significant positive correlation with the equivalent stress of the unstable model with collar contact assumed (0.846, $P < 0.0005$), as compared with the stress of the stable and the other unstable model.

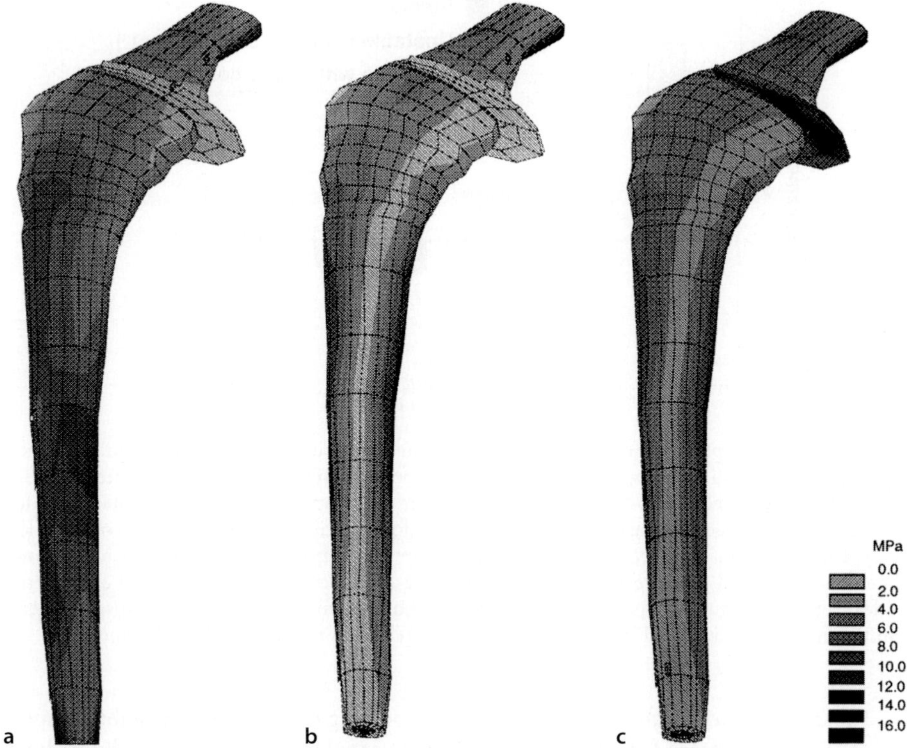

FIG. 4a–c. Plot of the magnitude of von Mises equivalent stresses at the stem surface as viewed from anterior to posterior direction. **a** Stable model. **b** Unstable model without collar contact. **c** Unstable model with collar contact

The strain energy density in the cortex showed a similar distribution pattern for the three models after the operation and the control model, respectively, as the von Mises equivalent stress.

Discussion

Many investigators have evaluated periprosthetic bone remodeling after cementless total hip arthroplasties with the use of DEXA. Some of these studies were intended to determine how long the bone remodeling proceeds after the operation [16]. Other studies aimed to explore the relationship between the degree of bone remodeling and some factors associated with femoral components and individual patients [7,17]. Most of those studies dealt with patients with clinically and radiographically satisfactory evaluations to avoid effects of ill-conditioning of femoral components on the DEXA results. We assumed, however, that those effects lead to another type of remodeling around the stem. To our knowledge, there are few reports concerning the effect of stem stability on periprosthetic bone remodeling with quantitative evaluation by DEXA.

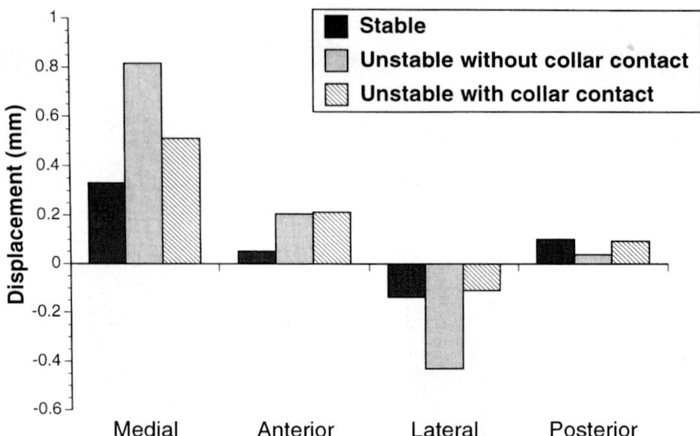

FIG. 5. Relative displacements at the stem-bone or stem-fibrous layer in the longitudinal direction along the medial, anterior, lateral, and posterior stem sides. Positive values mean subsidence of the stem relative to the bone or fibrous layer. The displacements in the unstable model without collar contact increased approximately threefold relative to the stable model on all sides except the posterior side. When the collar was in contact with the calcar, the subsidence and bending movement was prevented and the absolute displacements on the medial and lateral sides were reduced as compared to the models without collar contact. However, displacement on the medial side was still increased by approximately 50% relative to the stable model

Those factors which may influence bone remodeling other than stem stability, such as gender, age, disease for operation, and time interval since operation, did not show significant differences among the stable, loosening, and control groups. The proportion of implantations with larger stems was relatively high in the loosening group as compared to the stable group. It is reported that larger stems are subject to bone atrophy around the proximal femur to a greater extent [6,7]. Therefore, the difference of stem sizes should have resulted in a bias, if it existed, toward a relative BMD decrease around the proximal femur area versus the distal area and a decrease of BDR values at the proximal zones in the loosening group. The DEXA result showed relatively lower mean BDRs at the lateral and medial distal zones and higher mean BDR at the most proximal-medial zone in the loosening group as compared with the stable group. These distribution features were contrary to the bias assumed for the difference of stem sizes between the operated-on groups. We consider that the proximal femur provides salient features of BMD distribution mostly depending on the existence of a stem and the state of stem stability.

The biomechanical analysis using the FE models had some simplifications and difficulties. First, we compared three FE models for femora with the implant, varying only the mechanical condition of a thin layer around the stem-bone interface and collar contact condition. All other relevant parameters remained identical, as regards geometry and composition of the femoral bone, size and position of the femoral stem, and applied load. Clinical findings indicate that a loosening of the stem influences BMD distribution, or is likely to cause varus or valgus shift of the stem. Various loading conditions during gait or stair climbing are influential on the torsional moment or stress on the femoral bone and stem-bone interface. Accounting for

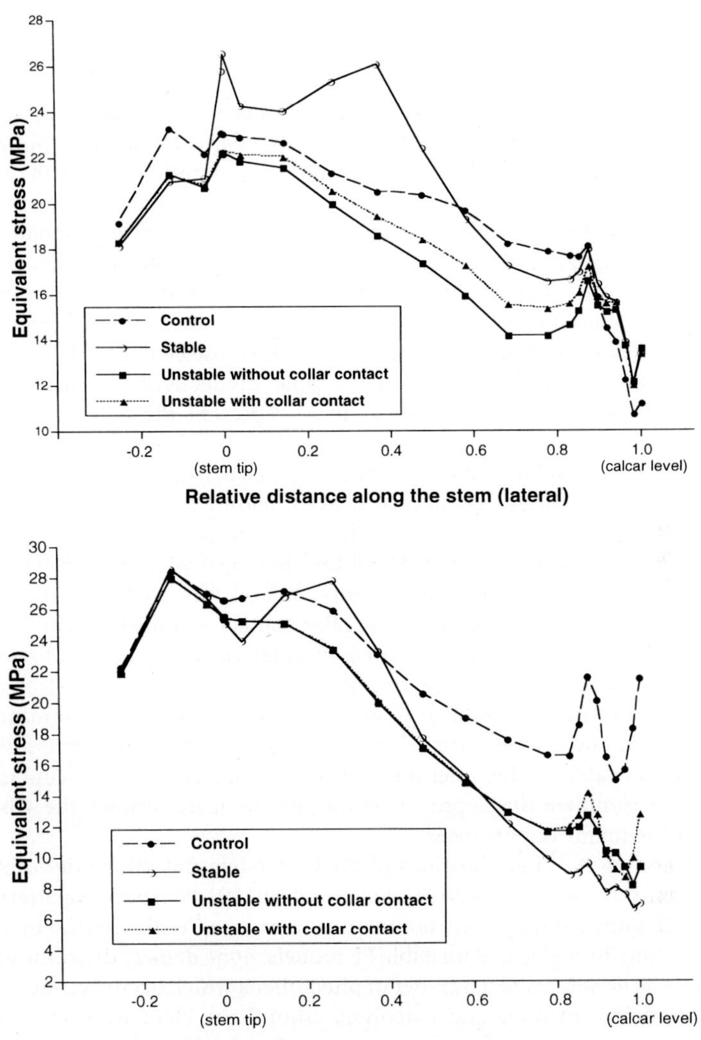

FIG. 6. Graph shows von Mises equivalent stress distribution in the lateral (a) and medial (b) cortex elements around the mid-frontal planes

those parameters for the FE models may lead to a detailed exploration of the mechanical condition of each case with a stable or loose stem. However, this could impede the understanding of the basic importance of stem stability on the mechanical condition. To evaluate conceptual mechanical features related to stem stability, we consider the use of the three models, under only one applied load case, representative of the common conditions during daily walking, and differing only in the most important parameters, to have been appropriate. In this context, care must be taken in extrapolating our results to each individual case after the arthroplasty.

Second, loosening of a femoral stem is a radiographic criterion with significant displacement of the stem, and may not be directly related to element configurations or materials of the FE model. In radiographic examinations of stem loosening, however, the appearance of extensive radiolucent lines is frequently observed around the stem [10]. At revision surgeries of stem loosening, thick fibrous membranes are commonly found surrounding the femoral component [14]. Weinans et al. [13] modeled a nonlinear contact interface between the stem and cement in combination with nonlinear material properties of the fibrous membrane in a two-dimensional FE model to investigate mechanical environment of the loose cemented femoral component. Therefore, we expected that our unstable model with fibrous tissue layer surrounding the entire surface of the stem to represent the condition of a loose cementless femoral stem.

Third, since a stem collar, if in contact with the calcar, increases load transfer to the medial calcar and decreases the effect of stress-shielding [18], modeling of the interface between the collar and calcar was another concern. In the unstable model without collar contact assumed, axial subsidence of the stem relative to the femoral bone was increased and the predominant load transmission area was developed over the whole stem surface. In the unstable model with collar contact assumed, on the other hand, axial subsidence of the stem was prevented by collar/calcar contact, and stress transfer between the stem and bone was concentrated at the collar and calcar interface. However, those two models resulted in an almost similar stress distribution pattern along the medial and lateral cortex (Fig. 6). Hence, the specific stress distribution pattern in our unstable models does not seem to be responsible for the contacted stem collar, but the complete development of the fibrous layer around the whole stem surface is of the major importance.

Notwithstanding the simplifications of the FE models and difficulties of modeling of stem stability in our FE analyses, the specific BMD distribution patterns in the operated-on groups from DEXA examinations correlated well with the biomechanical analysis using the stable and unstable FE models. Bone density distribution around loose stems may be subject to a number of phenomena which occur secondary to stem loosening. Radiolucent lines and osteolysis around the stem were often found in femora with loose stems [10], and these may influence the result of periprosthetic BMD examinations. However, our results proved that those specific patterns of BMD distribution with respect to the stem stability depend in a large part on biomechanical etiology. As long as the effects of biomechanical stimulus on bone remodeling is of great importance, the analysis of BMD distribution around the stem has a great possibility for providing information on stem stability.

For further investigations of the interrelationship between bone remodeling and biomechanical assessment, evaluation of geometrical changes of bone contour, such as distal bone hypertrophy, will be required, in addition to evaluation of BMD change. Bone remodeling proceeds in a very complicated, nonlinear process, under mechanical stimulus in the bone. Development of FE analysis in conjunction with adaptive bone remodeling theory will enhance the correlation of bone remodeling evaluation with biomechanical analysis.

References

1. Engh CA, Bobyn JD, Glassman AH (1987) Porous-coated hip replacement. The factors governing bone ingrowth, stress shielding, and clinical results. J Bone Joint Surg 69B:45–55
2. Sumner DR, Galante JO (1992) Determinants of stress shielding: Design versus materials versus interface. Clin Orthop 274:202–212
3. Huiskes R, van Rietbergen B (1995) Preclinical testing of total hip stems. The effects of coating placement. Clin Orthop 319:64–76
4. Keaveny TM, Bartel DL (1995) Mechanical consequences of bone ingrowth in a hip prosthesis inserted without cement. J Bone Joint Surg 77A:911–923
5. Van Rietbergen B, Huiskes R, Weinans H, Sumner DR, Turner TM, Galante JO (1993) The mechanism of bone remodeling and resorption around press-fitted THA stems. J Biomechanics 26:369–382
6. Bobyn JD, Mortimer ES, Glassman AH, Engh CA, Miller JE, Brooks CE (1992) Producing and avoiding stress shielding. Laboratory and clinical observations of non-cemented total hip arthroplasty. Clin Orthop 274:79–96
7. Kilgus DJ, Shimaoka EE, Tipton JS, Eberle RW (1993) Dual-energy X-ray absorptiometry measurement of bone mineral density around porous-coated cementless femoral implants. Methods and preliminary results. J Bone Joint Surg 75B:279–287
8. Skinner HB, Kim AS, Keyak JH, Mote Jr CD (1994) Femoral prosthesis implantation induces changes in bone stress that depend on the extent of porous coating. J Orthop Res 12:553–563
9. Korovessis P, Piperos G, Michael A (1994) Periprosthetic bone mineral density after Mueller and Zweymueller total hip arthroplasties. Clin Orthop 309:214–221
10. Nishii T, Sugano N, Masuhara K, Takaoka K (1995) Bipolar cup design may lead to osteolysis around the uncemented femoral componet. Clin Orthop 316:112–120
11. Marr D, Hildreth E (1980) Theory of edge detection. Proc Royal Soc Lond [Biol] 207:187–217
12. Huiskes R, Weinans H, Dalstra M (1989) Adaptive bone remodeling and biomechanical design considerations. Orthopedics 12:1255–1266
13. Weinans H, Huiskes R, Grootenboer HJ (1990) Trends of mechanical consequences and modeling of a fibrous membrane around femoral hip prostheses. J Biomechanics 23:991–1000
14. Duparc J, Massin P (1992) Results of 203 total hip replacements using a smooth, cementless femoral component. J Bone Joint Surg 74B:251–256
15. Brown TD, Vrahas MS (1984) The apparent elastic modulus of the juxtarticular subchondral bone of the femoral head. J Orthop Res 2:32–38
16. Steinberg GG, Kearns C, McCarthy C, Baran DT (1991) Quantification of bone loss of the proximal femur after total hip arthroplasty. Trans Orthop Res Soc 16:545
17. Hughes SS, Furia JP, Smith P, Pellegrini Jr VD (1995) Atrophy of the proximal part of the femur after total hip arthroplasty without cement. A quantitative comparison of cobalt-chromium and titanium femoral stems with use of dual x-ray absorptiometry. J Bone Joint Surg 77A:231–239
18. Djerf K, Gillquist J (1987) Calcar unloading after hip replacement. A cadaver study of femoral stem designs. Acta Orthop Scandinavica 58:97–103
19. Keaveny TM, Bartel DL (1993) Effects of porous coating and collar support on early load transfer for a cementless hip prosthesis. J Biomechanics 26:1205–1216
20. Paul JP (1996) Biomechanics. The biomechanics of the hip-joint and its clinical relevance. Proc Roy Soc Med 59:943–948

Abnormalities in Bone Marrow of Patients with Rheumatoid Arthritis

Tetsuya Tomita, Hideo Hashimoto, Eiji Takeuchi, Motoharu Kaneko, Hiroshi Takano, Kazuomi Sugamoto, and Takahiro Ochi

Summary. In a previous study we showed the presence of abnormal myeloid lineage cells in epiphyseal bone marrow (BM) adjacent to joints affected with severe rheumatoid arthritis (RA). In this study, we have investigated the abnormalities of the cellular population related to RA in the iliac BM, in vitro production and modulation of abnormal myeloid lineage cells, and the microenvironment in BM which may support these unique cellular changes specific to RA patients. Mononuclear cells (MNCs) were prepared from iliac BM aspirates from RA patients. Two-color flow cytometry was carried out to analyze the phenotypes of MNCs freshly isolated from BM aspirates, and the presence of abnormal myeloid cells under various cultured conditions. The absolute number of MNCs in the iliac BM was increased 3-fold in the RA patients compared with the non-RA controls. In CD8+ cell and myeloid cell fractions, significant differences were recognized between RA patients and non-RA controls. The production of abnormal myeloid cells was enhanced by granulocyte macrophage colony stimulating factor (GM-CSF) and interleukin-1β, but inhibited by T lymphocytes. Stromal cell lines from RA BM with nursing activity were established. Characteristic changes of the iliac BM suggest an important role of systemic BM in the pathogenesis of RA.

Key words. Rheumatoid arthritis, Bone marrow, Myeloid lineage cells, Stromal cells

Introduction

We consider that the major pathological site in RA may be the systemic bone marrow and that the synovial proliferation and infiltration of inflammatory cells in joints may be secondary changes. We have observed several characteristic BM changes related to experimental arthritis [1–4]. Our previous studies have demonstrated that preceding the induction of polyarthritis, maturation and proliferation of BM cells were observed, and IL-1 and IL-6 activity in BM serum were elevated in adjuvant and

Department of Orthopaedic Surgery, Osaka University Medical School, 2-2 Yamada-oka, Suita, Osaka 565, Japan collagen induced arthritis in rats. These pathological changes were maintained while arthritis continued. We have also reported the existence of abnormal myeloid cells, which strongly express the difucosyl or trifucosyl type 2 chain (dimetric or trimetric Lex, a specific marker of human undifferentiated cells) in the epiphyseal bone marrow adjacent to joints affected with severe RA [5]. Maintaining these cells in vitro could be achieved for only a short period by adding epiphyseal BM serum from severe RA patients [6]. Based upon these findings, in the present study we investigated the characteristic pathological changes of iliac BM, and in vitro production and modulation of abnormal myeloid cells.

Patients and Methods

Patients

Bone marrow blood samples were obtained from RA patients who met the American College of Rheumatology criteria [7], and healthy donors with who had given informed consent. According to our reported criteria [8], all RA patients were classified into three disease subsets: the subset with the least erosive disease (LES), the subset with more erosive disease (MES), and the subset with mutilating disease (MUD). In the LES, erosive articular changes were primarily limited to the smaller peripheral joints. In the MES, the large axial joints were also involved. In the most severely affected subset, MUD, almost all joints were extensively damaged.

Cell Preparations

Heparinized BM aspirate was obtained from the anterior iliac crest by needle puncture at the time of operation. MNCs from BM aspirate and venous blood were separated by density gradient centrifugation.

Cell Cultures

Cells were resuspended in HL-1 supplemented with 5% heat-inactivated fetal calf serum and cultured at 37°C in a humidified atmosphere of 5% CO_2 at cell densities $0.5 - 1.0 \times 10^6$/ml in various conditions.

Monoclonal Antibodies and Cytokines

The monoclonal antibodies (Mab) used were CD4, CD8, CD14, CD15, CD16, and HLA-DR. Recombinant human (rh) IL-1β, IL-3, IL-6, IL-8, monocyte colony stimulating factor, and GM-CSF were used in various culture conditions.

Two-Color Flowcytometry

The cells were collected and washed three times in PBS. The cells were incubated with fluorescent isothiocyanate conjugated Mab and phycoerythrin conjugated Mab. Two-color flow cytometric analysis was performed using a FACScan (Becton Dickinson, Mountain View, CA) equipped with an argon laser at 488 nm. The number of positive cells was expressed as a percentage of the total cell count.

Results

Number of Mononuclear Cells

There was a marked increase in the absolute number of MNCs in the iliac BM from RA patients compared with the non-RA controls. The means (±SEM) of the number of MNCs were 3122 ± 225 for RA patients and 1245 ± 311 for non-RA controls. There was a significant difference between RA patients and non-RA controls ($P <$ 0.01). The number of MNCs was increased according to the severity of RA ($P < 0.05$ for LES and $P < 0.01$ for MES and MUD vs. non-RA controls). In contrast, there was no significant difference in the absolute number of MNCs in tibial BM and peripheral blood between RA patients and non-RA controls.

Lymphocyte Subsets

In the iliac BM of RA patients, the percentage of lymphocytes subsets did not differ significantly from the non-RA controls, but the number of MNCs was increased 3-fold compared with the non-RA controls. Using anti-HLA-DR Mab, we analyzed the percentage of activated lymphocytes. The percentage of HLA-DR+CD4+ cells with respect to all CD4 cells did not differ significantly between RA patients and non-RA controls in the iliac BM and peripheral blood. In contrast, the percentage of HLA-DR+CD8+ cells to all CD8 cells differed significantly between RA patients and the non-RA controls in the iliac BM and peripheral blood ($P < 0.05$). In LES and MES, the percentage of HLA-DR+ CD8 cells to all CD8 cells in the iliac BM was increased significantly when compared with the non-RA controls ($P < 0.05$), whereas the percentage of HLA-DR+CD4 cells to all CD4 cells did not differ significantly between each RA subset and non-RA controls. In the most severely affected patients, MUD, the percentage of HLA-DR+CD8 cells to all CD8 cells varied so widely that no significant difference could be determined when compared with the non-RA controls (Fig. 1).

Myeloid Cell Population

Myeloid cells were analyzed using CD15 (MX-GA) Mab, which detects a broad range of myeloid lineage cells from myeloblasts to polymorphonuclear cells, and using CD16 Mab, which detects mature granulocytes (PMN) and natural killer (NK) cells. That is, the CD15+CD16– cells were considered to be panmyelocytes. In the iliac BM, the absolute number of myeloid cells in RA patients differed significantly from non-RA controls according to the severity of RA (Fig. 2).

Abnormal Myeloid Cells in BM

We found that abnormal and normal myeloid cells could be well separated using CD14 (MY4) Mab, which reacts with abnormal myeloid cells as well as monocyte-macrophages, but not with normal myeloid cells. These CD14 positive myeloid cells were confirmed to be the same population beaning oncofetal mono- or di-fucosylated type 2 chain inepiphyseal bone marrow adjacent to the affected joints in patients with severe RA [5]. It was characteristic that myeloid cells in the iliac BM could be separated into CD14+CD15+ cells and CD14–CD15+ cells in severe RA. But in the non-RA

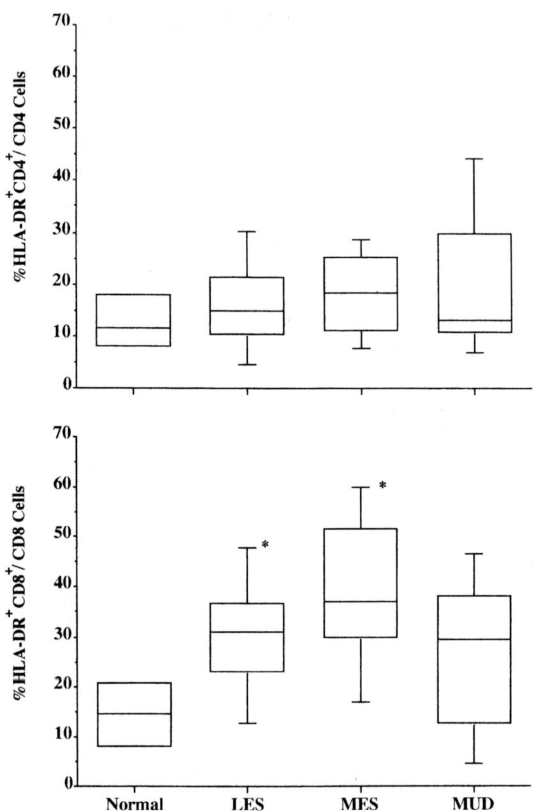

Fig. 1. HLA-DR antigen expression by CD4 and CD8 cells from the iliac bone marrow (BM) of rheumatoid arthritis (RA) patients and non-RA controls. *$P < 0.05$ as compared with the non-RA controls. *LES*, least erosive disease subset; *MES*, more erosive disease subset; *MUD*, mutilating disease subset

controls or LES, all myeloid cells in the iliac BM were CD14−CD15+. In the tibial epiphyseal BM of severe RA, all myeloid cells were CD14+CD15+. On the other hand no myeloid cells could be found in the tibial epiphyseal BM of non-RA controls or LES (Fig. 3).

Production and Modulation of Abnormal Myeloid Cells in Vitro

To assess in vitro production of CD14+CD15+ cells, BM MNCs from various donors were incubated for 5 days under various conditions. Adding autologous iliac BM serum, CD14+CD15+ cells were induced from CD14−CD15+ cells derived from severe RA patients. To study the effect of T lymphocytes in producing CD14+CD15+ cells, we compared the production of CD14+CD15+ cells in the presence of T lymphocytes and without T lymphocytes. This demonstrated the inhibitory effect of T lymphocytes on the production of CD14+CD15+ cells (Fig. 4a). To measure the effect of various cytokines on the production of CD14+CD15+ cells, CD14−CD15+ cells derived from severe RA patients were cultured in the presence of IL-1β, IL-3, IL-6, IL-8, G-CSF, M-CSF, and GM-CSF. With GM-CSF and IL-1β, CD14+CD15+ cells were produced in a dose-dependent manner (Fig. 4b).

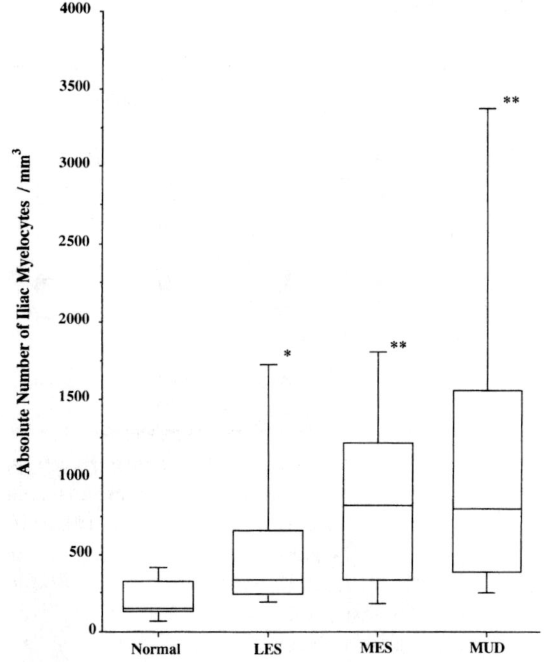

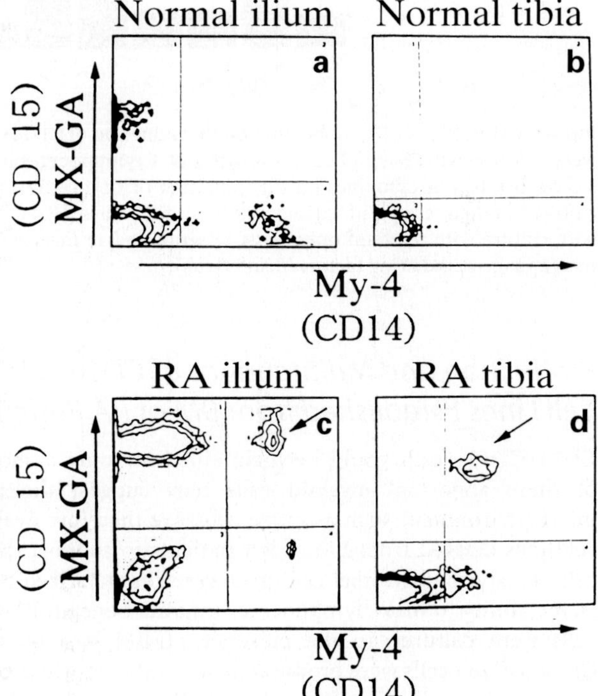

FIG. 3. The existence of abnormal myeloid cells in BM of severe RA patient. **a** Cells in the iliac BM of a normal donor. **b** Cells in the tibial epiphyseal BM of a normal donor. **c** Cells in the iliac BM of a severe RA patient. **d** Cells in the tibial epiphyseal BM of a severe RA patient. *Arrows* in **c** and **d** indicate the abnormal myeloid cell population

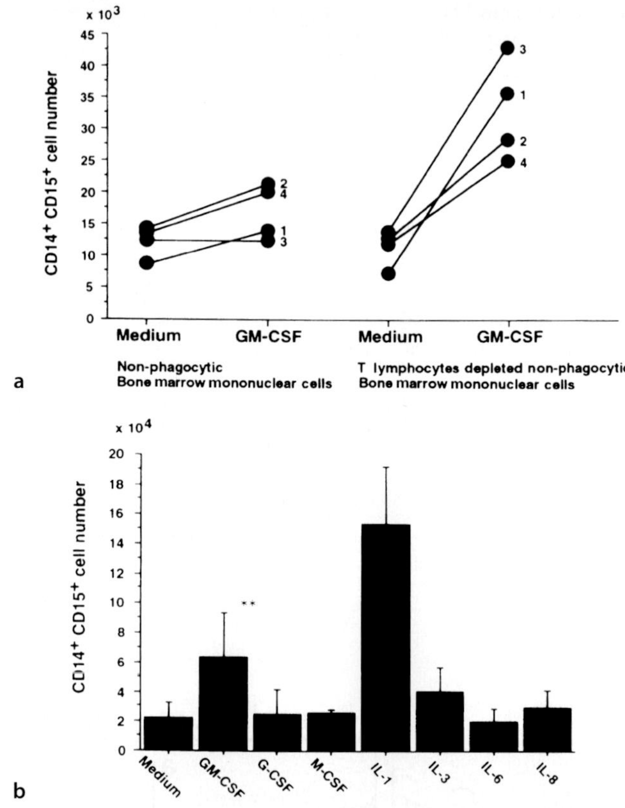

FIG. 4. **a** The effect of T lymphocytes on the induction of CD14+CD15+ cells, CD14−CD15+ cells were cultured with T lymphocytes or without T lymphocytes in the presence of rhGM-CSF for 5 days. **b** Effect of cytokines on the induction of CD14+CD15+ cells. CD14−CD15+ cells were cultured in the presence of various cytokines for 5 days. *$P < 0.0001$ and **$P = 0.0037$ compared with culture with medium only. *GM-CSF*, granulocyte macrophage stimulating factor; *M-CSF*, macrophage stimulating factor; *IL*, interleukin

Production and Maintenance of CD14+CD15+ Cells by Stromal Cell Lines Established from BM of RA Patients

CD14+CD15+ cells could be maintained for only a short period in vitro. Survival of these abnormal myeloid cells may suggest the presence of a unique BM microenvironment such as nurse cells. We therefore evaluated the ability of stromal cell lines derived from BM of RA patients to support these abnormal CD14+CD15+ cells. Established stromal cell lines were characterized by pseudoemperipolesis, that is, the ability to make lymphocytes migrate beneath BM stromal cells. CD14−CD15+ cells were cultured in the presence of BM stromal cells for 5 days. Abnormal CD14+CD15+ cells were produced in a significantly higher ratio when cocultured with BM stromal cells as compared with those cocultured with BM stromal cells but without contact ($P < 0.05$). When cocultured with BM stromal cells, CD14+CD15+ cells maintained a significantly higher ratio compared with those cocultured with BM stromal cells derived from a healthy donor ($P < 0.01$).

Discussion

In this study, we reported several abnormalities of BM cells of RA patients. The increase of MNCs was recognized in the iliac BM of RA patients. Peripheral blood white cell count was not significantly increased, so the rapid turnover and functional enhancement of white blood cells in peripheral organs of RA patients was suggested. The characteristic findings of RA patients were a significant enhancement of CD8+ cell activation, an increase of myeloid cells, and induction of abnormal myeloid cells. These abnormal myeloid cells were shown to develop into polymorphonuclear (PMN) cells [9]. Our previous studies revealed PMN cells with remarkably high levels of IL-1 in the same epiphyseal BM as accumulations of CD14+CD15+ cells [10]. Therefore, these abnormal myeloid cells may contribute to the tissue destruction in severe RA patients. To induce and maintain these abnormal myeloid cells, BM stromal cells might play an important role. Pherhaps BM stromal cells may also contribute to the activation of lymphocytes or other hematopoietic cells in BM of RA patients. These results suggest that hematopoietic BM may play an important role in the pathogenesis of RA.

References

1. Hayashida K, Ochi T, Fujimoto M (1992) Interleukin-1 and interleukin-6 activity and abnormal myelopoiesis. Arthritis Rheum 35:241–245
2. Fujimoto M, Ochi T, Owaki H, Wakitani S, Suzuki R, Takai M, Ono K (1988) Elevated activity of interleukins-1, -2 and -3 in the bone marrow of collagen-induced arthritis rats. Biomed Res 9:401–407
3. Fujimoto M, Hayashida K, Ochi T, Shimaoka Y, Ono K (1992) Fluctuation of inter-leukin-1 and -6 activity in the bone marrow serum in collagen-induced arthritis in rats. Biomed Res 13:243–251
4. Nakagawa S, Toritsuka Y, Wakitani S, Denno K, Tomita T, Owaki H, Kimura T, Shino K, Ochi T (1996) Bone marrow stromal cells contribute to synovial cell proliferation in rats with collagen induced arthritis. J Rheumatol 23:2098–2103
5. Ochi T, Hakomori S, Adachi M, Owaki H, Okamura M, Ono Y, Yamasaki K, Fujimoto M, Wakitani S, Ono K (1988) The presence of a myeloid cell population showing strong reactivity with monoclonal antibody directed to difucosyl type 2 chain in epiphyseal bone marrow adjacent to joints affected with rheumatoid arthritis (RA) and its absence in the corresponding normal and non-RA bone marrow. J Rheumatol 15:1609–1615
6. Owaki H, Ochi T, Yamasaki KV, Wakitani S, Ono K (1989) Elevated activity of myeloid growth factor in bone marrow adjacent to joints affected by rheumatoid arthritis. J Rheumatol 16:572–577
7. Arnett FC, Edworthy SM, Bloch DA, McShane DJ, Fries JF, Cooper NS, Healey LA, Kaplan SR, Liang MH, Luthra HS, Medsger TA, Mitchell DM, Neustadt DH, Pinals RS, Schaller JG, Sharp JT, Wilder RL, Hunder GG (1988) The American Rheumatism

Association 1987 revised criteria for the classification of rheumatoid arthritis. Arthritis Rheum 31:315–324
8. Ochi T, Iwase R, Yonemasu K, Matsukawa M, Yoneda M, Yukioka M, Ono K (1988) Natural course of joint destruction and fluctuation of serum C1q levels in patients with rheumatoid arthritis. Arthritis Rheum 31:37–43
9. Ochi T, Tomita T, Shimaoka Y, Owaki H, Tanabe M, Nakagawa S, Kawamura S, Denno K, Lee K (1994) Production of unusual (di-Lex+, CD14+) myeloid cells in the bone marrow of patients with rheumatoid arthritis. Arthritis Rheum 37 (suppl):S248
10. Wakitani S, Ochi T, Ono K (1994) Elevated interleukin-1 level in polymorphonuclear cells accumulating in bone marrow adjacent to the affected joints with severe rheumatoid arthritis. Jpn J Rheumatol 5:243–250

Extrathymic Differentiation of Resident T Cells in the Joint and Rheumatoid Arthritis

Tadamasa Hanyu[1], Katsumitsu Arai[1], and Toru Abo[2]

Summary. Murine collagen-induced arthritis (CIA) is known as a T cell-mediated autoimmune disease. We have demonstrated that the joints always comprise T cell populations, including IL-2R$\alpha^-\beta^+$ T cells, $\gamma\delta$ T cells, CD8$\alpha^+\beta^-$ cells, and CD44$^+$L-selectin$^-$ cells. All these properties coincide with those of extrathymic T cells in liver and intestine. In vivo treatment with various monoclonal antibodies, indicates that the $\gamma\delta$ T cells and CD8$\alpha\alpha^+$ cells are associated with the suppression of disease, especially after its onset. Furthermore, in patients with rheumatoid arthritis (RA), CD57$^+$ T cells levels were found to be elevated, and were especially high in joints and the adjacent bone marrow. The CD57$^+$ T cells contained higher proportions of double-negative CD4$^-$CD8$^-$ cells and $\gamma\delta$ T cells than CD57$^-$ T cells. We have suggested that the CD57$^+$ T cells with a natural killer (NK) cell marker probably are a counterpart to extrathymic T cells in humans and have unique immunosuppressive functions which are different from those of conventional T cells and NK cells. In rats with CIA, a great increase in the number of granulocytes was observed before the onset of arthritis. Furthermore, many clinicians know that active RA patients always show an increase in granulocytes in peripheral blood and joints. We have speculated that the interaction between the granulocytes and extrathymic T cells of the joints is important, since extrathymic T cells are activated in parallel with granulocytes in mice. We suspect that extrathymic T cells can exert potent anti-rheumatic effects when stimulated by some chemical mediator.

Key words. Extrathymic T cells, Rheumatoid arthritis, Collagen-induced arthritis, Mice, Granulocytes

Introduction

It is well known that T cells differentiate in the thymus [1,2], where positive and negative selections of T cell clones take place. As a result, most mature T cells after

Departments of [1]Orthopedic Surgery and [2]Immunology, Niigata University School of Medicine, 1 Asahimachi-dori, Niigata 951-8510, Japan maturation in the thymus comprise cells that recognize foreign antigens in the context of major histocompatibility complex (MHC) antigens. In recent studies, it was demonstrated that extrathymic pathways of T cell differentiation exist in the liver [3,4] and intestine [5].

Identification of Extrathymic T Cells in the Liver

Hepatic mononuclear cells (MNC) can be isolated using an improved method as described by Watanabe et al. [6]. Briefly, mice anesthetized with ether are killed by total bleeding with a cardiac puncture. To obtain the MNC, the liver is removed, pressed through a 200-gauge stainless steel mesh, and then suspended in phosphate-buffered solution (PBS) (0.1 M, pH 7.2). After washing once with PBS, MNC are isolated from both hepatocytes and the nuclei of hepatocytes by Ficoll-Isopaque density (1.090) gradient centrifugation. To avoid a selective loss of specific subsets, the meshed liver samples are then suspended in minimum essential medium (MEM) supplemented with 2% fetal calf serum (FCS).

The surface phenotypes of the cells are identified using monoclonal antibodies (mAbs) in conjunction with the two-color immunofluorescence test. The reagents included FITC-conjugated anti-CD3 mAb and phycoerythrin (PE)-conjugated anti-interleukin-2 receptor β-chain (IL-2Rβ) mAb. In this staining, natural killer (NK) cells are estimated as CD3$^-$IL-2Rβ^+, extrathymic T cells in the liver as intermediate-CD3$^+$IL-2Rβ^+, thymus-derived T cells as high-CD3$^+$IL-2Rβ^-, mainly B cells as CD3$^-$IL-2Rβ^-.

The number of T cell receptors (TCR) of these hepatic T cells is less than that of thymus-derived T cells, and the former is 1/5 of the latter [7]. In this regard, the extrathymic hepatic T cells have been termed "intermediate TCR cells". It is well established that regular T cells differentiate in the thymus, passing through a stage at which dull TCR are carried, and then acquiring high TCRs at maturity. The intensity of intermediate TCR on extrathymic T cells in the liver is at an intermediate position between those of dull and high TCR on thymocytes.

Since T cells with these properties were preferentially generated in the hepatic sinusoids of normal and athymic nude mice, and comprised all-T cell populations in athymic nude mice, they were thought to be of extrathymic origin [8]. Moroda et al. [9] reported that in liver MNC in control mice there was a mixture of NK cells, intermediate CD3 cells, and high CD3 cells, whereas those in athymic nude mice lacked high CD3 cells. Although liver MNC in neonatal thymectomy (NTx) mice comprised only intermediate CD3 cells among CD3$^+$ cells at young (6–10 weeks), a significant proportion of intermediate CD3 cells appeared thereafter (Fig. 1). In a later study, it was evident that the liver of the adult mice contained c-kit$^+$ stem cells [10]. The consistent expression of recombination activating gene-1 (RAG-1) and RAG-2 mRNA in B220$^-$ T cells in the liver has also suggested the existence of extrathymic pathways of T cell differentiation in this organ [11]. It is known that the thymic medulla comprises endodermal epithelial cells originating from gills. It seems likely therefore that in contrast to the cortex of the thymus, the thymic medulla supports primitive T cell differentiation as do the hepatic sinusoids [12].

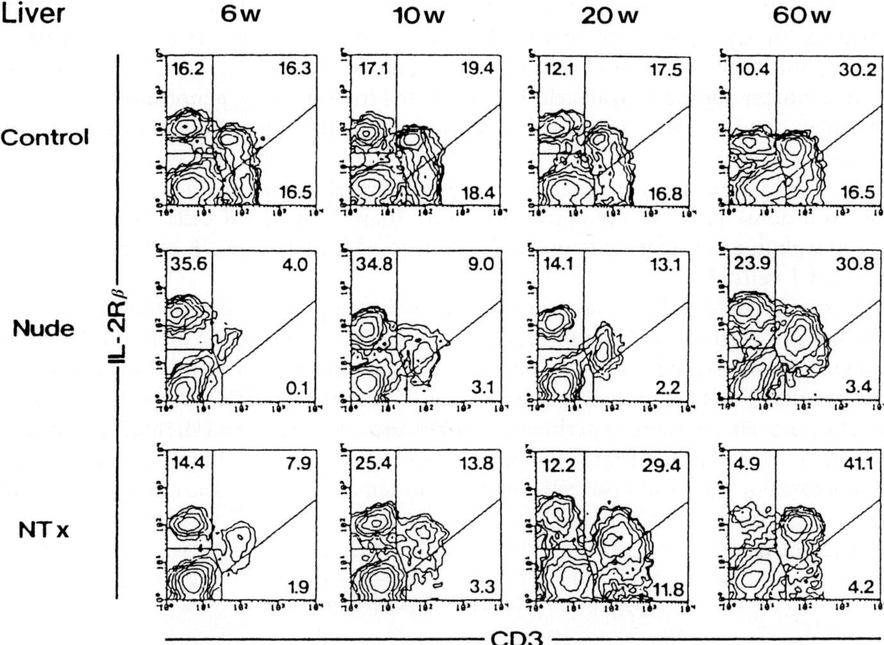

FIG. 1. Age-associated variation of lymphocyte subsets in the liver of various mice. In liver mononuclear cells (*MNC*) in control mice there was a mixture of natural killer (NK) cells, intermediate CD3 cells, and high CD3 cells, whereas those in athymic nude mice lacked high CD3 cells. Although liver MNC in neonatal thymectomy (*NTx*) mice comprised only intermediate CD3 cells among CD3$^+$ cells at 6–10 weeks, a significant proportion of intermediate CD3 cells appeared thereafter. (From [9], with permission)

Characteristics of Extrathymic T Cells in the Liver

Using mAbs in conjunction with either a single-, two-, or three-color immunofluorescence test, these differences between intermediate levels of TCR and thymus-derived T cells with high levels of TCR have been demonstrated. It is characteristic that these hepatic T cells express constantly the same IL-2Rβ as NK cells. As to the NK1.1 subset that NK cells express constantly, intermediate TCR cells comprise both NK1.1$^+$ and NK1.1$^-$ subsets. The NK1.1$^+$IL-2Rβ$^-$ subset is extremely rare among high TCR cells. Among intermediate TCR cells, double-negative CD4$^-$CD8$^-$ cells and/or CD4$^+$ are abundant in the NK1.1$^+$ subset, whereas CD8$^+$ cells are generally abundant in the NK1.1$^-$ subset [13]. It is also characteristic of the intermediate T cells that the double-negative CD4$^-$CD8$^-$ cells comprise about 30% of the population and γδ T cells comprise about 20%. We think that due to the lack of a double-positive stage for negative selection, double-negative CD4$^-$CD8$^-$ cells are abundant in the liver, in comparison with thymus-derived T cells.

The intermediate T cells in the liver have a CD44$^+$L-selectin$^-$ pattern of adhesion molecules, which is also found on NK cells. In contrast, the pattern of adhesion molecules on thymus-derived T cells is the reverse (CD44⁻L-selectin⁺) [14]. Two-color staining for anti-CD8α and anti-CD8β also revealed that high TCR cells consist of CDαβ, but in intermediate T cells CD8αα eventually exists.

In a morphologic study, all cells of the NK cell fraction show a morphology of large granular lymphocytes. On the other hand, cells of the intermediate T cell fraction contain granular or agranular lymphocytes. It has been demonstrated that intermediate T cells apparently belong to a family of granular lymphocytes. However, their electron-dense granules are apparently fewer than those of NK cells. More precisely, the morphology of intermediate T cells is intermediate between NK cells and thymus-derived T cells [13].

Self-reactive forbidden clones are eliminated by a process of negative selection at the stage of maturation from low levels of TCR cells to high levels of TCR cells in the thymus. However, self-reactive clones are consistently produced by the pathways of intermediate TCR cell differentiation [15]. For example, C3H/He mice at the age of 15 weeks were used in these experiments. Three-color staining for CD3, IL-2Rβ, and each Vβ was performed to estimate the proportion of Vβ⁺ cells in each population (Fig. 2). In the cases of Vβ2⁺ and Vβ6⁺ cells (non-forbidden clones for this strain), positive cells

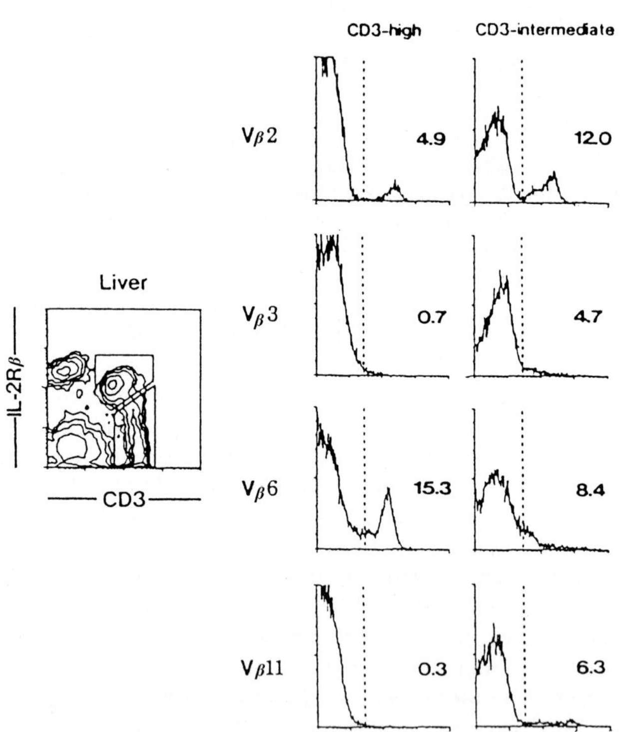

FIG. 2. Self-reactive forbidden T cell clones restricted to a population of intermediate *CD3* cells (C3H/He mice at the age of 15 weeks). Forbidden *Vβ3⁺ and Vβ11⁺* clones in C3H/He mice were diluted and detected in the intermediate CD3 cells, and did not exist in the high CD3 cells. (From [15], with permission)

existed in all populations. However, a large population of self-reactive forbidden clones, Vβ3$^+$ and Vβ11$^+$, was restricted to the intermediate TCR (CD3) population, but was not found in high TCR cells derived from thymus. This finding is one of the points of difference between T cell differentiation in the liver and that in the thymus. It is postulated that high TCR cells generated by the major intrathymic pathways may be important for the interaction with foreign antigens, while intermediate TCR cells generated by the primordial pathways may interact with abnormal self antigens.

Functions of Extrathymic T Cells

Studying the surface markers reveals that extrathymic T cells have the morphology of large granular lymphocytes, express IL-2Rβ similar to NK cells, and include double-negative CD4$^-$CD8$^-$ cells. It is therefore conceivable that their cells have functions like those of NK cells. Intermediate CD3 (CD3$^+$IL-2Rβ^+), high CD3 (CD3$^+$IL-2Rβ^-), and NK (CD3$^-$IL-2Rβ^+) cells are purified by cell sorters. Using YAC-1 which is a sensitive target of NK cells, cytotoxic activity can be measured by a specific ^{51}Cr-release assay. Kawachi et al. [15] reported that NK cells had strong cytotoxicity against NK-sensitive YAC-1 targets, and high CD3 cells did not have it. However, intermediate CD3 cells showed lower cytotoxicity against YAC-1 targets than did NK cells.

As to self-reactivity, cytotoxicity against MH134 hepatoma (originated from self-hepatic cells) in the presence of anti-CD3 mAb is measured using similar methods. Only intermediate CD3 cells could exert a cytotoxic effect against MH134 cells [15] (Fig. 3). Neither sorted NK cells nor sorted high CD3 cells had such activity. Since anti-CD3 mAb bound to T cells during the sorting procedure, it is not necessary to add the mAb for the induction of cytotoxicity. Intermediate T cells have strong NK activity and cytotoxic activity against a self tumor. It is therefore suggested that abnormal self cells may be eliminated promptly by intermediate T cells.

As shown in Fig. 1, intermediate T cells expand with aging when the thymus becomes involuted. Iiai et al. [16] reported that transgenic mice that carried a metallothionein/*ret* fusion gene, and which spontaneously developed melanomas in adulthood, displayed the predominant activation of intermediate TCR cells in the liver and tumor lesions. Seki et al. [17] reported that tumor-bearing mice were found to be at the activation stage of intermediate T cells, at least at an early phase after tumor inoculation. We speculate that the intermediate T cells are increased by recognizing abnormal self cells. Thymic atrophy, a well-known phenomenon, seen in tumor-bearing individuals, might appear as a reciprocal response to the suppression of the intrathymic T cell differentiation pathway. Hashimoto et al. [18] reported that administration of IL-12 to mice caused an elevation of the NK1 and CD2 expression of NK1$^+$ intermediate TCR cells in the liver. Experimental hepatic metastasis of EL4 (moderately NK-resistant) cells were greatly inhibited by systematic IL-12 administration.

MRL-*lpr/lpr* mice have the *lpr* gene and display a spontaneous onset of autoimmune disease similar to human systemic lupus erythematosus. With aging, these mice also show severe lymphadenopathy and splenomegaly, and exhibit the clinical features of immune disease, with glomerulo-nephritis, vasculitis, dermatitis, and arthritis. The proliferated T cells of these mice comprise abnormal double-negative CD4$^-$CD8$^-$ T cells after onset of the disease. It has been demonstrated that these double-negative

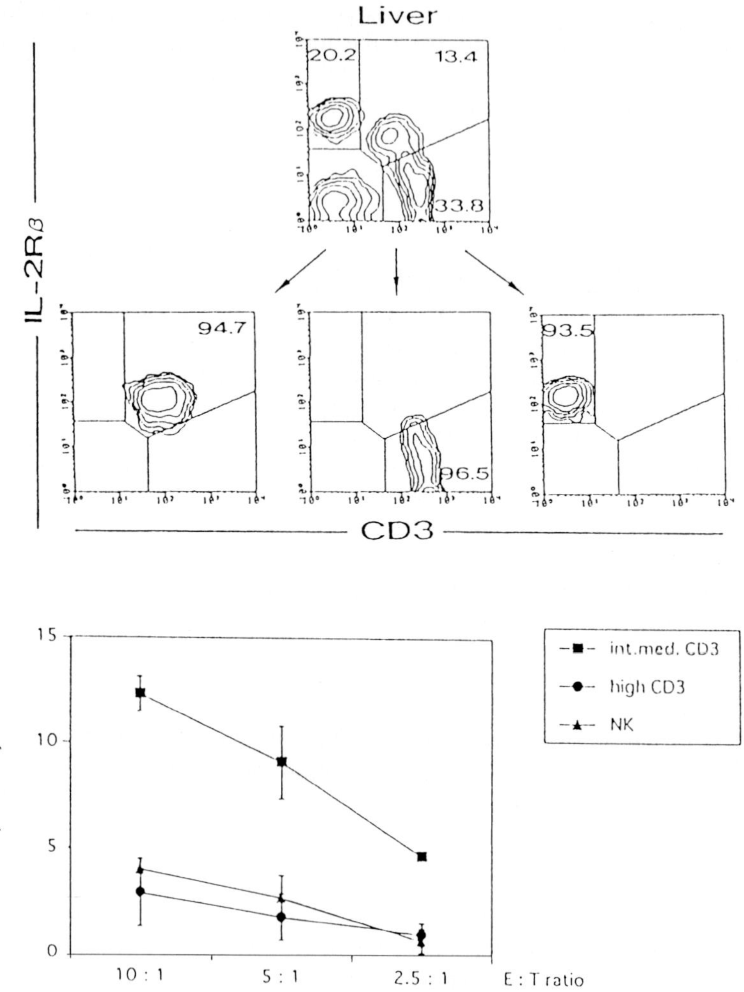

FIG. 3. Self-reactive and cytotoxic activity against hepatic lymphocytes. Sorting liver MNC into intermediate *CD3* cells, high CD3 cells, and NK cells. Cytotoxic activity against MN134 cells in the presence of anti-CD3 mAb was measured by a specific ^{51}Cr-release assay. Only intermediate CD3 cells could exert a cytotoxic effect against MH134 cells. (From [15], with permission)

CD4$^-$CD8$^-$ T cells correspond to the intermediate TCR cells in the liver [12]. Due to the apoptotic failure caused by abnormal Fas molecules in mice carrying the *lpr* gene, abnormal lymphocyte proliferation, especially of NK1$^-$ subset of intermediate TCR cells with a double-negative CD4$^-$CD8$^-$ phenotype, occurs as a function of age. However, a small population of normal NK1$^+$ subset of intermediate TCR cells was also found to exist in all tested organs. Moreover, these cells preferentially produced normal Fas mRNA and Fas molecules from the *lpr* gene [19,20].

Extrathymic T Cells in the Periphery of Humans

In humans, intermediate T cells such as those in mice do not exist. However, a small number of T cells with CD56 or CD57 are normally present in the periphery of humans [21,22]. These T cells, similar to the extrathymic T cells in mice, are abundant in the liver, including double-negative CD4⁻CD8⁻ cells and γδ T cells. These T cell with NK markers are present in tumor-infiltrating lymphocytes. Their proportion in the peripheral blood also increased in patients with colorectal cancer [23,24]. CD57⁺ T cells reportedly increased in patients with AIDS [25] and those subjected to kidney, heart, and bone marrow transplantation [26]. It is suggested that these T cells with NK cell markers may be counterparts of extrathymic T cells in mice, which have intermediate TCR (a major proportion also have the NK cell marker, NK1.1) and contain potentially self-minor lymphocyte stimulatory antigen reactive clones and thereby may play a role in inducing autoimmune disease [13].

Extrathymic T Cells in the Joints of Mice with Collagen-Induced Arthritis

Murine collagen-induced arthritis (CIA) is known as a T cell-mediated autoimmune disease and is one of the experimental models of rheumatoid arthritis (RA) [27], although autoantibodies are also thought to be associated with the onset of the disease. To determine the origin of such T cells in the joints of mice with CIA, Arai et al. [28] examined their phenotypic properties as well as those of T cells in other immune organs in DBA/1 mice. Since a significant number of MNC was also yielded by the joints of normal DBA/1 mice, the properties of these T cells were examined in parallel. We obtained the following results.

When CIA was induced by an intradermal injection of type II collagen (K-42, Cosmo-Bio, Tokyo, Japan) at the base of the tail, the numbers of MNC yielded by the liver and spleen were unchanged, while that yielded by the thymus decreased by 50%. However, the numbers of MNC yielded by the regional lymph nodes and foot joints were doubled. In mice with CIA, some difference in the staining pattern emerged, showing an increase in the proportion of intermediate CD3 cells in the liver and lymph nodes and an increase in IL-2Rβ⁺CD3⁺ cells in joints (Fig. 4).

Interestingly, regardless of the onset of CIA, the joints always comprised unique T cell populations, including IL-2Rα⁻β⁺ T cells, γδ T cells (Fig. 5a), CD8α⁺β⁻ cells (Fig. 5b), and CD44⁺L-selectin⁻ cells. All these properties coincide with those of extrathymic T cells in the liver and intestine. In the case of γδ T cells in joints, Vγ and Vδ usage were unique and different from those in the other organs. More importantly, Vγ and Vδ usage in γδ T cells in the joints of normal mice and in those of mice with CIA were essentially the same. Since the joint tissue is surrounded by various other tissue, such as bone marrow and peripheral blood, we had to distinguish between the staining pattern in joints from those in bone marrow and blood.

In contrast to the results in the joints of both control mice and mice with CIA, TCR-γδ⁺ cells and CD8αα⁺ cells were not found in these organs. A further confirmation was performed to identify CD8αα⁺ cells in the joints of both groups of mice. Immunohistochemical staining for CD8α clearly demonstrated that CD8α⁺ cells

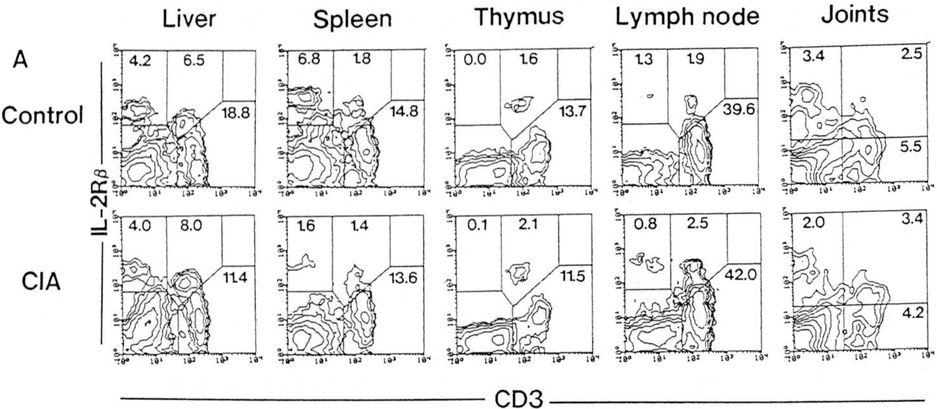

FIG. 4. Two-color staining of MNC for *CD3* and *IL-2Rβ* in various organs of control mice and mice with collagin-induced arthritis (*CIA*). Numbers indicate the percentage of fluorescence-positive cells in the corresponding areas. In liver of mice with CIA, there was a tendency for intermediate TCR cells (CD3$^+$IL-2Rβ$^+$) to increase while high TCR cells (CD3$^+$IL-2Rβ$^-$) decreased. The expression of IL-2Rβ increased among CD3$^+$ cells in joints of mice with CIA. (From [28], with permission)

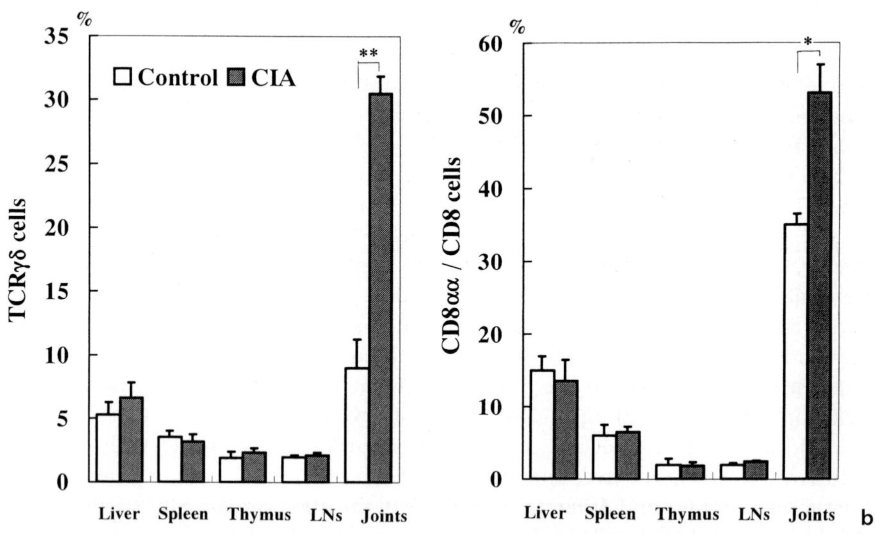

FIG. 5. **a** Increased levels of γδ T cells in joints of mice with CIA. Repeated experiments ($n = 6$). **b** Abundance of CD8α$^+$β$^-$ cells in joints of mice with or without CIA. Repeated experiments to identify the ratios of CD8αα/total CD8 ($n = 6$). *LNs*, lymph nodes. *$P < 0.05$, **$P < 0.01$ (From [28], with permission)

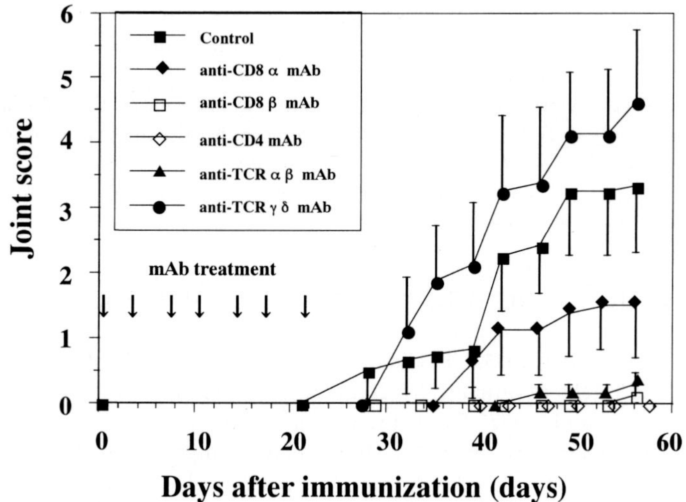

FIG. 6. Effects of in vivo treatments with various mAbs on the onset of CIA.
Various mAbs were injected into the collagen-immunized mice 7 times in 21 days. The onset and the progression of disease were estimated by the joint score of CIA. (From [28], with permission)

eventually existed in the synovial tissue. Although there were few CD8α^+ cells in the joints of control mice, CD8α^+ cells were abundant in the synovial tissue of mice with CIA. Taken together with the expression of recombination-activating gene-1 and -2 mRNAs by MNC in mice with CIA, these findings raise the possibility that the joints have their own resident T cells that are extrathymically generated in situ.

The predominant cells in the joints of mice with CIA were $\alpha\beta$ T cells, with or without CD8, and $\gamma\delta$ T cells. To determine the functional role of these T cells in the onset of CIA, in vivo treatment with available mAbs was conducted (Fig. 6). Each mAb was repeatedly injected (7 times in 21 days). Treatment with anti-TCR-$\alpha\beta$ mAb inhibited the onset of CIA, whereas anti-TCR-$\gamma\delta$ mAb had no such effect. More precisely, there was a tendency for the treatment with anti-TCR-$\gamma\delta$ mAb to somewhat retard the onset of disease, but later suppress the disease. In other words, $\gamma\delta$ T cells seem to be associated with the onset of disease but then suppress it in its late phase. In the case of treatments with anti-CD4 and anti-CD8β mAbs, the onset of CIA was completely suppressed. In other words, both CD4$^+$ and CD8$\alpha\beta^+$ cells among $\alpha\beta$ T cells are important for the onset of disease, possibly because of their mutual interaction. On the other hand, treatment with anti-CD8α mAb partially suppressed the disease. This treatment eliminated all CD8$^+$ cells, but after treatment with anti-CD8β mAb, CD8$\alpha\alpha^+$ cells remained. This raised the possibility that CD8$\alpha\alpha^+$ cells have the ability to suppress the onset of disease, similar to $\gamma\delta$ T cells.

In vivo treatments with various mAbs have been conducted in the present study; $\gamma\delta$ T cells and CD8$\alpha\alpha^+$ cells were associated with suppression of the disease, especially after its onset. However, there is a possibility that they are also associated with the onset of disease. Similar results for $\gamma\delta$ T cells were obtained by Peterman et al. [29].

It has been suggested with many investigations of mice with CIA that CD4[+] cells are major effector cells [27,30,31]. However, if anti-CD8 mAb was repeatedly injected, as in the present study, suppression of disease became prominent. In this experiment, >90% of CD8[+] cells were eliminated in the periphery. Therefore, the mutual interaction between CD4[+] and CD8[+] cells might be important for the onset of CIA. Additional studies are required to determine the interaction of conventional T cells with extrathymic T cells. It is still unknown whether there are resident, extrathymic T cells among CD4[+] cells in the joint.

Extrathymic T Cells and Rheumatoid Arthritis

We have postulated that CD57[+] T cells with a NK cell marker might be a counterpart of extrathymic T cells in humans. RA frequently occurs in patients with CD3[+]CD57[+] cell leukemia [32] and CD57[+] T cells increase in the peripheral blood of RA patients [33]. These findings suggest that CD57[+] T cells play an important role in the onset and pathogenesis of RA.

The distribution of CD57[+] and CD56[+] T cells in patients with RA has been examined [34]. Two-color staining of MNC for CD3 and CD57 is shown in Fig. 7. In control osteoarthritis patients, these cells existed as a minor population in the peripheral blood. In patients with RA, CD57[+] T cells were abundant in knee joint fluid (25.6 ± 3.2%, mean ± SE) and joint-adjacent bone marrow (36.8 ± 8.5) as compared with peripheral blood (18.2 ± 2.0) (Fig. 8). CD57[+] T cells were significantly more abundant

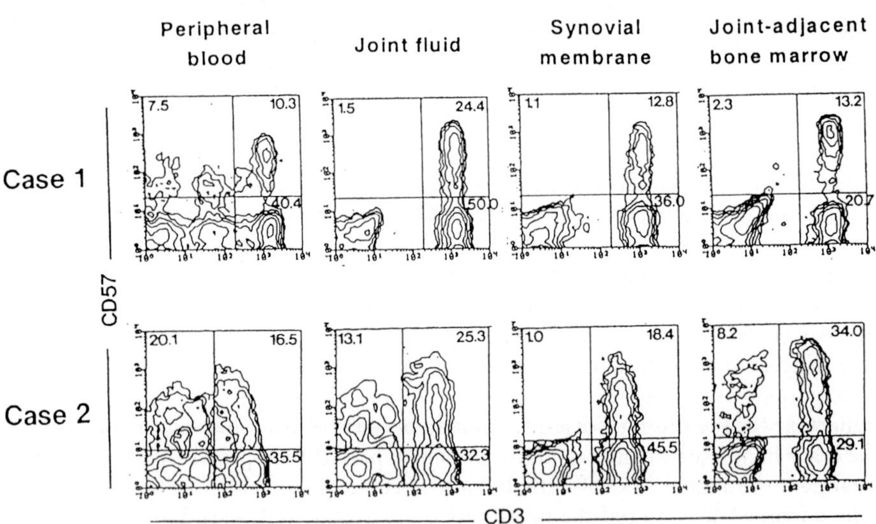

FIG. 7. Two-color staining of MNC for *CD3* and *CD57* was examined in peripheral blood, joint fluid, synovial membrane and joint-adjacent bone marrow in patients with RA. Numbers indicate the percentage of fluorescence-positive cells in the corresponding areas. *Case 1*: 57-year-old woman, disease duration 4.5 years, *Case 2*: 68-year-old woman, disease duration 12 years. (From [34], with permission)

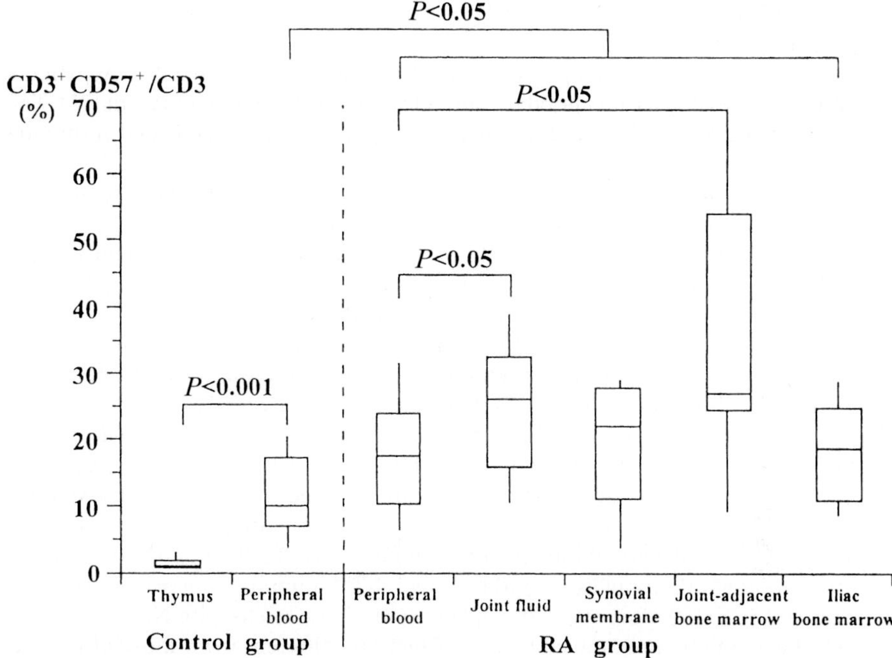

FIG. 8. The population of CD3$^+$CD57$^+$ cells among CD3$^+$ cells. The population of CD3$^+$CD57$^+$ cells among CD3$^+$ cells in peripheral blood ($n = 31$), joint fluid ($n = 21$), synovial membrane ($n = 11$), joint-adjacent bone marrow ($n = 10$), and iliac bone marrow ($n = 13$) in patients with RA, and compared with control peripheral blood ($n = 17$) and thymus ($n = 5$). The *line* in the middle of the box represents the median. The *top* of the box represents the 75th percentile, and *bottom* of the box the 25th percentile

in every RA patient site as compared with the peripheral blood of controls (11.7 ± 1.5), while CD56$^+$ T cells showed no such increase.

In peripheral blood, CD57$^+$ T cells contained significantly ($P < 0.05$) more double-negative CD4$^-$CD8$^-$ cells (8.5 ± 1.6) than did CD57$^-$ T cells (3.5 ± 0.5), and γδ T cells were also significantly ($P < 0.05$) more abundant in CD57$^+$ T cells (16.3 ± 4.3) as compared with CD57$^-$ T cells (4.1 ± 1.0). In joint fluid, double-negative CD4$^-$CD8$^-$ cells (8.5 ± 1.6) were significantly ($P < 0.05$) more abundant in CD57$^+$ T cells (7.0 ± 1.5) than in CD57$^-$ T cells (2.9 ± 0.5). CD57$^+$ T cells in peripheral blood and joint fluid increase with the duration of disease. The erythrocyte sedimentation rate (ESR) was inversely correlated with the proportion of CD57$^+$ T cells in the joint fluid.

The present study reveals that the number of CD57$^+$ T cells is elevated in RA patients, especially in joint fluids and in joint-adjacent bone marrow but not iliac bone marrow. These cells are composed mainly of CD8$^+$ T cells and significantly high populations of CD4$^-$CD8$^-$ T cells and γδ T cells. Proportions of these cells in joint fluids are inversely correlated with the ESR of RA patients, which is well known as an inflammatory marker. We also find that granulocytosis is always observed in patients with active RA. On the other hand, CD56$^+$ T cells are unlikely to be involved in the pathogenesis of RA.

There are characteristic changes in joint-adjacent bone marrow of RA patients, because CD57$^+$αβ T cells are abundant and myeloid lineage cells are present [35]. This finding is consistent with a report that extrathymic T cells are activated in parallel with granulocytes in mice [36]. In mice with CIA, although extrathymic T cells are higher in joints and might play an important role in the onset of the disease, these cells seemed to have a suppressive effect on arthritis because in vivo treatment of mice with anti-γδ TCR antibody significantly increased the severity of the arthritis [28]. These findings suggest that some of the extrathymic T cell populations might expand to suppress inflammation rather than aggravate arthritis.

This situation may be applicable to humans. In fact, CD57$^+$ T cells in the joint fluid of RA patients show an agranular lymphocyte morphology, and the proportion of CD57$^+$ T cells within the joint fluid is inversely correlated with ESR. It was reported that CD57$^+$ T cells suppress the differentiation of hematopoietic stem cells [37], the proliferation of B cells [38], and induction of cytotoxic T lymphocytes [9,39]. It was also reported that populations of these cells are elevated in the peripheral blood of long-term survivors after organ transplantations [26], including bone marrow transplantation. It raises the possibility that these donor-derived cells suppress the immune function of other cell populations and thereby inhibit immune response graft-versus-host disease (GVHD) after organ transplantation. Thus, T cells with NK cell markers seem to have unique immunosuppressive functions different from those of conventional T cells and NK cells.

It should also be noted that in RA patients, the population of CD57$^+$ T cells is elevated in joint-adjacent bone marrow but not in iliac bone marrow. This finding suggests that these cells do not increase as a result of systemic inflammation, but may do so in response to a local inflammation of diseased joints. CD57$^+$ T cells may differentiate in adjacent bone marrow or joint cavities in situ and may suppress the local inflammation of RA. One might speculate that other cells, such as cytotoxic T cells or granulocytes, may be important in the pathogenesis of the acute phase of RA or RA with strong clinical features. In fact, many clinicians know that active RA patients always show an increase of granulocytes in peripheral blood and joints, a fact that has been shown to play an important role in damaging various tissues [36,39]. We propose that, although CD57$^+$ T cells are certainly associated with the onset of RA, these cells may in turn suppress strong inflammation rather than lead to a further deterioration in RA.

Conclusion

Extrathymic T cells differ from thymus-derived T cells, and they can recognize abnormal self cell and eliminate them. They become predominant with aging and under conditions of bacterial infection, pregnancy, malignancy, and autoimmune disease. These T cells play an important role in the onset and pathogenesis of disease. We suggest that these T cells may suppress the inflammation of RA, and other cellular components may govern the severity of the inflammation of RA. These T cells probably are generated extrathymically in the adjacent bone marrow or joint space. They can be potent anti-rheumatic effectors when stimulated by some chemical mediator. Since these T cells consist of heterogenous populations, the precise role of each population in RA remains to be elucidated in further investigations.

References

1. Finkel TH, Cambier JC, Kubo RT, Born WK, Marrack P, Kappler JW (1989) The thymus has two functionally distinct populations of immature $\alpha\beta^+$ T cells: one population is deleted by ligation of $\alpha\beta$ TCR. Cell 58:1047–1054
2. Kisielow P, Blüthmann H, Staerz UD, Steinmetz M, von Boehmer H (1988) Tolerance in T-cell receptor transgenic mice involves deletion of nonmature CD 4^+8^+ thymocytes. Nature 333:742–746
3. Ohteki T, Seki S, Abo T, Kumagai K (1990) Liver is a possible site for the proliferation of abnormal $CD3^+4^-8^-$ double negative lymphocytes in autoimmune MRL-lpr/lpr mice. J Exp Med 172:7–12
4. Seki S, Abo T, Masuda T, Ohteki T, Kanno A, Takeda K, Rikiishi H, Nagura H, Kumagai K (1990) Identification of activated T cell receptor $\gamma\delta$ lyphocytes in the liver of tumor-bearing hosts. J Clin Invest 86:409–415
5. Bandeira A, Itohara S, Bonneville M, Burlen-Defranoux O, Mota-Santos T, Coutinho A, Tonegawa S (1991) Extrathymic organ of intestinal intraepithelial lymphocytes bearing T-cell antigen receptor $\gamma\delta$. Pro Natl Acad Sci USA 88:43–47
6. Watanabe H, Ohtsuka M, Kimura M, Ikarashi Y, Ohmori K, Kusumi A, Ohteki T, Seki S, Abo T (1992) Details of an isolation method for hepatic lymphocytes in mice. J Immunol Methods 146:145–154
7. Watanabe H, Iiai T, Kimura M, Ohtsuka K, Tanaka T, Miyasaka M, Tsuchida M, Hanawa H, Abo T (1993) Characterization of intermediate TCR cells in the liver of mice with respect to their unique IL-2R expression. Cell Immmunol 149:331–342
8. Iiai T, Watanabe H, Seki S, Sugiura K, Hirokawa K, Utsuyama M, Iwanaga HT, Iwanaga T, Ohteki T, Abo T (1992) Ontogeny and development of extrathymic T cells in mouse liver. Immunol 77:556–563
9. Moroda T, Iiai T, Kawachi Y, Kawamura T, Hatakeyama K, Abo T (1996) Restricted appearance of self-reactive clones into T cell receptor intermediate cells in neonatally thymectomized mice with autoimmune disease. Eur J Immunol 26:3084–3091
10. Watanabe H, Miyaji C, Seki S, Abo T (1996) c-kit$^+$ stem cells and thymocyte precursors in the livers of adult mice. J Exp Med 184:687–693
11. Makino Y, Yamagata N, Sasho T, Adachi Y, Kanno R, Koseki H, Kanno M, Taniguchi M (1993) Extrathymic development of $V\alpha 14$-positive T cells. J Exp Med 177:1399–1408
12. Iiai T, Kimura M, Kawachi Y, Hirokawa K, Watanabe H, Hatakeyama K, Abo T (1995) Characterization of intermediate T-cell receptor cells expanding in the liver, thymus and other organs in autoimmune *lpr* mice: parallel analysis with their normal counterparts. Immunol 85:601–608
13. Watanabe H, Miyaji C, Kawachi Y, Iiai T, Ohtsuka K, Iwanaga T, Iwanaga HT, Abo T (1995) Relationships between intermediate TCR cells and NK1.1$^+$ T cells in various immune organs: NK1.1$^+$ T cells are present within a population of intermediate TCR cells. J Immunol 155:2972–2983
14. Arai K, Iiai T, Nakayama M, Hasegawa K, Sato K, Ohtsuka K, Watanabe H, Hanyu T, Takahashi HE, Abo T (1995) Adhesion molecules on intermediate TCR cells I. Unique expression of adhesion molecules, CD44$^+$, L-selectin$^-$, on intermediate TCR cells in the liver and the modulation of their adhesion by hyaluronic acid. Immunol 84:64–71
15. Kawachi Y, Watanabe H, Moroda T, Haga M, Iiai T, Hatakeyama K, Abo T (1995) Self-reactive T cell clones in a restricted population of interleukin-2 receptor β^+ cells

expressing intermediate levels of the T cell receptor in the liver and other immune organs. Eur J Immunol 25:2272–2278

16. Iiai T, Watanabe H, Iwamoto T, Nakashima I, Abo T (1994) Predominant activation of extrathymic T cells during melanoma development of metallothionein/*ret* transgenic mice. Cell Immunol 153:412–427

17. Seki S, Abo T, Sugiura K, Ohteki T, Kobata T, Yagita H, Okumura K, Rikiishi H, Masuda T, Kumagai K (1991) Reciprocal T cell responses in the liver and thymus of mice injected with syngeneic tumor cells. Cell Immunol 137:46–60

18. Hashimoto W, Takeda K, Anzai R, Ogasawara K, Sakihara H, Sugiura K, Seki S, Kumagai K (1995) Cytotoxic NK1.1$^{\pm}$ Ag$^+$ αβ T cells with intermediate TCR induced in the liver of mice by IL-12. J Immunol 154:4333–4340

19. Takeda K, Dennert G (1993) The development of autoimmunity in C57BL/6 *lpr* mice correlates with the disappearance of natural killer type 1-positive cells: evidence for their suppressive action on bone marrow stem cell proliferation, B cell immunoglobulin secretion, and autoimmune symptoms. J Exp Med 177:155–164

20. Yamagiwa S, Kuwano Y, Hasegawa K, Sato K, Ohtsuka K, Iiai T, Tomiyama K, Watanabe H, Sugahara S, Seki S, Asakura H, Abo T (1996) Existence of a small population of IL-2Rβ^{HI} TCR^{INT} cells in SCG and MRL-*lpr/lpr* mice which produce normal Fas mRNA and Fas molecules from the *lpr* gene. Eur J Immunol 26:1409–1416

21. Abo T, Cooper MD, Balch CM (1981) Characterization of HNK-1(Leu-7) human lymphocyte. I. Two distinct phenotypes of human NK cells with different cytotoxic capability. J Immunol 129:1752–1757

22. Schmidt RE, Murray C, Daley JF, Schlossman SF, Ritz J (1986) A subset of natural killer cells in peripheral blood displays a mature T-cell phenotype. J Exp Med 164:351–356

23. Takii Y, Hashimoto S, Iiai T, Watanabe H, Hatakeyama K, Abo T (1994) Increase in the proportion of granulated CD56$^+$ T cells in patients with malignancy. Clin Exp Immunol 97:522–527

24. Okada T, Iiai T, Kawachi Y, Moroda T, Takii Y, Hatakeyama K, Abo T (1995) Origin of CD57$^+$ T cells which increase at tumour sites in patients with colorectal cancer. Clin Exp Immunol 102:159–166

25. Sadat-Sowti B, Debré P, Mollet L, Quint L, Hadida F, Leblond V, Bismuth G, Autran B (1994) An inhibitor of cytotoxic functions produced by CD8$^+$CD57$^+$ T lymphocytes from patients suffering from AIDS and immunosuppressed BM recipients. Eur J Immunol 24:2882–2888

26. Leroy E, Calvo CF, Divine M, Gourdin MF, Baujean F, Ariba HM, Mishal Z, Vernant JP, Farcet JP, Senik A (1986) Persistence of T8$^+$/HNK1$^+$ suppressor lymphocytes in the blood of long-term surviving patients after allogeneic bone marrow transplantation. J Immunol 137:2180–2189

27. Holmdahl R, Jonsson R, Larsson P, Klareskog L (1988) Early appearance of activated CD4$^+$ T lymphocytes and class II antigen-expressing cells in joints of DBA/1 mice immunized with type II collagen. Lab Invest 58:53–60

28. Arai K, Yamamura S, Hanyu T, Takahashi HE, Umezu H, Watanabe H, Abo T (1996) Extrathymic differentiation of resident T cells in the joints of mice with collagen-induced arthritis. J Immunol 157:5170–5177

29. Peterman GM, Spencer C, Sperling AI, Bluestone JA (1993) Role of γδ T cells in murine collagen-induced arthritis. J Immunol 151:6546–6558

30. Ranges GE, Sriram S, Cooper SM (1985) Prevention of type II collagen-induced arthritis by in vivo treatment with anti-L3T4. J Exp Med 162:1105–1110

31. Kadowaki KM, Matsuno H, Tsuji H, Tunru I (1994) CD4$^+$ T cells from collagen-induced arthritic mice are essential to transfer arthritis into severe combined immunodeficient mice. Clin Exp Immunol 97:212–218

32. Loughran TP Jr (1993) Clonal diseases of large granular lymphocytes. Blood 82:1–14

33. d'Angeac AD, Monier S, Jorgensen C, Gao Q, Travaglio-Encinoza A, Bologna C, Combe B, Sany J, Rème T (1993) Increased percentage of CD3$^+$, CD57$^+$ lymphocytes in patients with rheumatoid arthritis: correlation with duration of disease. Arthritis Rheum 36:608–612

34. Arai K, Yamamura S, Seki S, Hanyu T, Takahashi HE, Abo T (1998) Increase of CD57$^+$ T cells in knee joints and adjacent bone marrow of rheumatoid arthritis (RA) patients: implication for an anti-inflammatory role. Clin Exp Immunol 111:345–352

35. Ochi T, Hakomori S, Adachi M, Owaki H, Okamura M, Ono Y, Yamasaki K, Fujimoto M, Wakitani S, Ono K (1988) The presence of a myeloid cell population showing strong reactivity with monoclonal antibody directed to difucosyl type 2 chain in epiphyseal bone marrow adjacent to joints affected with rheumatoid arthritis (RA) and its absent in the corresponding normal and non-RA bone marrow. J Rheumatol 15:1609–1615

36. Yamamura S, Arai K, Toyabe S, Takahashi HE, Abo T (1996) Simultaneous activation of granulocytes and extrathymic T cells in number and function by excessive administration of nonsteroidal anti-inflammatory drugs. Cell Immunol 173:303–311

37. Vinci G, Vernant J-P, Nakazawa M, Zohair M, Kartz A, Henri A, Rochant H, Breton-Gorius, Vainchenker W (1988) In vitro inhibition of normal human hematopoiesis by marrow CD3$^+$, CD8$^+$, HLA-DR$^+$, HNK1$^+$ lymphocytes. Blood 72:1616–1621

38. Clement LT, Grossi CE, Gartland GL (1984) Morphological and phenotypic features of the subpopulations of Leu2$^+$ cells that suppress B cell differentiation. J Immunol 133:2461–2468

39. Jopy P, Guillon J-M, Mayaud C, Plata F, Theodorou I, Denis M, Debré P, Autran B (1989) Cell-mediated suppression of HIV-specific cytotoxic T lymphocytes. J Immunol 143:2193–2201

Relationship Between HLA-DRB1-DQB1 Haplotypes and the Effect of Chicken Cartilage Soup Containing Type II Collagen on Rheumatoid Arthritis

Yoshitaka Toda[1], Seisuke Takemura[2], Tadanobu Morimoto[2], and Ryokei Ogawa[2]

Summary. The HLA-DQB1 and HLA-DRB1 genotypes were determined by a PCR-SSO technique in 65 Japanese outpatients with rheumatoid arthritis (RA). Group A consisted of patients having one or two HLA-DRB1*0405-HLA-DQB1*0401 haplotypes. Group B consisted of patients without the haplotype. Eighteen and 14 patients were given chicken cartilage soup containing type II collagen (32 mg/160 ml) daily for over 3 weeks in group A and B, respectively (CII group). Nineteen and 14 patients were not treated with the soup in groups A and B, respectively (non-CII group).

The median number of weeks required for the C-reactive protein (CRP) values to drop by one half and for the number of swollen joints to decrease by one half were 5 and 6 weeks in the A/CII group, 11 and 11 weeks in the A/non-CII group, 8 and 9 weeks in the B/CII group, and 9 and 8 weeks in the B/non-CII group, respectively. Statistically significant differences were found between the A/CII and A/non-CII groups ($P < 0.05$). Thus, orally administered type II collagen was more effective in RA patients with the HLA-DRB1*0405-DQB1*0401 haplotype than with other haplotypes.

Key words. Collagen, Genetics, Rheumatoid arthritis, Oral tolerance

Introduction

Rheumatoid arthritis (RA) is a chronic autoimmune inflammatory disorder that leads to the destruction of joints. The etiology of RA remains unknown. However, mice can be induced to generate an autoimmune inflammatory polyarthritis by injections of heterologous type II collagen (CII). Collagen-induced arthritis (CIA) in mice is an animal model that has several features similar to clinical RA [1]. Although CII elicits an inflammatory disorder in CIA mice, the administration of native CII or fragments of CII before immunization with CII results in a suppression or delay of the onset of arthritis [2–4]. Thus, in CIA mice, CII can have two opposite effects: the suppression or the induction of arthritis.

[1] Toda Orthopedic Rheumatology Clinic, 14-1 Toyotsu-cho, Suita, Osaka 564-0051, Japan
[2] Department of Orthopedic Surgery, Kansai Medical University, 10-15 Fumizoho-cho, Moriguchi, Osaka 570-8506, Japan

Trentham et al. reported that in active RA patients, there was a decrease in the number of swollen and tender joints in subjects who were fed chicken CII for 3 months, but not in those patients who received a placebo. Furthermore, they mentioned that an oral tolerance phenomenon was elicited in RA patients by the administration of CII [5].

Much like RA, the susceptibility of mice to CII is influenced by a major histocompatibility complex. Miguel et al. reported that the EB^d transgene, which is analogous to one of human HLA-DR genes, reduces the incidence of CIA in B10. RQB3 mice which express the CIA susceptible H-2A^q gene (HLA-DQ equivalent) [6]. Following the results of this experimental study using CIA mice, Zanelli et al. proposed that the HLA-DRB1 locus was associated with protection against RA and that the actual arthritogenic peptide-presenting molecule is HLA-DQ [7]. Based upon these reports, we proposed that in the assessment of the effect of CII on the RA patients, the HLA-DR-DQ haplotype would be important.

HLA-DQ alleles are in the linkage disequilibrium with HLA-DR alleles. For example, the HLA-DQB1*0401 allele is in the linkage with the HLA-DRB1*0405 allele which is the major susceptible HLA-DRB1 allele in the Japanese RA population [8–10].

We postulated that if the effects of CII on RA inflammation were associated with the reaction in the HLA-DQB1 locus which produces the actual arthrogenic peptide, then the effects of orally administered CII on RA patients with the HLA-DRB1*0405-DQB1*0401 haplotype might be different from RA patients with the other haplotype.

In this study, chicken cartilage soup containing a known amount of CII was given to outpatients with RA, and its effect was compared in patients who had at least one HLA-DRB1*0405-DQB1*0401 haplotype versus patients without such a haplotype.

Materials and Methods

The subjects consisted of 65 seropositive outpatients diagnosed with RA, based on the 1987 American Rheumatology Association (ARA) criteria [11]. With their informed consent, 32 patients whose birthdays were odd-numbered days were treated daily with 160 ml of chicken cartilage soup containing CII (CII group). Those patients' whose birthdays were on even-numbered days were given the placebo soup (non-CII group) and were used as controls.

A 100 g breast bone plus ribs from a chicken was crushed into small pieces. The crushed bone was mixed with 160 ml water and boiled for 10 min for sterilization. After the crushed bone was discarded, 160 ml of the soup was incubated at 37°C and seasoned with ginger and 1 g salt. The soup was then dispensed to the patients in the CII group. The CII content in the soup was estimated by comparing it against the purified CII as the standard materials (Elastin, Tokyo, Japan). The measurements were performed by Japan Food Research Laboratories (Tokyo, Japan); a sodium dodecyl sulfate (SDS) polyacrylamide gel electrophoresis method was used [12,13]. After the electrophoretic pattern was obtained by decoloring with a mixture of 10% methanol and 7.5% acetic acid, the absorbance in the soup was compared with that of the standard CII material using a dual wavelength absorption method (difference between 570 nm and 470 nm), (Fig. 1).

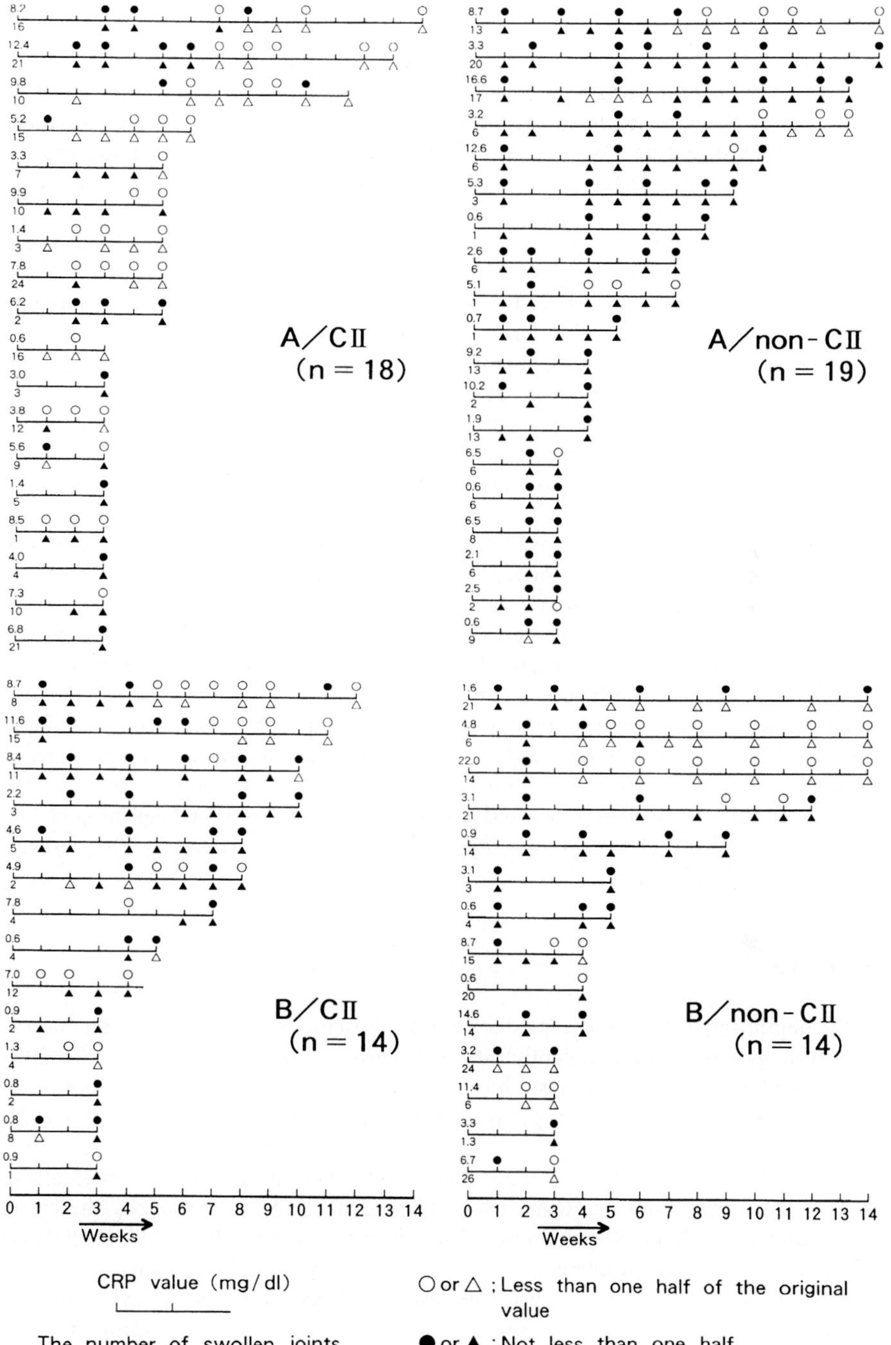

FIG. 1. "Life table" for changes in the C-reactive protein (CRP) value and the number of swollen joints. The numerical values on the *left* are the CRP values above the lines, and the number of swollen joints below the lines at the time of admission. When CRP value and the number of swollen joints were less than one half of the corresponding numerical value on admission, the *solid circles and triangles* were replaced *open* ones.

199

Genomic DNA was isolated from mononuclear cells in peripheral blood. The alleles were amplified with the primer sets by polymerase chain reaction. Each allele in HLA-DRB1 and HLA-DQB1 locus was genotyped by reverse dot blotting with a sequence-specific oligonucleotide [14]. Group A consisted of those patients having one or two HLA-DRB1*0405-DQB1*0401 haplotypes. Group B consisted of those patients possessing two haplotypes other than HLA-DRB1*0405-DQB1*0401 haplotype. According to the combination of the dispensation and genotype, the 65 patients were categorized into four groups: the A/CII group ($n = 18$), the B/CII group ($n = 14$), the A/non-CII group ($n = 19$) and the B/non-CII group ($n = 14$). Drugs that the patients had been taking before enrolling for this study were continued.

For the purpose of evaluating changes in inflammatory activity, measurements of C-reactive protein (CRP) value and the number of swollen joints were recorded regularly once each week. The number of swollen joints was assessed by three orthopedic surgeons before they were informed of the results of the genotyping. Changes with time in the CRP value and the number of swollen joints thus obtained for each patient are summarized in the "life table" (Fig. 1). In this "life table," if the CRP value and the number of swollen joints decreased to under one half of the original value (at the beginning of this study), then the solid symbols were replaced by an open circle or open triangle, respectively (Fig. 1).

Changes with time in the percentage of cases whose CRP value or number of swollen joints was one half or more of original value at the beginning of this study, which is analogous to the "survival" probability on the statistical life table, were calculated based on the Kaplan-Meier method (Fig. 2) [15]. Then comparisons were made between the four groups in the length of time (weeks) it took for the "survival" probability to reach 50%, which was the median number of weeks required for the CRP value or number of swollen joints to decrease by one half from the beginning of this study. Significant differences among the four groups were assessed by the log-rank test of Peto [16].

Results

At the beginning of this study, the distribution of demographic, clinical, and laboratory findings were not significantly different between the four groups ($P > 0.05$). In evaluating the results from this study, no significant difference in the distribution of background data and drug therapy were observed among the four groups ($P > 0.05$), (Table 1).

All of the patients with HLA-DQB1*0401 allele also had HLA-DRB1*0405 allele. None of patients without the HLA-DQB1*0401 had HLA-DRB1*0405 allele. Therefore, in this study, the relationship in linkage disequilibrium between HLA-DRB1*0405 and HLA-DQB1*0401 was complete.

The CII content of the soup was estimated by sodium dodcyl sulfate—polyacrylamide gel electrophoresis to be 0.02%: this means there was 32 mg of CII in the 160 ml of soup. By the same analysis, CII was not detected in soup made from the placebo (Fig. 3).

At the end of the study, the percentage of patients whose CRP value and number of swollen joints had decreased by over one half of the original value was 44.4% in the A/CII group (8/18 cases), 10.5% in the A/non-CII group (2/19 cases), 21.4% in the

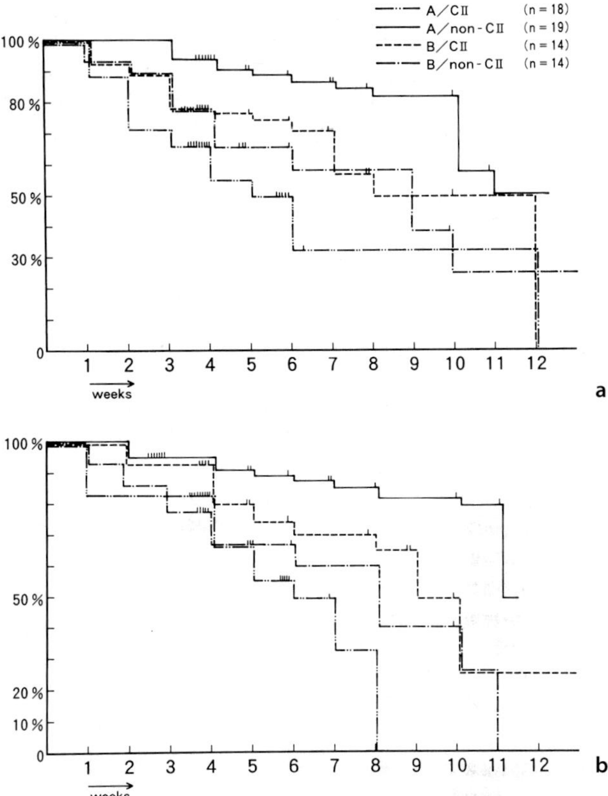

FIG. 2. The "survival" probability that **a** the CRP value and **b** the number of swollen joints did not decrease to below one half of their value at the time of admission

B/CII group (3/14 cases), and 28.5% in the B/non-CII group (4/14 cases). Using the Chi-square test, the difference was statistically significant between the A/CII versus A/non-CII groups ($P > 0.05$), but no significant differences were observed between any other combination of the groups ($P > 0.05$), (Fig. 1).

The median number of weeks that the CRP value took to decrease by one half was 5 weeks in the A/CII group, 11 weeks in the A/non-CII group, 8 weeks in the B/CII group, and 9 weeks in the B/non-CII group. The difference was statistically significant between the A/CII and A/non-CII groups ($P < 0.05$), but not between the B/CII and B/non-CII groups ($P > 0.05$) (Fig. 2a).

Similar statistical differences were observed for changes in the number of swollen joints. The median number of weeks required for the swollen joints to decrease by one half was 6 weeks in the A/CII group, 8 weeks in the A/non-CII group, 9 weeks in the B/CII group, and 11 weeks in the B/non-CII group (Fig. 2b).

Discussion

The relationship between the HLA-DRB1 genotypes and the pathology and clinical severity of RA has been further refined. It is now apparent that the shared amino acid

TABLE 1. Background data of subjects from the four groups

Group	Gender (number of cases)		Age (years)		Disease duration (years)		Morning stiffness (minutes)		CRP (mg/dl)		Swollen joints (Number)		Using drugs[a] (number of cases)
	male	female	mean	median	mean	median	mean	median	mean	median	mean	median	
A/CII	6	12	54.9	51	9.3	5	56.1	30	5.8	4.0	10.5	9	PMN(7), PDN(4), PN(2),PM(1), MN(4), DN(0)
B/CII	2	12	58.8	60	13.4	8	59.3	30	5.1	4.6	6.5	5	PMN(4), PDN(1), PM(0), MN(4), DN(2)
A/non-CII	5	14	57.5	50	9.3	6	74.7	30	5.2	3.3	7.3	6	PMN(7), PDN(3), PN(3), PM(2), MN(2), DN(2)
B/non-CII	2	12	61.2	64	14.3	9	87.9	40	5.9	3.1	12.3	8	PMN(4), PDN(1), PN(4), PM(0), MN(3), DN(2)

CII, type II collagen; CRP, C-reactive protein.
[a] Predonisolone (P): 2.5 mg orally twice a day. Disease-modifying antirheumatic drugs (DMARDs) (D): 3 mg auranofin or 100 mg bucillamine orally twice a day. Methotrexate (M): 2.5 mg. orally twice a day at 12 h intervals. NSAIDs (N): 5 mg acemetacin orally twice a day and/or 25 mg indomethacin rectally twice a day.

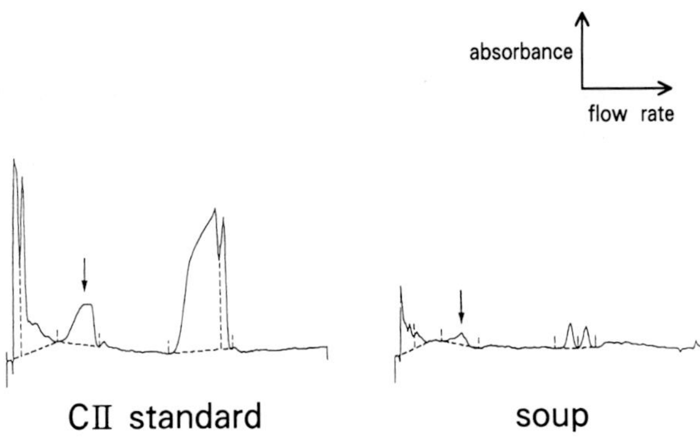

FIG. 3. Analysis of the CII content in the soup. For the assessment of the distribution of the relative rate of flow and absorbance, the soup was similar to CII standard material. An integration of the single wave (*downward-pointing arrow*) was formed and then compared between the soup and the standard CII. The CII content of the soup was estimated to be 0.02%

sequence, or epitope, is common to the DRB1 chains of all DR specificities associated with RA, which are the susceptible alleles (HLA-DRB1*0401, 0404, 0405, 0101, 1402 and 1001) [17–19]. Each susceptible HLA-DRB1 allele is in linkage disequilibrium with the different HLA-DQB1 alleles [9,10].

It has also been reported that the susceptible HLA-DRB1 alleles, which are HLA-DRB1*0101, 0401 and 0404 but not HLA-DRB1*0405 in the Caucasian population, were not related to the response to treatment with oral CII in RA patients [5,20]. However, if the effects of CII on RA-induced inflammation are associated with a reaction in the HLA-DQB1 locus, then it is likely that the HLA-DRB1/-DQB1 haplotype is more important than the susceptibility of HLA-DRB1 genotypes alone in this assessment.

Our data clearly indicate that treatment with oral CII suppressed both the CRP values and the number of swollen joints more prominently in patients with the HLA-DRB1*0405, -DQB1*0401 haplotype than in patients with the other haplotypes.

In the treatment of RA patients with HLA-DQB1*0405, an allele which is known as one of the major alleles affecting severity of RA in the Japanese, no effective method of treatment has yet been found [18]. In this study, all of the patients with the HLA-DRB1*0405 allele also had the HLA-DQB1*0401 allele. It is therefore worthwhile to further study this administration of CII for the treatment of RA patients with HLA-DRB1*0405 alleles.

Trentham et al. raised questions concerning the optimum dose for the treatment of RA with oral CII; these remain unanswered [5]. They reported that 5 mg of purified CII produced a detectable effect. In this study, however, 32 mg of thermally denatured CII was effective. The induction of CIA by thermally denatured CII has been reported to be more difficult than with native CII [21]. Even when non-native CII is used, CIA can be produced if the quantity of the fragment (CB-11) that is the specific epitope of the antigen that is recognized exclusively by either the T helper cell or the T suppressor cells remains [2].

As mentioned in the Introduction, CIA in mice and tolerance of CII in RA are caused by similar immunological mechanisms. Based upon the result of this study, we believe that even chicken cartilage soup containing thermally denatured CII can suppress the inflammatory activity with RA.

When a purified CII, an artificial substance, is to be administered to patients as a drug for RA, various tests have to be made to determine whether the patient is eligible for the drug. Another problem is that it is difficult and expensive to obtain pure CII. We are currently trying to evaluate the relationship between the HLA-DRB1, -DQB1 haplotypes and the effects of dispensing CII by assessing various parameters, increasing the number of subjects, and prolonging the observation period [22]. If both purified CII and the chicken cartilage soup described here can induce a tolerance in RA patients to HLA-DRB1*0405-DQB1*0401 haplotype, the soup generally taken as food is considered to be comparatively the more convenient and safer choice of treatment.

References

1. Trentham DE, Townes AS, Kang AH (1977) Autoimmunity to type II collagen: an experimental model of arthritis. J Exp Med 146:857–868
2. Kobayashi S, Terato K, Yoshida H, Moriya H, Taniguchi M (1991) Suppression of type II collagen-induced arthritis by monoclonal antibodies. Arthritis Rheum 34:48–54
3. Staines NA, Hardingham T, Smith M, Henderson B (1981) Collagen-induced arthritis in rat: modification of immune and arthritic responses by free collagen and immune anti-collagen antiserum. Immunology 44:737–744
4. Englert ME, Landes MJ, Oronsky AL, Kerwar SS (1984) Suppression of type II collagen-induced arthritis by the intravenous administration of type II collagen or its constituent peptide α-1 (II) CB10. Cell Immunol 87:357–365
5. Trentham DE, Dynesius-Trentham RA, Orav EJ, Combitchi D, Lorenzo C, Sewell KL, Halfer DA, Weiner HL (1993) Effect of oral administration of type II collagen on rheumatoid arthritis. Science 261:1727–1730
6. Gonzalez-Gay MA, Nobozny GH, Bull MJ, Zanelli E, Douhan III J, Griffiths MM, Glimcher LH, Luthra HS, David CS (1994) Protective role of major histo-compatibility complex class II Eb^d transgene on collagen-induced arthritis. J Exp Med 180:1559–1564
7. Zanelli E, Gonzalez-Gay MA, David CS (1995) Could HLA-DRB1 be the protective locus in rheumatoid arthritis? Immunol Today 16:274–278
8. Nepom BS, Nepom GT (1995) Polyglot and polymorphism. Arthritis Rheum 38:1715–1721
9. Imanishi T, Akaza T, Kimura A, Tokunaga K, Gojobori T (1992) Allele and haplotype frequencies for HLA and complement loci in various ethnic groups. In: Tsuji K, Akaza M, Sasazuki T (eds) HLA 1991. Oxford University Press, Oxford, pp 1200–1203
10. Wakitani S, Murata N, Toda Y, Ogawa R, Kaneshige T, Nishimura Y, Ochi T (1997) The relationship between HLA-DRB1 alleles and disease subsets of rheumatoid arthritis. Br J Rheumatol 36:630–636
11. Armett FC, Edworthy SM, Bloch DA, McShane DJ, Fries JF, Cooper NS (1988) The American Rheumatism Association 1987. Revised criteria for classification of rheumatoid arthritis. Arthritis Rheum 31:315–324
12. Weber K, Osborn M (1969) The reliability of molecular weight determination by dodecyl sulfate-polyacrylamide gel Electro-phoresis. J Bio Chem 244:4406–4412
13. Laemmli UK (1970) Cleavage of structural proteins during the assembly of the head of bacteriophage. Nature 227:680–685
14. Kaneshige H, Murayama A, Hisawa T, Sawa M, Amemiya H, Uchida K (1992) Rapid and practical HLA class II geno-typing by reverse dot blotting. Transplant Proc 25:194–198
15. Kaplan EL, Meier P (1958) Non parametric estimation from incomplete observation. J AM Stat Assoc 53:457–481

16. Peto R, Pike MC, Armitage NE (1977) Design and analysis of randomized clinical trials requiring prolonged observation of each patient. II. Analysis and examples. Br J Cancer 35:1–39
17. Gregersen PK, Silver J, Winchester RJ (1987) The shared epitope hypothesis: an approach to understanding the molecular genetic susceptibility of rheumatoid arthritis. Arthritis Rheum 30:1205–1213
18. Toda Y, Minamikawa Y, Akagi S, Sugano H, Mori Y, Nishimura H, Arita S, Sugino Y, Ogawa R (1994) Rheumatoid-susceptible allele of HLA-DRB1 are genetically recessive to non-susceptible alleles in the progression of bone destruction in the wrists and fingers of patients with RA. Ann Rheum Dis 53:587–592
19. Weyand CM, Hicok KC, Conn DL, Goronzy JJ (1992) The influence of HLA-DRB1 gene on disease severity in rheumatoid arthritis. Ann Intern Med 117:801–806
20. Sieper J, Kary S, Sörensen H, Altten R, Mithison NA (1996) Oral type II collagen treatment in early rheumatoid arthritis. A double-blind, placebo-controlled, randomized trial. Arthritis Rheum 39:41–51
21. Terato K, Hasty KA, Cremer MA, Stuart M (1994) Collagen-induced arthritis in mice. Localization of an arthritogenic determinant to fragment of the type II collagen molecule. J Exp Med 162:637–646
22. Toda Y, Takemura S, Morimoto T, Ogawa R (1997) Relationship between HLA-DRB1 genotypes and efficacy of oral type II collagen treatment using chicken cartilage soup in rheumatoid arthritis (in Japanese). Jpn J Clin Immun 20:44–51

Notes on the Disease Mechanism and Genetics of Rheumatoid Arthritis

Shunichi Shiozawa[1], Hiroki Kawasaki[1], Yasuo Tsukamoto[1], Sachiko Hayashi[1], Yoshitake Konishi[1], Koichiro Komai[1], Naoko Mukae[1], Eri Yamamoto[1], Norishige Yoshikawa[1], and Kazuko Shiozawa[2]

Summary. Rheumatoid arthritis (RA) is a chronic polyarthritis of unknown etiology that affects about 1% of the population worldwide. The risk of the disease in the siblings of affected individuals (λ_s) is significantly increased in RA, suggesting that both genetic and environment factors are important in the pathogenesis of RA. Previous studies in this laboratory have shown that features characteristic to RA, synovial overgrowth and bone resorption, can be experimentally reproduced by augmenting the expression of the c-*fos* protooncogene. We have searched the human genome for genes that predispose to RA using fluorescence-based microsatellite marker analysis and affected sib-pair linkage study. A panel of 41 Japanese families, each with at least two affected siblings, was typed for genome-wide 358 polymorphic microsatellite marker loci. Three principal chromosome regions of linkage, D1S253/214, D8S556 and DXS1232, have been identified which we call *RA1*, *RA2* and *RA3* for rheumatoid arthritis disease loci.

Key words. Rheumatoid arthritis, c-*fos* gene, Microsatellite marker, Sib-pair study, Gene loci

Introduction

Both environmental and genetic factors contribute to the pathogenesis of rheumatoid arthritis (RA). We have previously shown that activation of synovial mesenchymal cells plays an essential role in the pathogenesis of rheumatoid joint destruction, and c-*fos* protooncogene when overexpressed drives these synovial cells to promote joint destruction. Although genetic predisposition has long been suspected in autoimmunity, a detailed manner of inheritance remains unclear. However, a combination of recent developments in molecular biology and a classical genetic linkage study has now opened the door to the genetics of autoimmunity. The recent evidence for the role of the shared epitope in the HLA-DR Beta 1 chain in the predisposition to RA has

[1] Kobe University School of Medicine Faculty of Health Science, 7-10-2 Tomogaoka, Sumaku, Kobe 654, Japan
[2] Center for Rheumatic Diseases, Kakogawa National Hospital, 1545-1 Saijo, Kakogawa 675, Japan

led to increased interest. This gene, however, clearly does not explain all cases. In this chapter, we will summarize our data on the study of the disease mechanism and genetics of RA. Readers who are interested may also refer to references 1 and 2 for a detailed discussion.

Process of Joint Destruction in RA

The pathologic sequence of events occurring in the rheumatoid joint may be divided into three stages (Fig. 1) [1]. In the first stage, an unknown antigen, reaching the synovial membrane from systemic circulation, initiates the local immune response. In the second, chronic inflammation subsequently takes place in the synovium, involving various kinds of cellular infiltrates and cytokines. In the third, destruction of cartilage and bone takes place, finally leading to irreversible joint destruction and deformities.

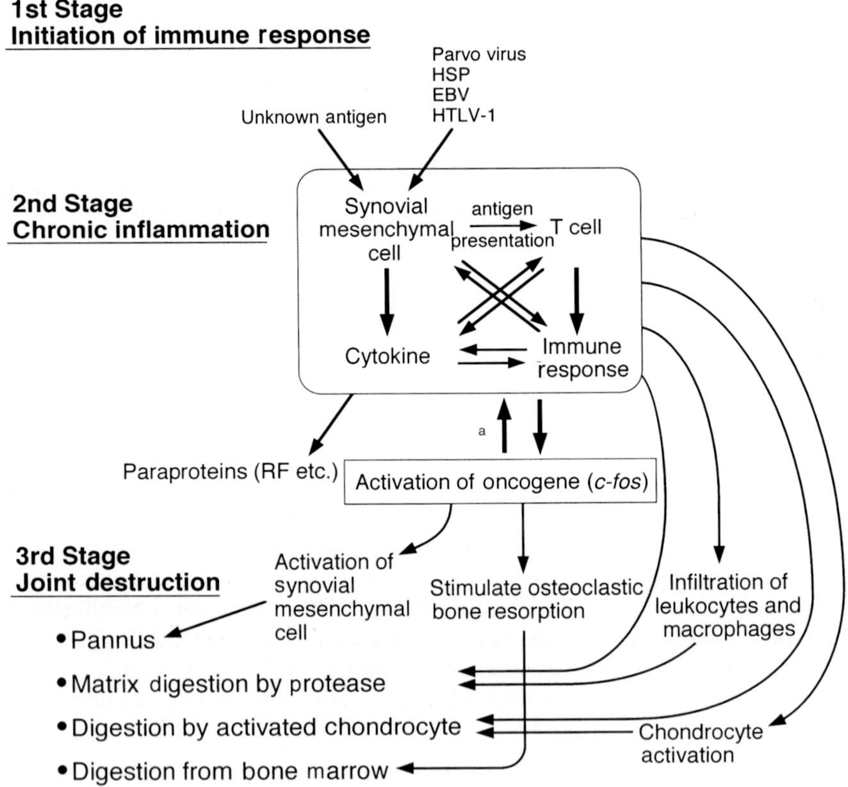

FIG. 1. Pathologic sequence of events occurring in rheumatoid arthritis. [a] activation of the oncogene is important for the continuation of chronic inflammation

T cell and Synovial Mesenchymal Cell

Previous studies have shown that both T cells and synovial mesenchymal cells are important in the initiation and progression of rheumatoid joint destruction [2]. T cells play a central role in initiating immune response against antigen coming to joints. It remains unclear whether or not the same antigen is responsible for the initiation and continuation of the rheumatoid inflammation.

Synovial mesenchymal cells not only produce important cytokines in arthritis such as IL-1, IL-6 and TNF-α but are also directly responsible for joint destruction as a major component of rheumatoid pannus [3]. Synovial mesenchymal cells as a major component of the synovial lining layer play an important role in the initiation of arthritis. Synovial lining fibroblast-like (Type B) and macrophage-like (Type A) cells possess HLA-DR antigen [4] and behave as antigen-presenting cells [5,6]. Because most intravenously injected antigens reach and pass through the joint space, thus having access to the synovial lining layer, antigen reaching the synovial lining layer from the systemic circulation is expected to be trapped, digested, and presented to T cells.

Synovial Mesenchymal Cell and Joint Destruction

Pannus, mainly composed of synovial mesenchymal cells, is defined as a vascular and fibrous granulation tissue arising from the perichondral synovial membrane, which clings tightly to the articular surface of cartilage. Pannus first extends onto the cartilage surface as a layer of morphologically quiescent fibroblast-like cells. Pannus subsequently invades the cartilage matrix with the appearance of macrophage-like cells [3]. Pannus formation is induced by the fibronectin deposited on the articular surface of rheumatoid cartilage in a disease-specific manner [7,8]. In particular, the splice variant form of fibronectin containing EDA or EDB portions, which are expressed in association with cellular proliferation and transformation, induces pannus extension onto the cartilage matrix. Interaction of synovial cells with the carboxyl-terminal heparin-binding (Hep 2) region of the fibronectin molecule is important in this process [9,10].

c-*fos*/AP-1 Drives Pannus to Promote Joint Destruction

Protooncogenes such as c-*fos* and c-*fos*/c-*jun* heterodimer (AP-1) are important in regulating the expression of IL-1β, IL-6, TNF-α, and collagenases that are essentially important in RA. In a previous study inducing collagen-induced arthritis in H2-c-*fos* transgenic mice, we have found that overexpression of the c-*fos* gene leads to joint destruction without lymphocyte infiltration into the joint in which the majority of cells invading the extensively eroded joint tissue were mesenchymal synovial cells. These had the potential for invading the cartilage matrix when cultured in vitro [11]. Subsequent transfection studies have shown that overexpression of c-*fos* gene in synovial cells potentiates the growth of synovial cells [12]. Overexpression of the c-*fos* gene in osteoblasts not only inhibited their collagen synthesis [13], but also stimulated osteoblasts to release factors to enhance osteoclastic bone resorption [14].

Osteoclastic bone resorption was also enhanced when the c-*fos* gene was overexpressed in osteoclasts [15]. Thus, osteoporosis, one of the characteristic features of RA [16,17], is experimentally produced by increasing c-*fos* expresssion.

Expression of the c-*fos* gene is indeed increased in RA [18], and arthritic joint destruction is inhibited in a sequence-specific manner by the double-stranded oligonucleotides that contained the AP-1 consensus sequence [19]. Thus, we may conclude that activation of c-*fos*/AP-1 is necessary and sufficient in arthritic joint destruction. In addition, two of the present authors (S.S. and H.K.) have shown that antigen-specific T cells overexpressing c-*fos* become resistant against anergy induction and are hyperresponsive against antigen challenge. Furthermore, those T cells overexpressing the c-*fos* gene came to reside in the 4C cell cycle state, and mitotic cell division was inhibited [20]. Thus, overexpression of the c-*fos* gene produces tumor-like cell growth, osteoporosis, and pannus formation that are characteristic of RA.

Genetic Predisposition to RA

Although the disease mechanism of RA has been clarified in some detail, these biochemical studies still do not reveal the whole picture of rheumatoid joint destruction; in particular, the contribution of genetic factors to the development of RA remains unclear. RA affects about 1% of the population worldwide, where genetic and environmental factors are suspected to be important in its pathogenesis [21]. Previous studies indicate that the risk of the disease in the siblings of affected individuals (λ_s) is much increased in RA [21,22], suggesting that genetic factors may be important as a cause of familial clustering. Genetic studies to date have focused primarily on the role of HLA molecules in RA. However, while the ratio of the risk for siblings of patients with a disease and the population prevalence of that disease (λ_s) was 8 for RA, the λ_s for HLA was significantly low at 1.6 in Caucasian patients with RA [23]. Thus, the HLA-linked susceptibility locus did not explain sufficiently the observed familial clustering of RA, and other non-HLA-linked disease loci have been proposed by genetic epidemiology studies [22,24].

Genome-wide Search for RA Disease Gene

We have searched for factors in the genetic predisposition of RA using fluorescence-based microsatellite marker analysis and an affected sib-pair linkage study (Fig. 2). A microsatellite marker is a portion of DNA characterized by the repeat of nucleotide sequences such as cytosine-adenine (CA) repeats. These microsatellite markers are genetically polymorphic, which means that the region in a human population is composed of more than four allotypes (in this case, DNA of a different size because of CA repeats). We can therefore identify which one of the allotypes is transmitted from mother or father to their children (Fig. 3). We call it identity-by-descent (IBD) when a marker from mother or father is distributed to both of their children. This is case "a" in Fig. 3. When a marker is distant from the true disease gene, the chance of sharing IBD between the affected sib-pair will be 0.25 for IBD = 0, 0.5 for IBD = 1, and 0.25 for IBD = 2.

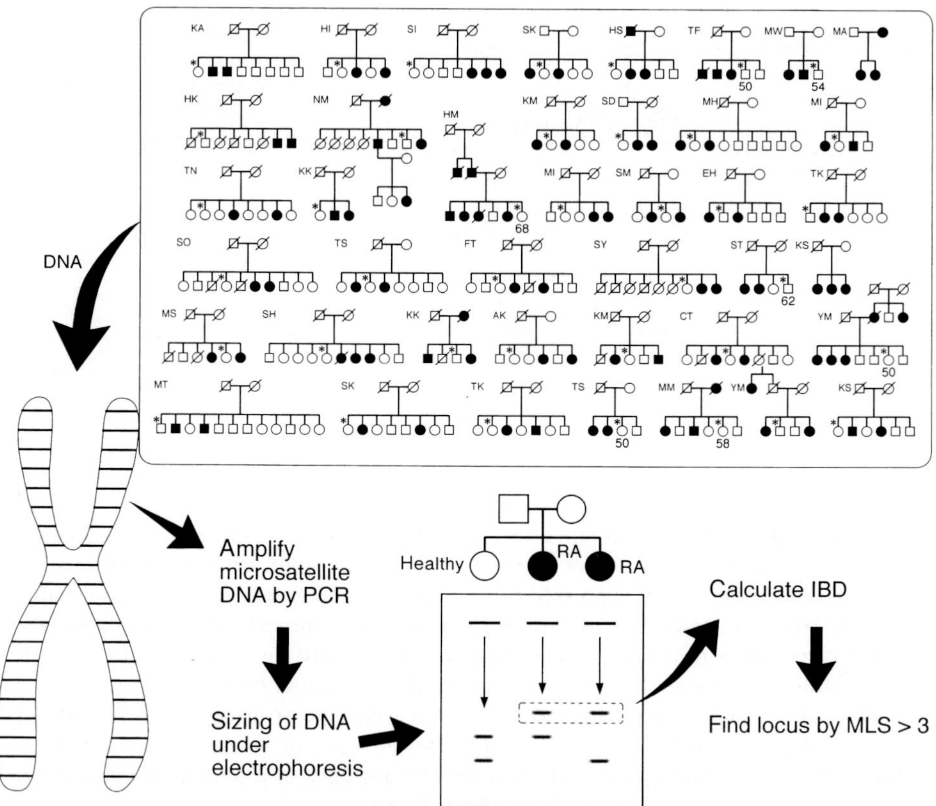

FIG. 2. Family trees of affected sib-pairs with rheumatoid arthritis. One unaffected elderly sibling (indicated by * with age) is typed in addition to the corresponding affected sib-pair for each family. DNA is extracted, amplified using polymerase chain reaction (PCR), and separated with electrophoresis. *MLS* (maximal lod score) of total families is calculated from their identity-by-descent (IBD) sharing states

However, when a particular marker is close (linked) to the disease gene, the IBD sharing state of families will be skewed to the direction of IBD = 2. This deviation can simply be analyzed using the chi-square test. The extent of deviation will also be expressed in an exact form as a lod (log odds) score and maximum lod score (MLS) as calculated in the classical sib-pair linkage analysis.

Since microsatellite markers are distributed evenly genome-wide throughout chromosomes 1 to X, when hundreds of microsatellite markers are analyzed one by one in each family for their IBD sharing states and such data are piled up, we can identify which locus (microsatellite marker) on the chromosomes is highly skewed (MLS value exceeding 3).

We have analyzed genome-wide 358 microsatellite markers, which is on average 10.8 cM (centi Morgan) apart, in families with RA. Microsatellite markers are amplified by the polymerase chain reaction (PCR) using fluorescence-tagged primers

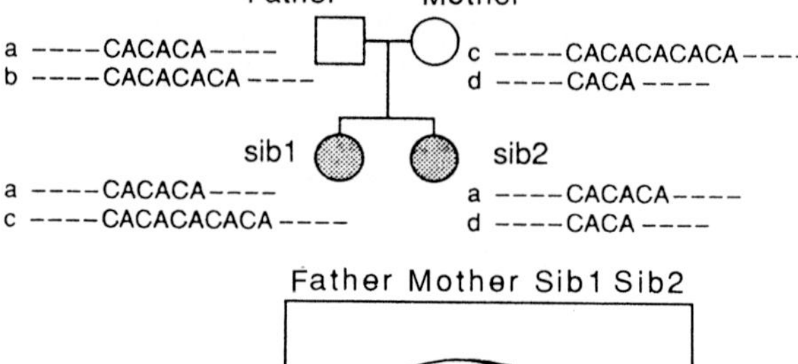

Fig. 3. Affected sib-pair linkage analysis. Gene "a" is transmitted from mother to both affected sibs. This is assigned IBD = 1. DNA of different size due to CA repeats can be differentiated using electrophoresis

and sized based on the difference in CA repeats on DNA using a computer-based ABI377 DNA sequencer. We have selected 41 families with an affected sib-pair where the affected sib-pairs have expressed full-blown clinical RA with clear and identifiable joint destruction identifiable in X-rays. This selection criterion was especially important because if one of the affected sib-pairs presented with transient arthritis without identifiable joint destruction, the subsequent analysis would be made difficult.

We also screened the unaffected siblings in a family. At least one of unaffected siblings should be older than one of the affected sib-pair within the family. If an unaffected sib was younger than both of the affected sibs, such a family was excluded from the study unless the age of the unaffected sib was greater than the time since the onset of the disease in the affected sibs. Seven out of 41 families were of this type and the youngest unaffected sibling in these families was 50 years old.

Identification of the Gene Loci that Predispose to RA

We have typed one unaffected sibling in addition to the affected sib-pair for each family—parents were not typed in most of the RA families at the time of the diagnosis of RA because of late onset of the disease [25]. Linkage analysis was made using the SIB-ADONE program which was developed by us according to the method of Holmans and Clayton [26]. This program is specified for the maximum likelihood analysis of sib-pairs for each of which parents are not typed but a pair of affected sib and an unaffected sib are typed. Probabilities of allele sharing of affected sibs but not those of other types of pairs were considered. The MAPMAKER/SIBS program was used to confirm and extend the result obtained by the SIB-ADONE [27].

Based on detailed microsatellite marker analyses on average of 2–3 cM resolution, linkage has been assigned to chromosome 1 at D1S253/214, chromosome 8 at D8S556 and chromosome X at DXS1232. The MLS for D1S253 and D1S214 was 3.77 and 3.58 respectively by the single point analysis and the MLS for D1S253 was 6.13 by the multipoint analysis of MAPMAKER/SIBS. The MLS for D8S556 and DXS1232 were 4.20 and

2.35, respectively, by single point analysis. The MLS was 3.03 at the locus 2 cM right to DXS1232 by multi-point analysis. Therefore, three principal chromosome regions of linkage, D1S253/214, D8S556 and DXS1232, have been identified which we call *RA1*, *RA2*, and *RA3* for rheumatoid arthritis disease loci [28,29].

The relative risks of RA for a sib of an affected proband versus population prevalence were estimated from the maximum likelihood of allele sharing proportions at autosomal loci to be 2.6 for D1S253/214 linked to *RA1* and 2.7 for D8S556 linked to *RA2*. The contribution of these loci, in addition to HLA-linked loci and *RA3* may explain the value of 8 previously estimated for the relative risk of sibs of RA.

However, we found that the MLS for the microsatellite markers in the vicinity of HLA-DRB1 regions was 1.98 for D6S299, 0.66 for D6S265, and 1.03 for D6S273, suggesting that the HLA-DR region was genetically not significant. This was in line with the calculation of MLS based on the classical HLA-DRB1 DNA typing using PCR-RFLP. The result may be consistent with the previous studies based on genetic epidemiology that the HLA-linked susceptibility locus accounted for less than 20% of RA cases in the general population [22] and the ratio of the risk for siblings of patients with a disease and the population prevalence of that disease (λ_s)was 8 for RA, whereas λ_s for HLA was less significant at 1.6 [21,23].

Acknowledgments. We thank Toyama Chemical Co., Ltd. (Tokyo) and Hayashibara Biochemical Co., Ltd. (Okayama) for supporting the genetic program.

References

1. Shiozawa S, Shiozawa K (1988) A review of the histopathological evidence on the pathogenesis of cartilage destruction in rheumatoid arthritis. Scand J Rheumatol Suppl 74:65–72
2. Shiozawa S, Tokuhisa T (1992) Contribution of synovial mesenchymal cells to the pathogenesis of rheumatoid arthritis. Sem Arthritis Rheum 21:267–273
3. Shiozawa S, Shiozawa K, Fujita T (1983) Morphologic observations of the early phase of the cartilage-pannus junction: light and electron microscopic studies of active cellular pannus. Arthritis Rheum 26:472–478
4. Shiozawa S, Shiozawa K, Fujita T (1983) Presence of HLA-DR antigens on the synovial type A and B cells: An immunoelectron microscopic studies in rheumatoid arthritis, osteoarthritis, and traumatic joints. Immunology 50:587–594
5. Tiku ML, Theodorescu M, Skosey JL (1985) Immunobiological function of normal rabbit synovial cells. Cell Immunol 91:415–424
6. Shimizu S, Shiozawa S, Shiozawa K, Imura S, Ishikawa H, Hirohata K, Fujita T (1988) The restoration of proliferation and differentiation of peripheral blood mononuclear non-adherent cells into immunoglobulin-secreting cells by autologous synovial adherent cells from patients with rheumatoid arthritis. Virchows Arch. [Cell Pathol] 54:350–356
7. Shiozawa K, Shiozawa S, Shimizu S, Fujita T (1984) Fibronectin on the surface of articular cartilage in rheumatoid arthritis. Arthritis Rheum 27:615–622
8. Shiozawa S, Yoshihara R, Kuroki Y, Fujita T, Shiozawa K, Imura S (1992) Pathogenic importance of fibronectin in the superficial region of articular cartilage as a local factor for the induction of pannus extension on rheumatoid articular cartilage. Ann Rheum Dis 51:869–873

214   S. Shiozawa et al.

9. Hino K, Shiozawa S, Kuroki Y, Ishikawa H, Shiozawa K, Sekiguchi K, Hirano H, Sakashita E, Miyashita K, Chihara K (1995) EDA-containing fibronectin is synthesized from rheumatoid synovial fibroblast-like cells. Arthritis Rheum 38:678–683
10. Hino K, Maeda T, Sekiguchi K, Shiozawa K, Hirano H, Sakashita E, Shiozawa S (1996) Adherence of synovial cells on EDA-containing fibronectin. Arthritis Rheum 39:1685–1692
11. Shiozawa S, Tanaka Y, Fujita T, Tokuhisa T (1992) Destructive arthritis without lymphocyte infiltration in H$_2$-c-*fos* transgenic mice. J Immunol 148:3100–3104
12. Kuroki Y, Shiozawa S, Yoshihara R, Hotta T (1993) The contribution of human c-*fos* DNA to cultured synovial cells: A transfection study. J Rheumatol 20:422–428
13. Kuroki Y, Shiozawa S, Sugimoto T, Fujita T (1992) Constitutive expression of c-*fos* gene inhibits type I collagen synthesis in transfected osteoblasts. Biochem Biophys Res Commun 182:1389–1394
14. Kuroki Y, Shiozawa S, Sugimoto T, Kanatani M, Kaji H, Miyauchi A, Chihara K (1994) Constitutive c-*fos* expression in osteoblastic MC3T3-E1 cells stimulates osteoclast maturation and osteoclastic bone resorption. Clin Exp Immunol 95:536–539
15. Miyauchi A, Shiozawa S, Kuroki Y, Fukasa M, Fujita T, Chihara K (1994) Persistent expression of proto-oncogene c-*fos* stimulates osteoclast differentiation. Biochem Biophys Res Commun 205:1547–1555
16. Shimizu S, Shiozawa S, Shiozawa K, Fujita T (1985) Quantitative histologic studies on the pathogenesis of periarticular osteoporosis in rheumatoid arthritis. Arthritis Rheum 28:25–31
17. Shiozawa S, Kuroki Y (1994) Osteoporosis in rheumatoid arthritis: A molecular biological aspect of connective tissue gene activation. Tohoku J Exp Med 173:189–198
18. Trabandt A, Aicher WK, Gay RE, Sukhatme VP, Fassbender HG, Gay S (1992) Spontaneous expression of immediately-early response genes c-*fos* and erg-1 in collagenase-producing rheumatoid synovial fibroblasts. Rheumatol Int 12:53–59
19. Shiozawa S, Shimizu K, Tanaka K, Hino K (1997) Studies on the contribution of c-*fos*/AP-1 to arthritic joint destruction. J Clin Invest 99:1210–1216
20. Kawasaki H, Hikasa M, Morisawa T, Ou Yang F, Shiozawa S (1998) Antigen-specific T cells overexpressing c-fos gene reside in G2/M(4c) state due to increased wee1 kinase and histone acetylation. Arthritis Rheum 41(9) Suppl:S35
21. Vyse T, Todd JA (1996) Genetic analysis of autoimmune disease. Cell 85:311–318
22. Lynn AH, Kwoh KC, Venglish CM, Aston CE, Chakravarti A (1995) Genetic epidemiology of rheumatoid arthritis. Am J Hum Genet 57:150–159
23. Wordsworth P (1995) Genes and arthritis. Br Med Bull 51:249–266
24. Rigby AS, Voelm L, Silman AJ (1993) Epistatic modeling in rheumatoid arthritis: an application of the Risch theory. Genet Epidemiol 10:311–320
25. Risch N (1990) Linkage strategies for genetically complex traits. III. The effect of marker polymorphism on analysis of affected relative pairs. Am J Hum Genet 46:242–253
26. Holmans P, Clayton D (1995) Efficiency of typing unaffected relatives in an affected-sib-pair linkage study with single-locus and multiple tightly linked markers. Am J Hum Genet 57:1221–1232
27. Kruglyak L, Lander ES (1995) Complete multipoint sib-pair analysis of qualitative and quantitative traits. Am J Hum Genet 57:439–454
28. Shiozawa S, Hayashi S, Tsukamoto Y, Yasuda N, Goko H, Kawasaki H, Wada T, Shimizu K, Kamatani N, Takasugi K, Tanaka Y, Shiozawa K, Imura S (1997) Identification of the gene loci that predispose to rheumatoid arthritis. Arthritis Rheum 40(9)Suppl:s329
29. Shiozawa S, Hayashi S, Tsukamoto Y, Yasuda N, Goko H, Kawasaki H, Wada T, Shimizu K, Kamatani N, Takasugi K, Tanaka Y, Shiozawa K, Imura S (1998) Identification of the gene loci that predispose to rheumatoid arthritis. Int. Immunol. 10:1891–1895

Apoptosis Is a Novel Therapeutic Strategy for RA: Investigations Using an Experimental Arthritis Animal Model

Hiroaki Matsuno[1], Kazuo Yudoh[1], Isaya Morita[1], Takashi Sawai[2], Miwa Uzuki[2], Tomoko Hasunuma[3], Kusuki Nishioka[3], Haruo Tsuji[1], and Tomoatsu Kimura[1]

Summary. To investigate the time at which apoptotic cells appear during the course of synovitis in rheumatoid arthritis (RA) patients, we conducted a time-course observation of changes of apoptotic cells in collagen-induced arthritis mice as a RA model. No apoptotic cells were detected before the onset of synovitis. The number of such cells increased parallel to the progress of the arthritis in its initial stages, and the number of cells decreased in the proliferative stage of arthritis. These results suggest that apoptotic cells appear to maintain homeostasis when there is synovium proliferation which is undesirable for the morphological maintenance of a joint. If the induction of apoptosis is possible in RA synovitis, this procedure might lead to a cure for RA. Based on this hypothesis, apoptosis therapeutic experiments using the anti-Fas mAb and Fas-ligand were performed in SCID-HuRAg mice implanted with human RA synovial tissues. It was found, that the synovitis implanted in mice was reduced markedly, suggesting that apoptosis induction therapy may be a novel treatment strategy for RA.

Key words. Rheumatoid arthritis, SCID mouse, Treatment, Apoptosis, Collagen-induced arthritis

What is Apoptosis?

"Apoptosis" is derived from the Greek terms *apo* ("off") and *ptosis* ("fall"). It is a medical term meaning "a falling off". The effects of apoptosis in cells vary widely, and are studied extensively in immunological and embryological research. Apoptosis is associated with the differentiation of the five fingers from the "mitt-like" paw, and has

---

[1] Department of Orthopaedic Surgery, Toyama Medical and Pharmaceutical University, 2630 Sugitani, Toyama 930-01, Japan
[2] Department of Pathology, Iwate Medical University School of Medicine, 19-1 Uchimaru, Morioka 020, Japan
[3] Institute of Medical of Science, St. Marianna University School of Medicine, 2-16-1 Sugaoi, Miyamae-ku, Kawasaki 216, Japan

been proven to provide thymic cell selection [1,2]. Apoptosis, which results in death of a cell (also referred to as programmed cell death), is also considered to be one of the consistent biological mechanisms for controlling cellularling proliferation. A form of cell death contrasting with apoptosis is necrosis, which is observed in the course of death of a cell in a pathological condition. Thus, while necrosis is an accidental cell death caused by swelling and rupture of a cell, apoptosis is regarded as death of a cell in a normal condition. These two forms of cell death are different also from a morphological point of view; apoptosis is accompanied by cell shrinkage, nuclear condensation, and aggregation of chromatin, but exhibits less change in the cytoplasm. The surface of the cell loses its microvilli and is flattened, and the resultant cell is then segmented into apoptosis corpuscles of various sizes. Thus apoptosis can be detected by agarose get electrophoresis [3] in which the DNA fragments formed by the biochemical segmentation are identified. In addition, the morphological characteristics of the cell can be observed by electron microscopy. As a histological approach, the TUNEL (TdT-mediated dUTP biotin nick end labeling) method using in situ endolabeling of DNA terminals can be employed for detecting apoptotic cells [4].

Why Does Apoptosis Occur in Rheumatoid Arthritis?

Apoptosis has been observed in the synovium of rheumatoid arthritis (RA) patients [5–7]. The pathology of RA thus presents an apparent paradox: Synovitis, a substantially chronic and proliferative condition leading to destruction of joints and bones, is observed in RA [8,9]. At the same time, there is the occurrence of apoptosis, which suppresses the proliferation of cells. We therefore have attempted to explain these apparently paradoxical phenomena in RA.

When considering the structure of a joint, the initial form at the embryonic stage is like a stick having no articular cavity. The formation of a joint is initiated when the part corresponding to a joint in this stick-like tissue, i.e., mesenchymal tissue also referred to as an interzone, is lost to form an articular cavity [10]. The formation of this articular cavity involves the occurrence of apoptosis, which causes the disappearance of the mesenchymal tissue. This process is similar to that which results in the disappearance of the webs between the fingers (Fig. 1). At the terminal phase of an advanced RA the bone has no articular cavity, and has changed into a form analogous to the stick-like structive observed at the early embryonic stage. This is synarthrophysis [11]. These findings lead to the conclusion that when this abnormal state of synarthrophysis induced by RA is reached, apoptosis may appear as one of a number of biological defense responses intended to maintain the structure of the joint cavity. In this chapter, the relationship between RA and apoptosis is discussed, referring to the results of the experiments we conducted to prove the hypothesis described above.

Time-Course Observation of Apoptosis in CIA Mice

To prove the hypothesis described above, we first conducted an experiment to investigate when apoptosis appears in the process of synovitis in RA and how the apoptosis which thus appears is changed thereafter [12]. For this purpose, collagen-

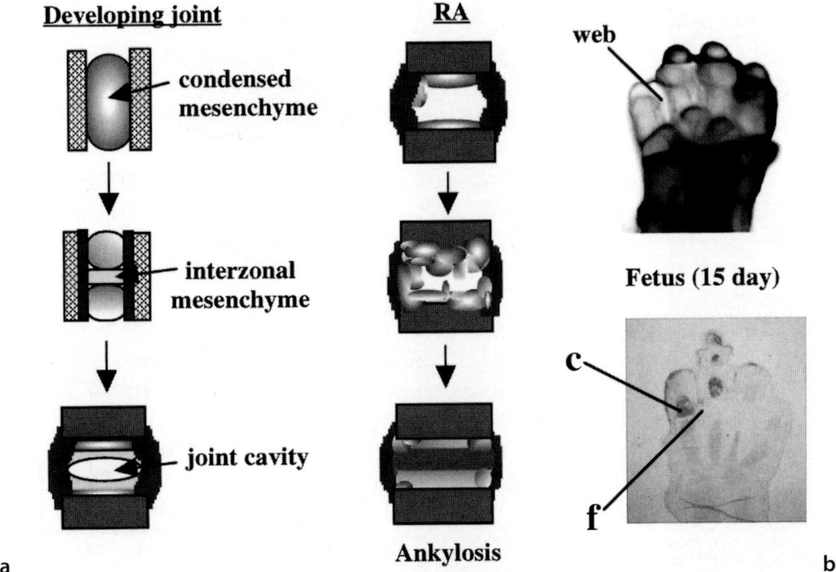

Fig. 1a, b. Articular cavity at apoptosis and embryonal stage. a The loss of mesenchymal tissue due to apoptosis forms the articular cavity. In the terminal stage of rheumatoid arthritis (RA), the articular cavity disappears due to ankylosis. b At the embryonal stage, apoptosis forms the fingers (*f*) and an articular cavity (*c*) (TUNEL-stained fetal mouse)

induced arthritis (CIA) mice were used to observe the course of pathological change at intervals over time before onset of the arthritis. The CIA mice were prepared according to the method reported previously [13,14], histological observations were performed using an electron microscope, and the presence of apoptotic cells was demonstrated using the TUNEL method.

It was shown that no apoptotic cells were present before the onset of the arthritis. However, apoptotic cells appeared concurrently with the occurrence of arthritis, and then increased in number depending on the degree of arthritic exacerbation. This was demonstrates by microscope observing histological specimens under the electron (data not shown). Nevertheless, subsequent observations revealed that the degree of the arthritis remained exacerbated while the number of apoptotic cells decreased gradually (Fig. 2). These findings supported our novel hypothesis that the advent of apoptosis is designed to maintain the homeostasis that is a stationary phase in tissues during an emergency, such as synovium proliferation caused by RA, and that the synovitis is exacerbated when local rescue at the joint by apoptosis is insufficient or unsuccessful. In other words, if apoptosis can be induced exogenously in the synovium of RA, this apoptosis induction therapy may be a novel approach for the treatment of RA (Fig. 3).

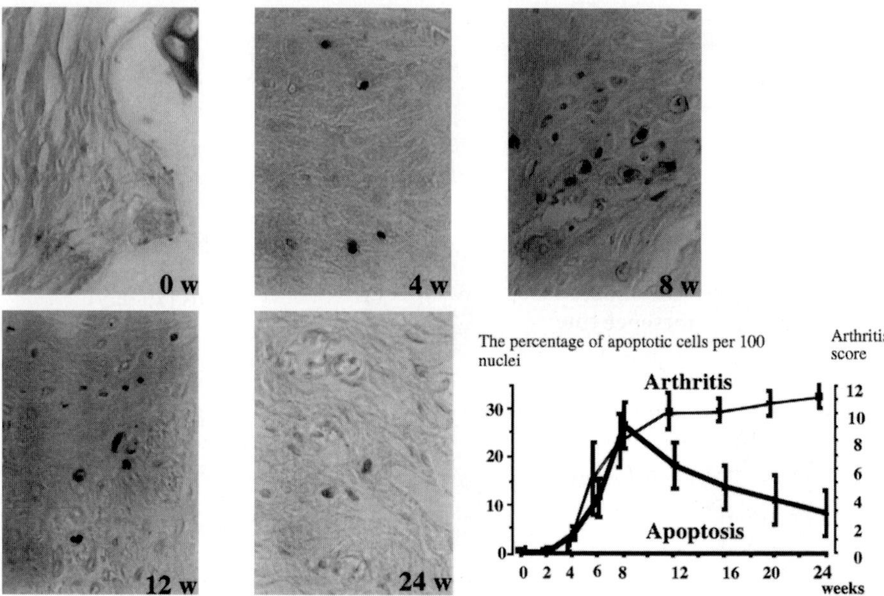

FIG. 2. Time-course observation of apoptotic cells in collagen-induced arthritis (CIA) mice. No synovial apoptotic cells were detected before the onset of arthritis, but upon the development of the arthritis the apoptotic cells appeared. The number of apoptotic cells increased parallel to the progress of arthritis in its initial stages, and the number of cells decreased in the proliferative stage of arthritis. (TUNEL staining and arthritic score). *W*, weeks. (Original magnification ×1,000.) With permission from [12]

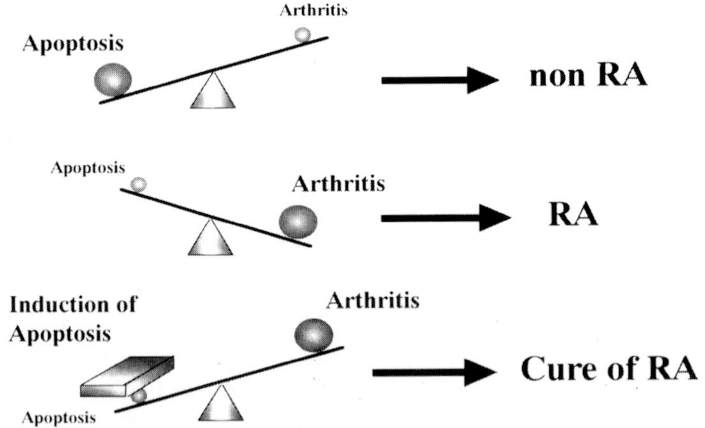

FIG. 3. Relationship between RA and apoptosis. RA and apoptosis are considered to be balanced in a seesaw-like equilibrium which maintains the homeostasis of a joint. RA is advanced when the degree of arthritis weighs greater, while RA is reduced when apoptosis weighs greater. If this hypothesis is correct, the therapeutic effects against arthritis can be obtained by inducing apoptosis in RA

SCID-HuRAg Model as an Experimental Animal Model

We proposed that apoptosis could be induced as a treatment, and then we conducted a therapeutic experiment. Conventional therapeutic experiments of drugs in RA model animals were reported to produce different therapeutic results from those observed in human RA [15]. Accordingly, we concluded that a model mouse whose pathological state is more analogous to that in humans should be developed. In addition, a screening animal model capable of being subjected to human monoclonal antibodies (mAb) was necessary. Our reasoning was that the mAbs that have been employed extensively in the development of novel treatment methods for RA may exhibit different effects, side effects, and antibody affinity upon conversion of the antibody from the mouse type to the human type [16–19].

We implanted the synovium, cartilage, and bone tissue of RA patients into severe combined immunodeficiency (SCID) mice to create SCID-HuRAg mice [20–24]. This form of model mouse preparation also has been attempted in other institutions [25–28]. However, our SCID-HuRAg mice differ somewhat from those in previous reports in terms of the characteristics of the tissues implanted. In the previous reports, the cells remaining even after implantation into the SCID mice were mainly RA synovial fibroblast, vessels, and macrophages, and other cells were reported to remain only in extremely small amounts. The reduction in the number of the cells was especially marked in T lymphocytes [25–28]. In addition, the examination of matrix metalloproteinase (MMP) revealed that almost no MMP-1,3 was detected in the implanted tissues [27]. These findings indicate that the pathological characteristics of the implanted tissues after implantation into the SCID mice involved a difference from those of the synovium of the human RA. Accordingly, we changed the implantation procedure and prepared a model animal whose synovium was as close histopathologically to that of the human RA as possible [20–24].

The resultant SCID-HuRAg mouse model is characterized by the morphology of the tissues implanted, which are almost identical to the tissues of the human RA as a donor [22]. The histological findings in RA such as villous proliferation of the synovium, multilayer formation of the superficial cells of the synovium, vascularization, infiltration of inflammatory cells, and lymph follicles were also found in the implanted tissues of the SCID-HuRAg mice. Pannus formation in which the implanted synovium was infiltrated into the cartilage was also observed as being maintained in the tissues implanted into the SCID mice. This pannus site exhibited a proliferation of fibroblasts, polynuclear giant cells, and inflammation cells which were infiltrated. TRAP positive osteoclasts were also observed, and hyaluronic acid was present in the implanted cartilage (Fig. 4). Immunocytes similar to those in the RA synovium of a human donor were observed, and immunostaining of the lymph follicles revealed a large number of CD4 positive cells around and in the center of the follicles, together with a small number of surrounding CD8 positive cells. In the center of the lymph follicles, CD20 positive cells were also observed [29]. CD68 positive cells, the markers of macrophages, were observed likewise and were especially extensive on the surface of the synovium.

While it was reported that cytokine developed extensively on the surface of human RA [30,31], a SCID-HuRAg mouse also exhibited tumor necrosis factor alpha (TNF-α) and interleukin 6 (IL-6) in the implanted tissues. MMP-1 and MMP-9 were also

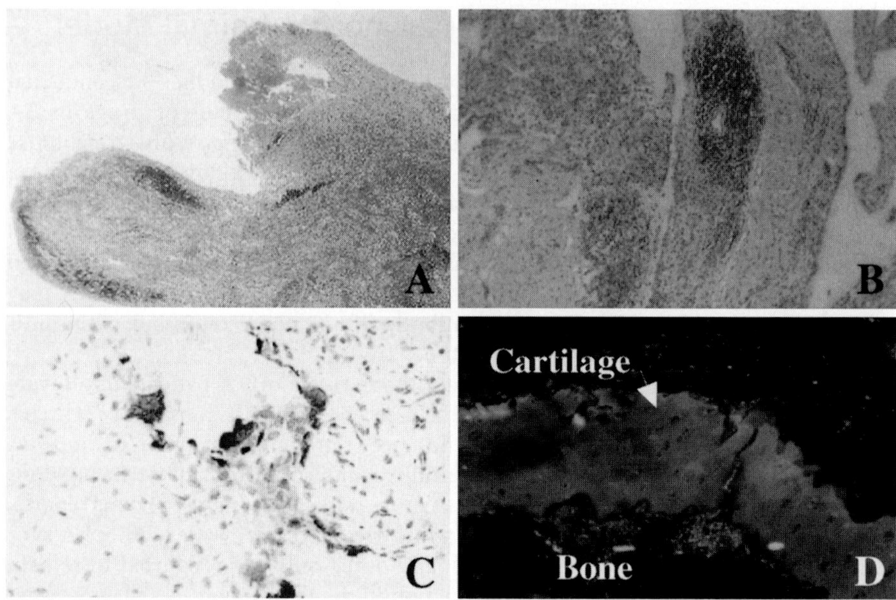

Fig. 4A–D. Human RA tissues implanted in SCID-huRAg mice (8 weeks after tissue implantation). **A, B** Villous proliferation of the synovium, multilayer of the superficial cells and infiltration of a large number of inflammatory cells and lymph follicles are observed. **C** In the pannus site, TRAP-positive osteoclasts are also observed. **D** In the implanted tissues, the cartilage tissue (*arrowhead*) is maintained and hyaluronic acid capable of being stained fluorescently is observed. (Original magnification ×100 in A, B, and C; ×75, D ×240.) With permission from [22]

observed (Fig. 5). Implanted tissues expanded to 1 to 1.5 times larger than the size of the tissues immediately after implantation and involved cell division mediated by the cycle of the cells capable of being stained positively with Ki-67 [22,32]. Human rheumatoid factor (RF) and IL-6 in mouse serum were also detected to be increased by implantation of the synovial tissues [22]. Based on the findings described above, the novel SCID-HuRAg mouse model we prepared was considered to resemble very closely the local pathological tissues of a human RA joint.

Therapeutic Experiment with Anti-RA Agents in SCID-HuRAg Model

Our SCID-HuRAg mouse model was subjected to a therapeutic experiment with anti-RA agents. Anti-TNF-α mAb and receptor monoclonal antibody (anti-IL-6R mAb) are potent anti-RA agents. Administration of these mAbs resulted in a reduction in the size of the implanted synovial tissues as well as a decrease in the number of inflammatory cells [22,23]. On the other hand, in the therapeutic experiment using conventional anti-RA agents, methotrexate (MTX) auranofin and salazosulfapyridine, a significant decrease in the number of inflammatory cells and reduction in the size of the syn-

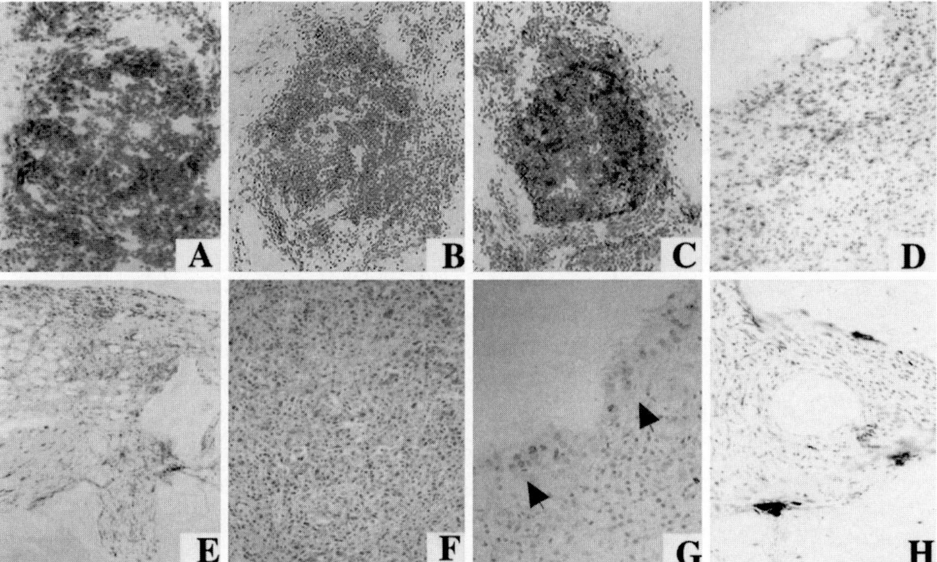

FIG. 5A–H. SCID-huRAg mouse immunohistochemical staining (8 weeks after tissue implantation). A large number of CD4 positive cells (**A**) and a small number of CD8 positive cells (**B**) are observed in the lymph follicle, while CD20 positive cells are observed in the center of the follicles (**C**). CD68 positive cells are observed widely throughout the entire synovium (**D**), with the development being especially intense in the superficial cells of the synovium. Both TNF-α (**E**) and IL-6 (**F**) are observed widely throughout the entire layer of the synovium. MMP-1 (**G**, *arrows*) develops in the superficial cells of the synovium. MMP-9 is observed widely throughout the entire layer of the synovium (**H**), with the development being especially marked in the pannus site. (Original magnification ×240 in A, B, C, and Hi ×100 in D, F, and G; ×180 in E.) With permission from [22]

ovial tissues were observed in the MTX group, but other agents caused no histologically significant change (Fig. 6). Since the clinical results of these conventional agents in the SCID-HuRAg mice were almost consistent with the efficacy rates of the anti-RA agents [33], our model was considered capable of being utilized as a model for screening the drugs.

Efficacy and Future Use of Apoptosis Induction Therapy in RA Synovitis

The SCID-HuRAg mouse model was subjected to a therapeutic experiment employing apoptosis induction therapy. TNF-Fas ligand (FasL) and anti-Fas mAb are known to be factors that transmit the signals of apoptosis into the cells (34,35). FasL and TNF bind to their specific receptors Fas/APO-1 and TNF receptor 1 (TNF-R$_1$) and TNF-R$_2$ to transmit the messages of apoptosis to cells. Accordingly, we employed anti-Fas mAb (clone CH-11) [36] and FasL to induce the Fas/FasL-mediated apoptosis in the synovia of the SCID-huRAg mice to investigate the synovitis-inhibiting effect of apoptosis

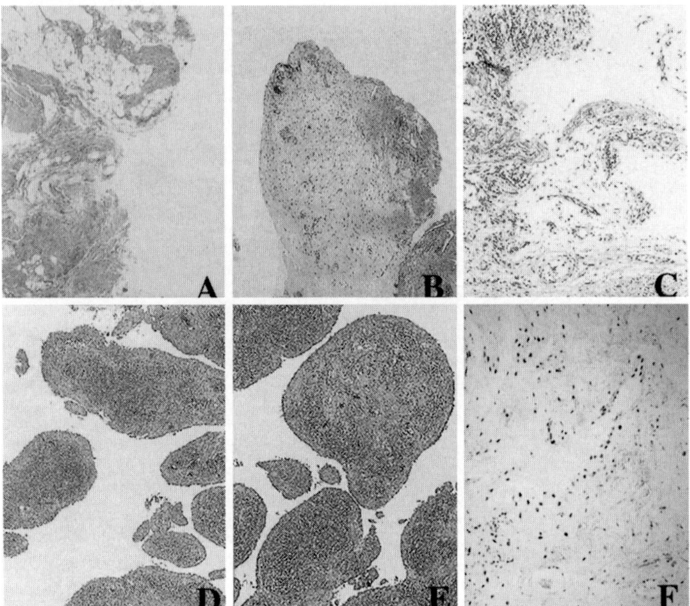

FIG. 6A–F. Histological characteristics in treatment groups. Anti-TNF-α mAb (A) and anti IL-6R mAb (B) treatments cause a marked decrease in the number of inflammation cells in the synovium. Decrease in the number of inflammation cells is also observed in the MTX treatment group (C). Auranofin (D) and salazosulfapyridine (E) treatment groups exhibited synovitis even after treatment. Administration of anti-TNF-α mAb induces apoptosis in the synovium (F). (TUNEL staining of the synovium 72 h after administration of anti-TNF-α mAb.) (Original magnification ×180 in A, B, C, D, E and F; ×240)

[20,24,29]. As a result, significantly attenuated inflammatory synovitis which had not been observed previously was observed after apoptosis induction (Fig. 7).

Induction of Apoptosis by Anti-RA Agents

Anti-TNF-α mAb therapy has come to be regarded as an potential method treatment of RA [37,38]. Administration of TNF-α mAb not only improves the clinical condition of the RA patient more effectively than conventional anti-RA agents, but it is expected to inhibit bone destruction as well [39]. Accordingly, we have investigated the relationship of anti-TNF-α therapy to apoptosis and found that apoptotic cells appeared as a result of the administration of anti-TNF-α mAb (Fig. 6). This appearance of apoptosis was confirmed by immunostaining with Fas/FasL pathway (data not shown). However, TNF-α, is a cytokine which serves to transmit apoptosis signals into the cells [40]. Further more, in RA apoptosis was reportedly induced by the addition of TNF-α in a synovial cell culture system [7].

Nevertheless, our results indicate that apoptos occurs in spite of the blockage of TNF-α by anti-TNF-α mAb. This seems to be unlikely when considering the pathway of TNF-α to apoptosis. However, a study conducted in another institute has indicated

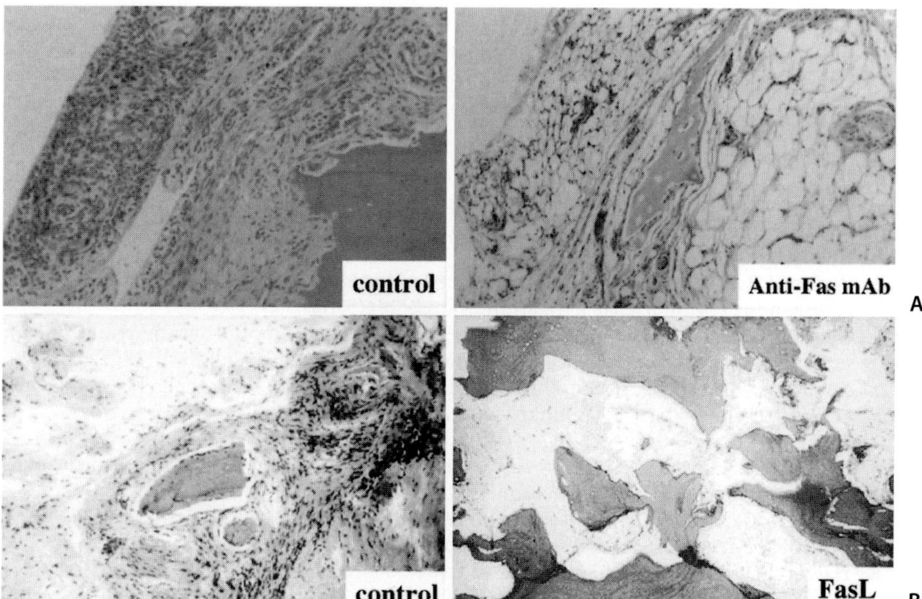

Fig. 7A,B. Histological characteristics after treatment with anti-Fas mAb and FasL **A** Administration of *anti-Fas mAb* causes significant inhibition of the synovitis when compared with the *control* group. **B** Treatment with *FasL* also causes an almost complete inhibition of synovitis similarly to anti-Fas mAb. (Original magnification ×100.) With permission from [22]

that addition of TNF-α to cultured RA synovial cells caused inhibition of apoptosis-induced cell death, which is consistent with our results [41]. This indicates that in RA there may be a signal pathway other than the ordinary pathway of TNF-α to apoptosis. In fact, our experimental system exhibited an increased appearance of Fas/FasL which is involved in the other apoptosis pathway of the TNF-α family. Since the RA synovium exhibited a higher sensitivity to Fas/FasL pathway than that in a normal condition [42], anti-TNF-α mAb may transmit some signals to Fas/FasL directly or indirectly (via a structure neutralized with TNF-α), thereby inducing apoptosis. Further investigation is required with regard to this issue. We also observed in our experimental system that apoptosis was induced after the treatment with MTX (data not shown). Thus, the effect of MTX in RA may also be a pharmacological effect mediated by apoptosis.

On the results of the study described above, it was concluded that the synovitis is caused when the formation of apoptosis at the onset of an inflammation in the synovial tissues in an RA patient is not sufficient to maintain homeostasis. It was also concluded that in RA, the induction of apoptosis served to inhibit synovitis.

Acknowledgment. This work was supported, in part, by grants from the research foundation of the Education Ministry (no. 08671646) and the Japan Orthopaedic and Traumatic Foundation (JOTF; no. 0091), and by a grant-in-aid for Fundamental

Comprehensive Research on Long-Term Chronic Disease (Department of Rheumatoid Arthritis) from the Japan Ministry of Health and Welfare.

References

1. Hurle JM, Ros MA, Garcia-Martinez V, Macias D, Ganan Y (1995) Cell death in the embryonic developing limb. Scan Microscop 9(2):519–534
2. von Boehmer H (1992) Thymic selection: a matter of life and death. Immunol Today 13(11):454–458
3. Wyllie AH (1980) Glucocorticoid-induced thymocyte apoptosis is associated with endogenous endonuclease activation. Nature 284(5756):555–556
4. Gavrieli Y, Sherman Y, Ben-Sasson SA (1992) Identification of programmed cell death in situ via specific labeling of nuclear DNA fragmentation. J Cell Biol 119(3):493–501
5. Nakajima T, Aono H, Hasunuma T, Yamamoto K, Shirai T, Hirohata K, Nishioka K (1995) Apoptosis and functional Fas antigen in rheumatoid arthritis synoviocytes. Arthritis Rheum 38(4):485–491
6. Hirohata S, Hirohata K (1994) Interactions between lymphocytes and type A synoviocytes in rheumatoid synovium (letter). Lancet 344(8930):1158
7. Firestein GS, Yeo M, Zvaifler NJ (1995) Apoptosis in rheumatoid arthritis synovium. J Clin Invest 96(3):1631–1638
8. Harris ED Jr (1990) Rheumatoid arthritis. Pathophysiology and implications for therapy. N Engl J Med 322(18):1277–1289
9. Stamenkovic I, Stegagno M, Wright KA, Krane SM, Amento EP, Colvin RB, Duquesnoy RJ, Kurnick JT (1988) Clonal dominance among T-lymphocyte infiltrates in arthritis. Proc Natl Acad Sci USA 85(4):1179–1183
10. Ogden JA, Grogan DP (1987) Prenatal development and growth of the musculoskeletal system. In: Albright JA, Brand RA (eds) The scientific basis of orthopaedics (2nd edn). Appleton & Lange, New York, pp 47–89
11. Steinbroker O, Traeger CH, Batterman RC (1949) Therapeutic criteria in rheumatoid arthritis. JAMA 140:659–662
12. Morita I, Matsuno H, Sakai K, Nezuka T, Tsuji H, Shirai T, Nishioka K (1998) Time course of apoptosis in collagen-induced arthritis. Int J Tissue React 20(2):37–43
13. Matsuno H, Matsushita I, Okada C, Suzuki M, Tsuji H, Ochiai H (1991) Role of lymphocytes in collagen induced arthritis. J Rheumatol 18:1344–1349
14. Kadowaki KM, Matsuno H, Tsuji H, Tunru I (1994) CD4+ T cells from collagen induced arthritic mice are essential to transfer arthritis into severe combined immunodeficient mice. Clin Exp Immunol 97:212–218
15. Jones SA, Kennedy AJ, Roberts NA (1982) Assessment of drugs for activity in established type II collagen arthritis. Agents Actions 12:650–656
16. Horneff G, Burmester GR, Emmrich F, Kalden JR (1991) Treatment of rheumatoid arthritis with an anti-CD4 monoclonal antibody. Arthritis Rheum 34(2):129–140
17. Choy EH, Chikanza IC, Kingsley GH, Corrigall V, Panayi GS (1992) Treatment of rheumatoid arthritis with single dose or weekly pulses of chimaeric anti-CD4 monoclonal antibody. Scand J Immunol 36(2):291–298
18. Verhoeyen M, Milstein C, Winter G (1988) Reshaping human antibodies: grafting an antilysozyme activity. Science 239(4847):1534–1536
19. Riechmann L, Clark M, Waldmann H, Winter G (1988) Reshaping human antibodies for therapy. Nature 332(6162):323–327
20. Sakai K, Matsuno H, Nezuka T, Tsuji H, Nishioka K, Shirai T, Yonehara S (1996) Inhibitory effect on rheumatoid synovitis by induction of apoptosis using in vivo model of human rheumatoid arthritis. 8th APLAR Congress of Rheumatology s25, Melbourne

21. Matsuno H, Nezuka T, Sakai K, Morita I, Nishioka K, Shirai T, Tsuji H (1997) Etiology and treatment effects of apoptosis in RA patients using animal model study. Arthritis Rheum 40(9):S294

22. Matsuno H, Sawai T, Nezuka T, Uzuki M, Tsuji H, Nishimoto N, Yoshizaki K (1998) Treatment of RA synovitis with anti-reshaping human IL-6 receptor monoclonal antibody: using a RA tissue implants in SCID mouse model. Rheum 41(11):2014–2021

23. Nezuka T, Matsuno H, Sawai T, Saeki Y, Uzuki M, Tsuji H (1997) Inhibitory effects of TNF-α in engraftment RA synovium into SCID model. Arthritis Rheum 40(9): S79

24. Okamoto K, Asahara T, Kobayashi H, Matsuno H, Hasunuma T, Kobata T, Sumida T, Nishioka K (1998) Fas ligand transfectants induce apoptosis in human rheumatoid synoviocytes. Gene Therapy, 5:331–338

25. Rendt KE, Barry TS, Jones DM, Richter CB, McCachren SS, Haynes BF (1993) Engraftment of human synovium into severe combined immune deficient mice. Migration of human peripheral blood T cells to engrafted human synovium and to mouse lymph nodes. J Immunol 151:7324–7336

26. Geiler T, Kriegsmann J, Keyszer GM, Gay RE, Gay S (1994) A new model for rheumatoid arthritis generated by engraftment of rheumatoid synovial tissue and normal human cartilage into SCID mice. Arthritis Rheum 37:1664–1671

27. Sack U, Kuhn H, Ermann J, Kinne RW, Vogt S, Jungmichel D, Emmrich F (1994) Synovial tissue implants from patients with rheumatoid arthritis cause cartilage destruction in knee joints of SCID. bg mice. J Rheumatol 21:10–16

28. Sack U, Kuhn H, Kampfer I, Genest M, Arnold S, Pfeiffer G, Emmrich F (1996) Orthotopic implantation of inflamed synovial tissue from RA patients induces a characteristic arthritis in immunodeficient (SCID) mice. J Autoimmun 9:51–58

29. Sakai K, Matsuno H, Morita I, Nezuka T, Tsuji H, Shirai T, Yonehara S, Hasunuma T, Nishioka K (1998) Potential withdrawal of rheumatoid synovium by the induction of apoptosis using a novel in vivo model of rheumatoid arthritis. Arthritis Rheum 41(7):1251–1257

30. Deleuran BW, Chu CQ, Field M, Brennan FM, Mitchell T, Feldmann M, Maini RN (1992) Localization of tumor necrosis factor receptors in the synovial tissue and cartilage-pannus junction in patients with rheumatoid arthritis—Implication for local actions of tumor necrosis factor-α. Arthritis Rheum 35:1170–1178

31. Fukamachi T, Uzuki M, Tamura H, Nakai H, Koishihara Y, Sawai T (1994) Interleukin-6 receptor (IL-6R) dynamics in patients with rheumatoid arthritis (in Japanese with English abstract). Jpn J Inflamm 14:489–496

32. Gerdes J, Lemke H, Baisch H, Wacker HH, Schwab U, Stein H (1984) Cell cycle analysis of a proliferation-associated human nuclear antigen defined by the monoclonal antibody Ki-67. J Immunol 133.1710–1715

33. Tokano Y, Kobayashi S (1997) Methotrexate therapy (in Japanese). Rheumatology 17(3):288–292

34. Nagata S, Golstein P (1995) The Fas death factor. Science 267(5203):1449–1456

35. Fujisawa K, Asahara H, Okamoto K, Aono H, Hasunuma T, Kobata T, Iwakura Y, Yonehara S, Sumida T, Nishioka K (1996) Therapeutic effect of the anti-Fas antibody on arthritis in HTLV-1 tax transgenic mice. J Clin Invest 98(2):271–278

36. Fadeel B, Thorpe CJ, Yonehara S, Chiodi F (1997) Anti-Fas IgG1 antibodies recognizing the same epitope of Fas/APO-1 mediate different biological effects in vitro. Int Immunol 9(2):201–209

37. Elliott MJ, Maini RN, Feldmann M, Kalden JR, Antoni C, Smolen JS, Leeb B, Breedveld FC, Macfarlane JD, Bijl H, Woody JN (1994) Randomised double-blind comparison of chimeric monoclonal antibody to tumor necrosis factor alpha (cA2) versus placebo in rheumatoid arthritis. Lancet 344(8930):1105–1110

38. Elliott MJ, Maini RN, Feldmann M, Long-Fox A, Charles P, Bijl H, Woody JN (1994) Repeated therapy with monoclonal antibody to tumor necrosis factor alpha (cA2) in patients with rheumatoid arthritis. Lancet 344(8930):1125–1127
39. Brennan FM, Browne KA, Green PA, Jaspar JM, Maini RN, Feldmann M (1997) Reduction of serum matrix metalloproteinase 1 and matrix metalloproteinase 3 in rheumatoid arthritis patients following anti-tumor necrosis factor-alpha (cA2) therapy. Brit J Rheumatol 36(6):643–650
40. Yuan J. Transducing signals of life and death. Curr Opin Cell Biol 9(2):247–251
41. Ohsima S, Saeki Y, Mima T, Sasai M, Shimizu M, Murata N, Nakanishi K, Suemura M, McCloskey RV, Kishimoto T (1997) Tumor necrosis factor-α (TNF-α)interferes with Fas mediated apoptotic cell death on RA synovial cells. Arthritis Rheum 40(9):S289
42. Asahara H, Hasunuma T, Kobata T, Inoue H, Muller-Ladner U, Gay S, Sumida T, Nishioka K (1997) In situ expression of protooncogenes and Fas/Fas ligand in rheumatoid arthritis synovium. J Rheumatol 24(3):430–305

Part 4
Response of Spinal Cord and Cauda Equina to Dynamic Stress

Evaluation of Dynamic Stress of the Cervical Spinal Cord Using a High-Resolution Positron Emission Tomography

HISATOSHI BABA[1], YASUHISA MAEZAWA[1], KENZO UCHIDA[1], NOBUAKI FURUSAWA[1], YASUO KOKUBO[1], NORIHIRO SADATO[2], and YOSHIHARU YONEKURA[2]

Summary. We assessed the use of high-resolution ^{18}F-2-fluoro-deoxy-D-glucose (^{18}FDG)-positron emission tomography (PET) in evaluating the presence of variable degrees of dynamic stress of the cervical spinal cord in 22 patients with cervical myelopathy. For this purpose, we examined the correlation between the average standardized uptake value (SUV) of ^{18}FDG utilization rate of the cervical cord and neurological functional score before and after surgery. The average preoperative SUV of ^{18}FDG utilization correlated significantly with the preoperative neurological score ($P < 0.05$) but did not correlate with the postoperative score ($P = 0.08$). The average SUV correlated with the rate of neurological improvement ($P < 0.05$) after surgery. Although the results suggest that high-resolution ^{18}FDG-PET imaging may provide qualitative and quantitative estimates of impaired metabolic activity of the compromised cervical cord, at present, ^{18}FDG-PET imaging does not provide a clear visualization of the cervical cord injury caused by dynamic stress of the cord.

Key words. Cervical myelopathy, Dynamic stress, ^{18}F-2-fluoro-deoxy-D-glucose, Positron emission tomography

Introduction

Application of dynamic stress to the spinal cord may cause a progressive compromise of its function, and ultimately may lead to the appearance of clinical symptoms such as myelopathy. Mechanical compression of the cervical cord is a major cause of myelopathy; however, as Panjabi and White [1] have suggested, the spinal cord is damaged when certain dynamic forces are applied, particularly in the presence of

---

[1] Department of Orthopaedic Surgery, School of Medicine, Fukui Medical University, Shimoaizuki 23, Matsuoka, Fukui 910-1193, Japan
[2] Biomedical Imaging Research Center, Fukui Medical University, Shimoaizuki 23, Matsuoka, Fukui 910-1193, Japan

certain structural abnormalities of the cervical spine, such as excessive kyphosis or multiple subluxation, or ossification of the posterior longitudinal ligament (OPLL). Further stresses may result in serious functional damage of the spinal cord. Several groups, including ours [2–6], have used various methods to evaluate neural conductivity across the compromised cord as well as functional recovery following surgical treatment.

Budinger and Taylor [7] suggested the usefulness of positron emission tomography (PET) imaging for assessing the functional activity of damaged tissues, including the spinal cord. Di Chiro et al. [8] were the first group to visualize and quantify ^{18}F-2-deoxyglucose utilization rate of the cervical cord in 34 normal volunteers and patients, using a high-resolution PET scanner (Neuro-PET, NIH, Bethesda, MD USA). More recently, Higano et al. [9] used the ^{11}C-methionine-PET technique to identify the pathological viability of a cervical intramedullary ependymoma, and stressed the potential usefulness of PET for assessing spinal cord function. The present study was designed to assess the use of ^{18}F-2-fluoro-deoxy-D-glucose (^{18}FDG)-PET in evaluating the presence of dynamic stress of the cervical spinal cord in patients with compressive myelopathy requiring surgical decompression.

Patients and Methods

Patients and Neurological Assessment

Twenty-two patients with cervical compressive myelopathy volunteered for ^{18}FDG-PET study (3 patients with OPLL and 19 patients with spondylosis). Their age at operation averaged 56.7 years (range, 42–71 years). PET studies were also repeated in seven patients, 2.0–2.5 years postoperatively. Three patients underwent C3-C7 laminoplasty while 19 were treated with anterior decompression and fusion. Neurological assessment was conducted in accordance with the scoring system of the Japanese Orthopaedic Association (JOA) [3,5,6]. In this system, a 17-point score represents the normal (maximum) score, and the extent (rate) of relative neurological improvement was obtained by:

$$\text{Rate }(\%) = \frac{\text{postoperative score} - \text{preoperative score}}{17 - \text{preoperative score}} \times 100$$

Recording of Epidural Spinal Cord Evoked Potentials

Epidural spinal cord evoked potentials (SCEPs) were recorded intraoperatively in all patients using the method described previously [4,6]. Using a five-pole epidural catheter electrode (UKG-100-2PMW, Unique Medical, Tokyo, Japan), unipolar SCEPs were recorded simultaneously at five different segments of the cervical spinal cord following electrical stimulation of the thoracic spinal cord. Abnormalities of the first negative component (N1) of SCEP were graded into four types, including type I (normal or 30% reduction of N1 amplitude relative to control), type II (30–50% reduction in the amplitude of N1), type III (>50% reduction in the amplitude of N1 spike or total disappearance), and type IV (a positive-deflection evoked potential, designated as a spinal cord evoked injury potential [6]).

Radiological Examination

Radiological assessment of dynamic stress was based on the presence of the following abnormalities: (a) clinical instability at the affected segment(s) or neighboring intervertebral levels, indicating sagittal plane vertebral translation ≥ 3 mm and/or sagittal plane rotation $\geq 20°$ [1,10], (b) dynamic spinal canal stenosis, a distance of <12 mm between the posterior inferior edge of the vertebral body and superior edge of the caudal lamina, in the extension position [10], and (c) kyphosis ($\theta < -10°$), or loss of lordosis $\geq 15°$ of the vertebral column in neutral position of the neck [5,10]. Magnetic resonance imaging (1.5 Tesla Signa; General Electrics, Milwaukee, WI, USA) was performed to estimate changes in the intensity signal on T2-weighted spin-echo image (TR, 2000–5000 ms, TE, 50–98 ms), rated conveniently as isointense, mildly or severely hyperintense, or cyst formation, as we have reported previously [2].

Positron Emission Tomography

We used the GE Advance system (GE-YMS, Tokyo, Japan) for the tracer technique of PET scanning. The system allows simultaneous acquisition of 35 transverse slices with interslice spacing of 4.25 mm with septa (two-dimensional mode). Images were reconstructed to a full width at half maximum of 4.2 mm in both transaxial and sagittal directions. The field of view and pixel size of the reconstructed images were 256 mm and 2 mm, respectively. Transmission scans were obtained over 10 min using a standard pin source of 68Ge/68Ga for attenuation correction of the emission images. A dose of 244–488 MBq of ^{18}FDG was injected into the antecubital vein over a period of 10 s. Dynamic scans were obtained up to 60 min after the injection with arterial sampling. Arterial blood was withdrawn from the distal artery on the opposite side of the injection. Following injection, blood samples (2 ml each) were obtained every 15 s in the first 2 min, and then at 2.5, 3, 5, 10, 15, 20, 30, 45, 60 min after injection. Plasma radioactivity was measured by the scintillation counter against which the PET camera was cross-calibrated, using a cylindrical phantom filled with the ^{18}FDG solution.

Using the DoctorView software (Asahikasei, Nobeoka, Japan), the PET image was processed on SUN SPARC 20 workstation (SUN Microsystems, Mountain View, CA, USA). For quantitative analysis during data processing, the tissue activity was normalized to the injected dose and bodyweight (Standardized Uptake Value; SUV in mg/ml), as described by Sokoloff et al. [11]. A significant correlation between SUV and glucose metabolic rate in the normal cervical cord was described recently by Kamoto et al. [12], and SUV is thought to reflect the level of glucose utilization of the cervical cord [13–16]. A round region of interest (ROI, 10.3 mm in diameter, 21 pixels) was selected at the level of the injured spinal cord, which was slightly larger than the anteroposterior diameter of the cervical cord of normal Japanese subjects. During placement of ROI on the cord in every transaxial slice, a sagittal image of MRI served as "on-line" reference to match the level of ROI placed on the spinal cord. The maximal count in the ROI was then used as the tissue radioactivity to minimize the partial volume effect of ROI.

We then examined the correlation between SUV and JOA scores by Pearson's correlation analysis using the StatView II program (Abacus Concepts, Berkeley, CA, USA) with the level of significance set at $P < 0.05$.

Results

Neurological Findings

Patients showed symptoms and signs of myelopathy with an average JOA score of 12.5 ± 3.4 points preoperatively (range, 8–15 points). Postoperative neurological improvement was noted in all patients and the average score at follow-up increased to 15.6 ± 1.7 points (range, 12–17 points). The postoperative rate of neurological improvement was thus determined to be 68.9 ± 21.4%.

Radiological and Spinal Cord Evoked Potential Findings

On lateral radiographs, dynamic spinal canal stenosis was detected in 13 of 19 patients with spondylosis (4 patients at C3–4 level; 7 patients at C4–5; and 2 patients at C5–6). Clinical instability at the level of dynamic stenosis was found in 2 of these 13 patients (1 at C3–4 level and 1 at C4–5 level). On preoperative MRIs, six of these 13 patients showed hyperintense intensity signal at the level of dynamic spinal stenosis. The other seven cases showed an isointense intensity signal on MRIs. Four patients showed kyphotic alignment ($\theta < 0°$) of the cervical spine. None of the other three cases with OPLL had dynamic spinal stenosis or clinical instability on preoperative radiographs. In these three cases, the cervical spine kyphotic angle (θ) was <+10°, showing relative kyphotic alignment.

Qualitative SCEPs were recorded intraoperatively in 20 patients (17 with spondylosis and 3 with OPLL). In 17 cases, abnormal SCEPs (type III and/or IV) were recorded at the level causing myelopathy (at C3–4 level in 5 cases, at C4–5 level in 12 patients, and at C5–6 level in 8 patients).

Positron Emission Tomography Findings

The average SUV at the level of injury of the spinal cord correlated significantly with the preoperative JOA score ($r^2 = 0.331$, $P < 0.05$). Postoperative improvement in JOA scores tended to correlate with high preoperative SUV values ($r^2 = 0.253$, $P = 0.0794$). However, the average SUV in patients with myelopathy correlated significantly with the postoperative rate of neurological improvement ($r^2 = 0.335$, $P < 0.05$). The second PET examination conducted postoperatively in seven patients showed increased (normalization) average SUV at the level of injury of the cervical cord.

Dynamic Stress to the Cervical Cord and Positron Emission Tomography Findings

The average SUV at the level of spinal dynamic stenosis was high in five patients, normal in five and low in three cases. In two patients with spondylosis who showed clinical instability on radiographs, the average SUV was markedly low. Three patients with OPLL and loss of lordosis showed low average SUV at the level where the ossified lesion was most extensive. Figure 1a–c shows radiological, MRI, and PET images of a 58-year-old male patient with extensive OPLL, complaining of slight numbness in the bilateral forearms (JOA score, 16 points). In this patient, the kyphotic angle of the cervical spine was −5° with the neck in the neutral position, and the spinal cord was

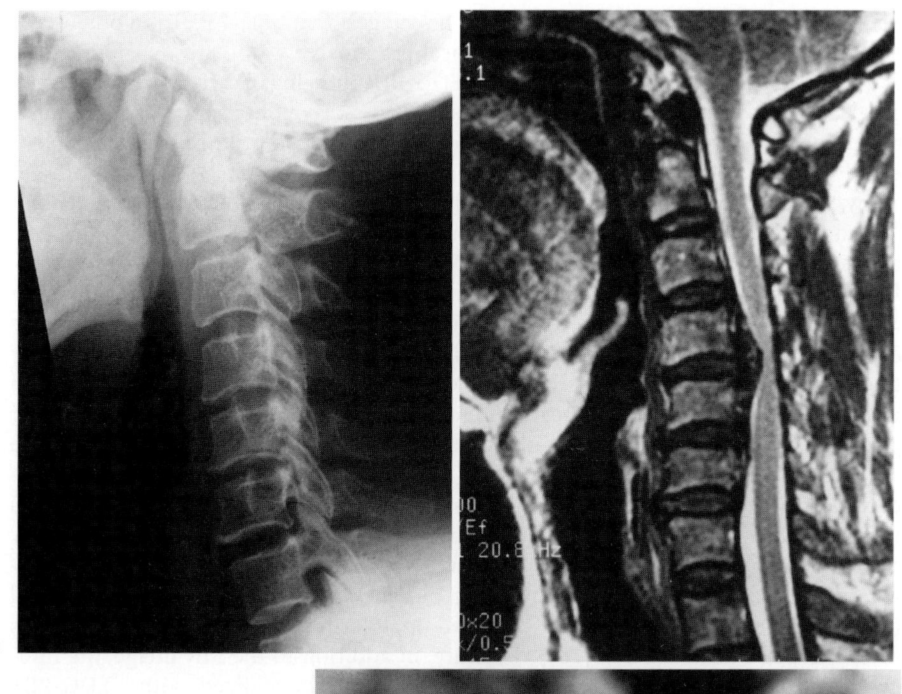

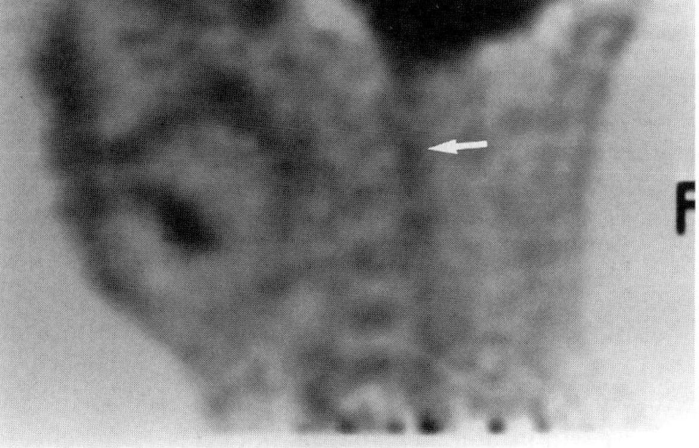

Fig. 1. Images of a 58-year old man with extensive ossification of the posterior longitudinal ligament (OPLL). a Lateral radiograph showing mixed-type OPLL between C3 and C7 levels. b T2-weighted (TR, 5000 ms; TE, 84 ms) MR image. c Sagittal ^{18}FDG-PET image (SUV, 2.0 mg/ml; *arrow*, C4 vertebral level)

severely impinged anteriorly between C4 and C6 levels. The average SUV at these levels slightly increased to 2.0 mg/ml.

Discussion

We demonstrated in the present study the usefulness of PET in assessing spinal cord function in patients with compressive myelopathy. Low glucose utilization rates were present in our patients relative to those in normal subjects. The average SUV in patients with myelopathy also correlated significantly with the rate of postoperative neurological improvement. Thus, our findings suggest that [18]FDG-PET is a potentially useful tool for the assessment of neurological prognosis.

There is a clinical concern of whether [18]FDG-PET imaging can visualize a damaged cervical cord secondary to a variable dynamic stress. Dynamic spinal canal stenosis occurring during neck extension is a major factor that compromises the cord posteriorly in association with buckling of the ligamentum flavum [10]. In the present study, dynamic canal stenosis was not always visualized by PET, but in a patient with a long history of such stress, the cervical cord at the level of injury was associated with a low glucose utilization. On the other hand, the spinal cord is infrequently encroached upon ventrally where the cervical spine appears flexed within the canal. When the neck is in a flexion position, the spinal cord is biomechanically extended longitudinally [1] resulting in increased tension within the cord. Under these circumstances of a tight dural tube, the spinal cord may be easily damaged ventrally even by a small osteocartilaginous tissue. More importantly, the anterior gray matter (which is mechanically more fragile than the white matter) or the anterior nerve roots are at a high risk of injury in these patients. Under these circumstances, motor paresis can be more profound than sensory dysfunction. Studies from our group have previously shown that stretch of the spinal cord longitudinally results in a significant damage of the middle portion of the cord [17]. A representative case was reported previously by our group [18]. In our patient, a small herniated intervertebral disc at C3–4 caused upper arm paresis when the patient was forced to hyperflex her neck [18]. Therefore, in addition to the MR image, the mid-cervical area of the spinal cord should be carefully visualized with [18]FDG-PET imaging. The presented case (Fig. 1a–c) having OPLL without significant neurological symptoms and signs showed an increased glucose utilization at the cord level where the most severe longitudinally tensile stress on the gray matter was highly possible, particularly anteriorly. The PET result may suggest a certain neurobiological reaction of the gray matter neurons to such a tensile as well as compressive stress, increasing the neuronal activity [19]. If we are able to visualize such a neuronal response of neurons to various stresses, PET imaging would be worth more clinically during a patient's neurological assessment. Our results, however, did not show a significant correlation between reduced [18]FDG utilization and a specific level of spinal cord compromise pertaining to such dynamic stress. However, we are confident that with further technical improvements as well as increased clinical experience using PET, we will be able to visualize more clearly the effect of dynamic stress on the cervical spinal cord by [18]FDG-PET imaging.

We conclude that PET imaging using [18]FDG provides a qualitative and quantitative measure of low metabolic activity of the compromised cervical cord in patients with myelopathy due to a fixed compression as well as dynamic stress, and correlates with the score of neurological deficit. [18]FDG-PET imaging appears to be of value in evaluating the metabolic activity of the compromised cervical cord.

Acknowledgments. This work was supported by grants from the Japanese Orthopaedics and Traumatology Foundation Incorporated (grant no. 0082; 1996) and the Investigation Committee on Ossification of the Spinal Ligaments, Public Health Bureau of the Japanese Ministry of Health and Welfare.

References

1. Panjabi MM, White AA III (1990) Physical properties and functional biomechanics of the spine. In: White AA III, Panjabi MM (eds) Clinical biomechanics of the spine, 2nd edn. J.B. Lippincott, Philadelphia, pp 67–71
2. Baba H, Furusawa N, Chen Q, Imura S, Tomita K (1995) Anterior decompressive surgery for cervical ossified posterior longitudinal ligament causing myeloradiculopathy. Paraplegia 33:18–24
3. Baba H, Maezawa Y, Uchida K, Furusawa N, Wada M, Imura S (1997) Plasticity of the spinal cord contributes to neurological improvement in patients treated by cervical decompression: a magnetic resonance imaging study. J Neurol 244:455–460
4. Baba H, Kawahara N (1995) Spinal cord evoked potential monitoring in orthopaedic spinal surgery. In: Dimitrijevic MR, Halter JA (eds) Atlas of human spinal cord evoked potentials. Butterworth-Heinemann, Boston, Massachusetts, pp 123–131
5. Baba H, Uchida K, Maezawa Y, Furusawa N, Azuchi M, Imura S (1996) Lordotic alignment and posterior migration of the spinal cord following en bloc open-door laminoplasty for cervical myelopathy: a magnetic resonance imaging study. J Neurol 243:626–632
6. Baba H, Maezawa Y, Imura S, Kawahara N, Tomita K (1996) Spinal cord evoked potential for cervical and thoracic compressive myelopathy. Paraplegia 34:100–106
7. Budinger TF, Taylor SE (1995) New approaches to targeting arthritis with radiopharmaceuticals. J Rheumatol 22 (Suppl 43):62–67
8. Di Chiro G, Oldfield E, Bairamian D, Brooks RA, Patronas NJ, Mansi L, Kornblith PL, Smith BH, Sank VJ, Margolin RA (1985) In vivo glucose utilisation of tumors of the brain stem and spinal cord. In: Greitz T, Ingvar DH, Widén L (eds). The mechanism of the human brain studied with positron emission tomography. Raven, New York, pp 351–361
9. Higano S, Shishido F, Nagashima M, Tomura N, Murakami M, Inugami A, Tabata K, Yasui N, Uemura K (1990) PET evaluation of spinal cord tumor using [^{11}C]-methionine. J Comput Assist Tomogr 14:297–299
10. Baba H, Furusawa N, Imura S, Kawahara N, Tsuchiya H, Tomita K (1993) Late radiographic findings after anterior cervical fusion for spondylotic myeloradiculopathy. Spine 18:2167–2173
11. Sokoloff L, Reivich M, Kennedy C, Des Rosiers H, Patlak CS, Pettigrew KD, Sakurada O, Shinohara M (1977) The [^{14}C]deoxyglucose method for the measurement of local cerebral glucose utilisation: theory, procedure, and normal values in the conscious and anesthetized albino rat. J Neurochem 28:897–916
12. Kamoto Y, Sadato N, Yonekura Y, Tsuchiya T, Uematsu H, Waki A, Uchida K, Baba H, Imura S, Konishi J (1998) Visualization of cervical spinal cord with ^{18}FDG and high resolution PET. J Comput Assist Tomogr 22:487–491
13. Huang S-C, Phelps ME, Hoffman EJ, Sideris K, Selin CJ, Kuhl DE (1980) Noninvasive determination of local cerebral metabolic rate of glucose in man. Am J Physiol 238:69–82
14. Kim CK, Gupta NC, Chandramouli B, Alavi A (1994) Standardized uptake values of FDG: body surface area correction is preferable to body weight correction. J Nucl Med 35:164–167
15. Mazziotta JC, Phelps ME, Plummer D, Kuhl DE (1981) Quantitation in positron emission computed tomography: 5. Physical-anatomical effects. J Comput Assist Tomogr 5:734–743
16. Mazziotta JC, Phelps ME, Miller J, Kuhl DE (1981) Tomographic mapping of human cerebral metabolism: normal unstimulated state. Neurology 31:503–516

17. Kawahara N, Baba H, Nagata S, Kikuchi Y, Tomita K, Nomura S (1991) Experimental studies on the spinal cord evoked potentials in cervical spine distraction injuries. In: Shimoji K, Kurokawa T, Tamaki T, Willis WD Jr (eds) Spinal cord monitoring and electrodiagnosis. Springer, Berlin Heidelberg, pp 107–115
18. Murakami H, Tomita K, Baba H, Yamada Y, Morikawa S, Horii T (1995) Central cord syndrome secondary to hyperflexion injury of the cervical spine in a child. A case report. J Spinal Disord 8:494–498
19. Baba H, Maezawa Y, Uchida K, Imura S, Kawahara N, Tomita K, Kudo M (1997) Three-dimensional topographic analysis of spinal accessory motoneurons under chronic mechanical compression: an experimental study in the mouse. J Neurol 244:222–229

Dynamics of Cauda Equina Compression in Lumbar Spinal Stenosis

KEISUKE TAKAHASHI and IWAO SHIMA

Summary. The effects of mechanical loading to the lumbar spine on the cauda equina in patients with lumbar spinal stenosis were assessed by epidural pressure measurements. The study of epidural pressure measurements demonstrated that the local extradural pressure at the stenotic level is changed by posture and walking. The pressure was low on lying and sitting, and high on standing. Notably, The pressure was increased by lumbar extension, but decreased by forward flexion. Changes in the epidural pressure correlated with the occurrence of clinical symptoms of nerve root compression. These pressure changes may explain the postural dependency of symptoms in lumbar spinal stenosis. The epidural pressure also changed at walking in patients with neurogenic claudication. The change in epidural pressure had a pattern of increase and decrease, and this oscillation was repeated during walking. The degree of pressure increase was related to lumbar posture during walking. The epidural pressure was high at simple walking, and low at walking with lumbar flexion. Intermittent compression to the nerve roots during walking might have an important role in the pathogenesis of neurogenic intermittent claudication.

Key words. Lumbar spine, Cauda equina, Lumbar spinal stenosis, Epidural pressure, Neurogenic claudication

Introduction

Motion and loading of the lumbar spine induce a bulging disc and a buckling ligamentum flavum, which influence the size of the spinal canal. These changes do not influence the nerve roots in the normal spine, but influence the compression level to the nerve root in spinal stenosis. As we know from the results of functional myelogram, the dural sac is more compressed by lumbar extension at intervertebral disc level than lumbar flexion in lumbar spinal stenosis. Cauda equina and radicular symptoms with lumbar spinal stenosis are often related to certain posture. Pain and numbness in the buttock, thigh, and leg are provoked either by walking or by prolonged

Department of Orthopaedic Surgery, Ishikawa Prefectural Central Hospital, 153 Minami-shinbo Kanazawa, Ishikawa 920-8350 Japan standing in the upright posture. On the contrary, symptomatic relief can be obtained by lying, sitting, or standing with lumbar flexion.

Neurogenic claudication is the most common presenting symptom in lumbar spinal stenosis. Patients with neurogenic claudication also complain of posture-related pain. Patients feel more comfortable walking in a stooped posture [1,2]. For example, patients could ride a bicycle without symptoms [3]. Walking behind a shopping cart or lawn mower or walking up an incline or stairs is generally better tolerated than simple walking or walking down an incline or stairs [4]. These phenomena suggest that there are probably dynamic factors that are important in the pathogenesis of the clinical presentation of cauda equina and radicular symptoms in spinal stenosis. However, the exact mechanisms for there symptoms developing or being relieved by lumbar posture are uncertain. Furthermore, the pathogenesis of neurogenic claudication remains obscure. It is postulated that the pressure to the nerve root may change as a function of posture and walking. We could measure compressive forces to the dural sac at a stenotic level by inserting the pressure transducer into the epidural space. In this chapter we demonstrate the changes in epidural pressure with various postures and walking in patients with lumbar spinal stenosis.

Epidural Pressure Measurements

Epidural pressure was measured in 50 patients who had cauda equina and/or radicular symptoms at L4-5 level with lumbar spinal stenosis. All patients' myelograms showed hourglass defects or incomplete blocks at this level. As control subjects, there were seven individuals who had a normal spinal canal.

A flexible pressure transducer was used for the measurements and continuous measuring of epidural pressure in various forms of motion was possible. A Mikro-tip catheter transducer (SPC 330A, Millar Instruments Houston, Tx, USA) was used as a pressure transducer; This transducer is flexible with a diameter of 1.2mm. A Tuohy needle was inserted into the epidural space by loss-of-resistance method through the L5/S1 interlaminar space. The catheter transducer was inserted into the epidural space and the tip of transducer was placed at the L4/5 disc level. The course was monitored by TV fluoroscopy. The transducer was connected to a pressure amplifier (AP-641G, Nihon Koden, Tokyo, Japan) and a thermal recorder (WR-7300, Graphtech Tokyo, Japan). Epidural pressure was measured continuously.

Various postures were studied: supine, supine with knee flexion, prone, prone with lumbar sitting extension, sitting in a chair, sitting cross-legged, Kneeling, standing upright, standing with lumbar extension, and standing with lumbar flexion. In another study, patients walked on treadmill at a velocity of 2km/h, and the epidural pressure was continuously measured during walking. The pressure was measured during two different kinds of walking: simple walking (without lumbar flexion) and walking with lumbar flexion.

Postural Influences on Epidural Pressure

Epidural pressure was found to be affected by posture. Epidural pressure was 18.0 ± 6.9mmHg in supine posture, and 17.0 ± 8.1mmHg in supine with knee flexion. There was no difference statistically between the epidural pressure of supine with and

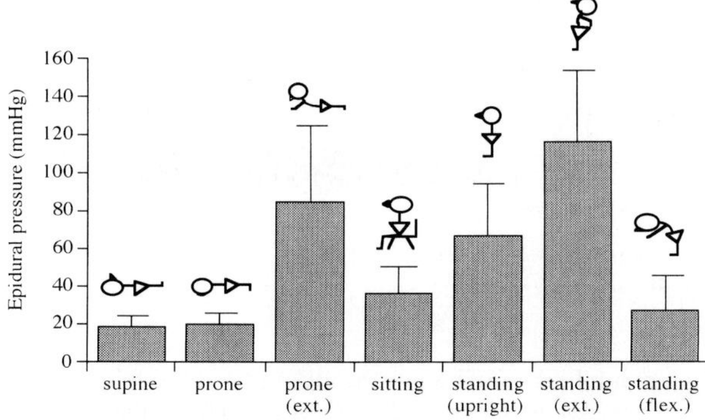

Fig. 1. Summary of epidural pressure in various postures. The pressure was low in the lying and sitting posture, and high in the standing posture. The pressure was increased especially by lumbar extension in the prone and standing position

without knee flexion. In prone posture the pressure was 13.1 ± 6.0 mmHg, and was remarkably increased by maximum extension to 85.0 ± 39.2 mmHg. There was a significant difference between the pressure with or without lumbar extension in prone posture ($P < 0.001$). Three kinds of sitting posture were investigated. The epidural pressure was 36.4 ± 15.1 mmHg when sitting in a chair, 41.6 ± 19.4 mmHg when Kneeling, and 34.9 ± 19.3 mmHg when seated cross-legged. There were no differences statistically between the three forms of sitting. In standing posture the epidural pressure was 66.9 ± 27.5 mmHg at upright position, and was markedly increased by a maximum extension to 116.5 ± 38.4 mmHg, but decreased by a 30° forward flexion to 27.3 ± 19.7 mmHg. There was a significant difference between the epidural pressure resulting from standing with extension and standing with flexion ($P < 0.001$) and between upright standing and standing with flexion ($P < 0.01$). The epidural pressure on standing with lumbar extension was 116 mmHg, which was about six times higher than lying posture. A summary of epidural pressures caused by various postures is shown in Fig. 1 [5].

Changes in Epidural Pressure During Walking

The change in epidural pressure had a pattern of increase and decrease, and this pattern was repeated during walking [6] (Fig. 2). Intermittent pressure increase was seen about 90 times per minute when walking at a velocity of 2 km/h. The epidural pressure was high with simple walking and low at walking with lumbar flexion [6] (Fig. 3). In simple walking with upright lumbar posture, peak values of pressure increase were 82.8 ± 14.2 mmHg in patients with spinal stenosis, and 34.2 ± 4.9 mmHg in individuals with a normal canal. Peak values of the pressure increase were significantly different ($P < 0.01$) between spinal stenosis and normal individuals. In walking with lumbar flexion, peak values of pressure increase decreased to 36.8 ± 8.2 mmHg in patients with spinal stenosis, and 27.4 ± 11 mmHg in individuals with a normal canal. The peak value of the pressure increase was significantly different ($P < 0.01$) between the simple walking and walking with lumbar flexion in patients

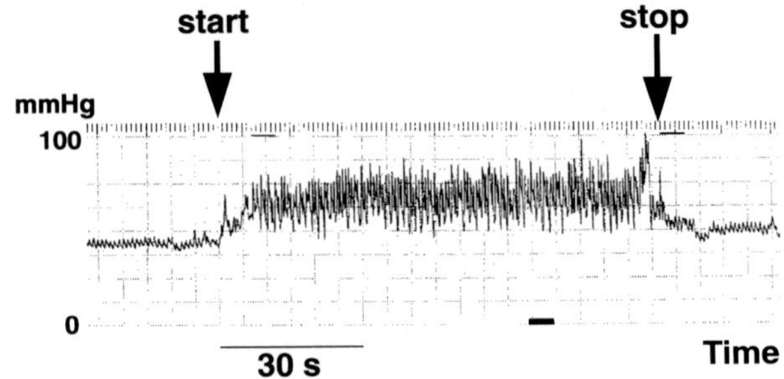

FIG. 2. Changes in epidural pressure before, during, and after walking. When simple walking was started, epidural pressure was increased and during walking there was a repeated pattern of increase and decrease. The patient could not walk when leg pain developed. When walking, was stopped, the epidural pressure immediately decreased and the leg pain subsided

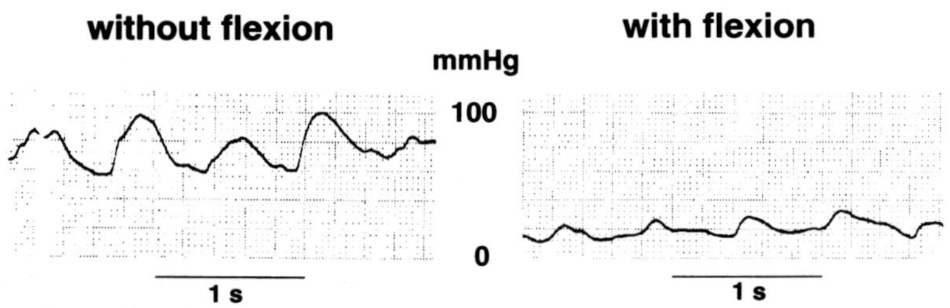

FIG. 3. Changes in epidural pressure during simple walking (*left*) and stooped walking (*right*) in the same patient with spinal stenosis. Oscillation of the epidural pressure during simple walking was significantly higher than when the patient walked with lumbar flexion

with lumbar spinal stenosis. There was no statistical difference between simple walking in normal individuals and walking with lumbar flexion in patients with lumbar spinal stenosis.

This pattern of changes in pressure might be explained by spinal movement during walking. It was the response of the pelvis and the spine to the action of the lower limbs that produced the characteristic movements during walking. Thurston and Harris [7] showed a spinal movement in a wave pattern in the sagittal plane during walking. The increase of epidural pressure during walking was seen at the double supporting phase in the gait cycle [8]. This result corresponded to the data showing that maximum backwards tilt of the pelvis occurred at the double supporting phase. Flexion and extension of the lumbar spine in the sagittal plane was continuously repeated during walking. There was a significant difference between epidural pressure in standing with forward flexion (27.3 ± 19.7 mmHg) and with maximum extension (116.5 ± 38.4 mmHg). These repeated movements of the lumbar spine during walking thus induce epidural pressure changes with a pattern of increase and decrease.

Postural Dependency of Clinical Symptoms in Lumbar Spinal Stenosis

As a cause of the symptoms of spinal stenosis, mechanical compression has a direct effect on the nerve roots. The size of the spinal canal significantly changes when the spine is extended or loaded [9,10]. These size variations might explain the postural dependency of the stenotic symptoms in some patients. The results of epidural pressure measurements revealed the magnitude of the epidural pressure of patients with spinal stenosis in various posture. According to this study, the most important factor that will lead to an increase of epidural pressure is lumbar extension. In standing with extension, the epidural pressure was 116 mmHg, and cauda equina and radicular symptoms were generally elicited in patients with spinal stenosis. The increase of epidural pressure with posture may induce compression of the cauda equina and impair, for example, the blood supply to the cauda equina, so that cauda equina and radicular symptoms may appear.

Pathogenesis of Neurogenic Claudication

Mechanisms of neurogenic claudication have been debated by various authors. Some authors have suggested that as a cause of neurogenic claudication mechanical compression which can be induced by standing and walking might directly affect the nerve roots [11–13]. Other have supported the theory that an ischemic mechanism intervenes at root level. [14–17] Currently, these two processes are accepted to explains the pathogenesis of neurogenic claudication. However, the specific causes of the neurogenic claudication in an individual patient are uncertain, because both of these causes are dynamic in nature [18].

In this study we have been able to monitor the dynamic changes within the spinal canal during walking. When a patient was standing in a stooped posture, epidural pressure was low. Epidural pressure was quickly increased when simple walking started, and a repeated pattern of increased and decreased pressure occurred during walking. A pattern of increase and decrease and the magnitude of the increase were not changed even after symptoms appeared with walking. The patient had to stop walking as a result of pain. By stopping walking and by standing with lumbar flexion, epidural pressure was immediately decreased to the level before walking commenced. The magnitude of epidural pressure was significantly different in walking with or without lumbar flexion. The magnitude of the pressure and the degree of the pressure increase during walking with lumbar flexion were lower than without lumbar flexion. Walking with lumbar flexion might be associated with few or no symptoms because of low pressure and low degree of increase. However, neurogenic claudication occurs on simple walking. This may be caused by a frequent repeated increase in epidural pressure. An intermittent increase in the epidural pressure at the stenotic level may induce intermittent compression of the cauda equina. It has been reported that intermittent compression to the cauda equina also reduces nerve conduction properties [19]. This supports the theory that intermittent compression of the nerve roots during walking in patients with spinal stenosis might induce physiological changes in the nerve roots, as in nerve root ischemia. An intermittent increase of the epidural pressure during walking may have a important role in the pathogenesis of neurogenic claudication.

Conclusion

The study of epidural pressure measurements in patients with lumbar spinal stenosis revealed that the compression level on the cauda equina is not stable but varied depending upon the posture and walking. There was a close relationship between the increase in epidural pressure and the symptom appearance. Continuous compression to the cauda equina in an upright standing position and intermittent compression to the cauda equina during walking were found to provoke symptoms in lumbar spinal stenosis.

References

1. Dyck P (1979) The stoop-test in lumbar entrapment radiculopathy. Spine 4:89–92
2. Dong GX, Porter RW (1989) Walking and cycling tests in neurogenic and intermittent claudication. Spine 14:965–969
3. Dyck P, Doyle JB (1977) Bicycle test of Van Gelderen in diagnosis of intermittent cauda equina compression syndrome. J Neurosurg 46:667–670
4. Porter RW (1989) Spinal stenosis. Semin Orthop 1:97–111
5. Takahashi K, Miyazaki T, Takino T, Matsui T, Tomita K (1995) Epidural pressure measurements in patients with lumbar spinal stenosis. Spine 20:450–453
6. Takahashi K (1996) Dynamic influences of posture and walking on the stenotic spinal canal. In: Weinstein JN, Gordon SL (eds) Low back pain: a scientific and clinical overview. American Academy of Orthopaedic Surgeons, Rosemont, pp 741–750
7. Thurston AJ, Harris JD (1983) Normal kinematics of the lumbar spine and pelvis. Spine 8:199–205
8. Takahashi K, Kagechika K, Takino T, Matsui T, Miyazaki T, Shima I (1995) Changes in epidural pressure during walking in patients with lumbar spinal stenosis. Spine 20:2746–2749
9. Pening L, Wilmink JT (1981) Biomechanics of lumbosacral dural sac. A study of flexion-extension myelography. Spine 6:398–408
10. Wilmink JT, Pening L (1983) Influence of spinal posture on abnormalities demonstrated by lumbar myelography. AJNR 4:656–658
11. Ehni G (1969) Significance of the small lumbar canal: Cauda equina compression syndrome due to spondylosis. J Neurosurg 31:490–494
12. Verbiest H (1955) Further experiences on the pathologic influence of a developmental narrowness of the bony lumbar vertebral canal. J Bone Joint Surg (Br) 37:576–583
13. Wilson CB (1969) Significance of the small lumbar spinal canal: Cauda equina compression syndromes due to spondylosis. J Neurosurg 31:499–506
14. Blau JN, Louge V (1961) Intermittent claudication of the cauda equina. Lancet 1:1081–1086
15. Cavanaugh GJ, Svein J, Holman CB, Jonson RM (1968) "Pseudoclaudication" syndrome produced by compression of cauda equina. JAMA 206:2477–2481
16. Watanabe R, Parke WW (1986) Vascular and neural pathology of lumbosacral spinal stenosis. J Neurosurg 64:64–70
17. Porter RW, Ward D (1992) Cauda equina dysfunction, the significance of multilevel pathology. Spine 17:9–15

18. Andersson GBJ, McNeill TW (1992) Definition and classification of lumbar spinal stenosis. In: Andersson GBJ, McNeill TW (eds) Lumbar spinal stenosis. Mosby Year Book, St Louis, pp 9–15
19. Konno S, Olmarker K, Byrod G, Rydevik B, Kikuchi S (1995) Intermittent cauda equina compression: An experimental study on the porcine cauda equina with analyses of nerve impulse conduction properties. Spine 20:1223–1226

Neurophysiological Changes of the Nerve Root Induced by Mechanical Compression

SHIGERU KOBAYASHI, HIDEZO YOSHIZAWA, SADAAKI NAKAI, and MASATO NAKAGAWA

Summary. Physiological investigations of nerve root compression were performed experimentally using dog models. The blood flow, partial oxygen pressure, tissue pH, and action potential were more severely affected at the proximal side than at the distal side when the nerve root was compressed. When the clamp was released, the blood flow at the proximal side and the partial oxygen pressure at both sides were almost completely restored, whereas the blood flow at the distal side and the tissue pH at both sides after 60 g and 30 g force compression did not recover and persisted at the reduced level. These functional changes induced by compression not only can be caused by mechanical nerve fiber deformation, but also may be a consequence of changes in the microcirculation and endoneurial (cerebrospinal fluid) flow in the nerve root due to formation of intraradicular edema. This intraradicular edema may then lead to acidosis, with subsequent impairment of the nerve function. This suggests that intraradicular inflammatory reactions are critical factors in the development of pain associated with nerve root compression.

Key words. Nerve root, Compression, Radiculopathy, Cerebrospinal fluid, Intraradicular edema

Introduction

Compression of the lumbar nerve root is a frequent clinical problem. An important manifestation of the degenerative lumbar spine is pain radiating to the legs, also called sciatica. In 1926, Schmorl [1] reported the existence of nodules originating from the intervertebral disc tissue that protruded into the adjacent vertebrae, the abnormal cavity, or the spinal canal. However, it was not until 1934 that Mixter and Barr [2] found a correlation between these intraspinal nodules and sciatica. Since then, the main research efforts in the field of low back pain have been focused on the intervertebral disc, thus leading to substantial knowledge about the physiology and pathology of intervertebral discs.

Department of Orthopaedic Surgery, Fujita Health University School of Medicine, 1-98 Dengakugakubo, Kutsukake-cho, Toyoake, Aichi 470-1192, Japan

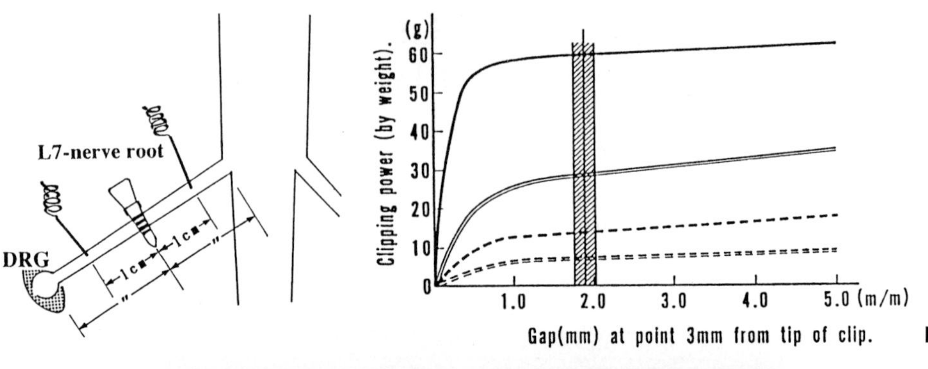

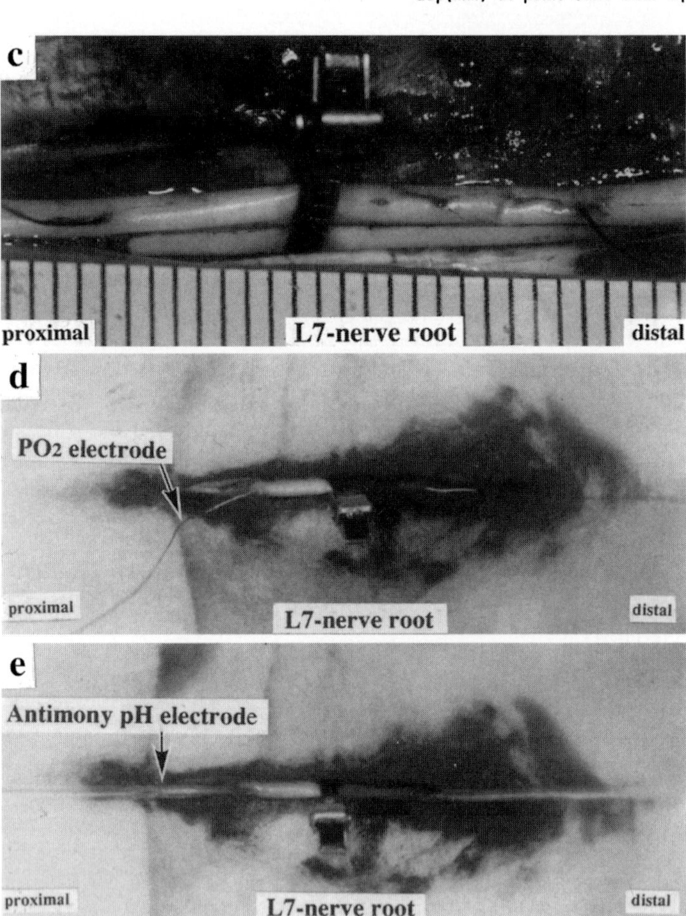

Fig. 1. a–e

FIG. 1. **a** Clamping of the seventh lumbar nerve root. The nerve root was clamped with a clip for microvascular suturing at the midpoint between the dural sac and the dorsal root ganglion (*DRG*). **b** A clip for microvascular suturing and its natural curve. The compression forces used in this study were 60, 30, 15, and 7.5 gram force (gf). **c** Two electrodes measuring the intraradicular blood flow at the proximal and distal sides of the clip. **d** Two electrodes measuring the intraradicular partial oxygen pressure (PO$_2$) at the proximal and distal sides of the clip. **e** Two electrodes measuring the intraradicular pH at the proximal and distal sides of the clip. **f** Four electrodes measuring the action potential of the nerve root at the proximal and distal sides of the clip

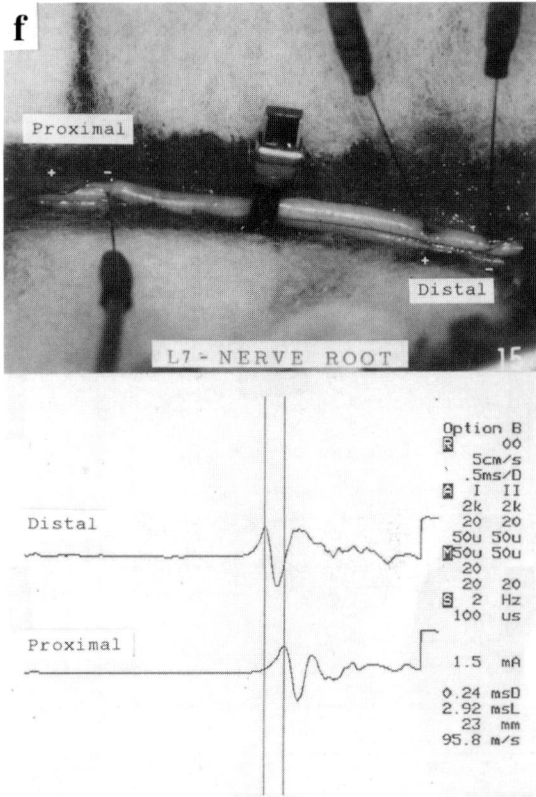

Many papers about the reaction pattern of nerve roots to experimentally applied compression have been published [3–14]. Consequently, it has been considered that development of radiculopathy associated with degenerative diseases of the spine is related to the circulation and metabolism in the nerve root. However, the basic pathophysiology of these conditions is not fully understood. The aim of the present experimental investigation was to study the effects of mechanical compression on the blood flow, partial oxygen pressure (PO$_2$), tissue pH, and action potential of the nerve root.

Materials and Methods

Ninety-eight adult dogs, weighing 15 kg to 25 kg, were anesthetized with an intramuscular injection of 3 ml of ketalar (ketamine 50 mg/ml; Warner-Lambert, Morris Plains, NJ, USA) and ventilated with a respirator under general anesthesia (O$_2$: 3 ml/min, N$_2$O: 3 ml/min, halothane: 1.5 ml/min). The femoral artery was cannulated, and the systemic arterial blood pressure and blood gases were monitored in all animals throughout the experiment. The body temperature was recorded with a rectal thermometer. Each animal was thus maintained at a constant physiologic level.

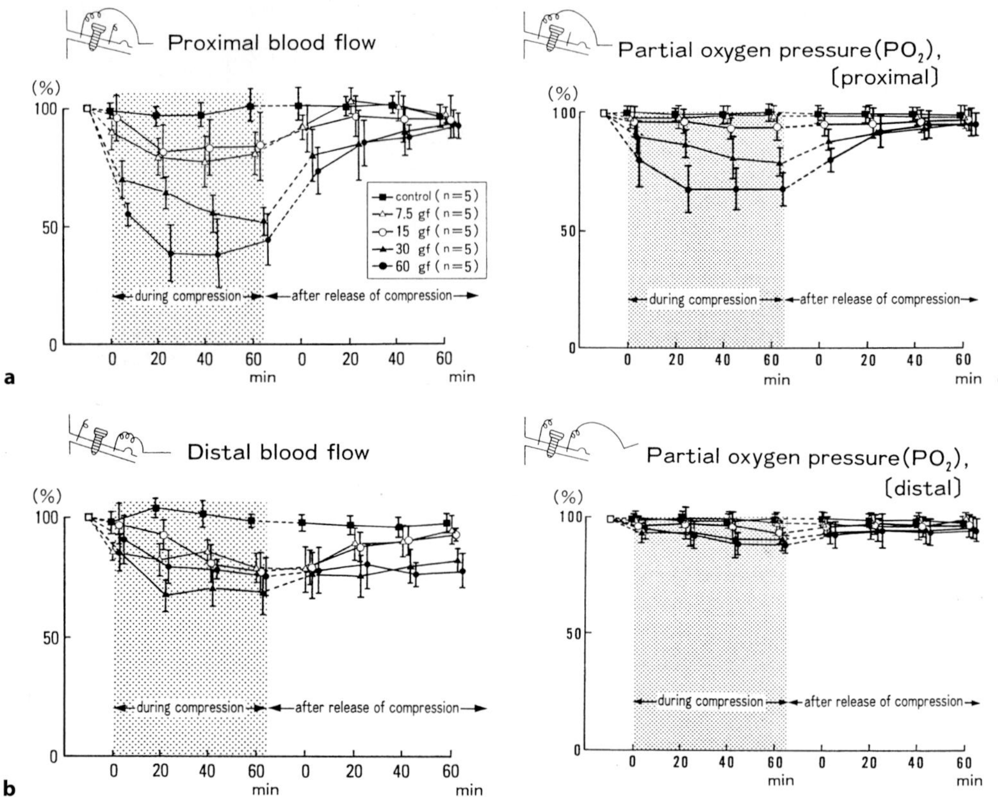

FIG. 2. **a–d**

The animal was placed in the prone position on a frame. The sixth and seventh lumbar laminae were removed, and the seventh lumbar nerve root was exposed widely on the left side. The nerve root was clamped with a clip for microvascular suturing at the midpoint between the dural sac and the dorsal root ganglion (Fig. 1a). The nerve root was exposed to compression for one hour at 7.5, 15, 30, and 60 g force (gf) clipping power (Fig. 1b). Measurements of the blood flow ($n = 25$), partial oxygen pressure; (PO$_2$) ($n = 25$), tissue pH ($n = 25$), and nerve root action potential ($n = 23$) were repeated over a period of 1 h after release of clipping. These measurements were performed in the posterior root at both the proximal and distal sides of the clip.

The electrochemically generated hydrogen washout method [15] (Model DHM-3001 Tissue Blood Flow Meter: M.T. Giken, Tokyo, Japan) was used to measure the blood flow in the posterior nerve root. A small electrode with a diameter of 200 μm (MHD-60: M.T. Giken) was inserted into the nerve root (Fig. 1c). We used a polarized voltage of 600 mV and a direct current of 20 A for 25 s to electrochemically generate hydrogen in the nerve root. PO$_2$ in the nerve root was measured by the polarographical method (Model POG-5000S PO$_2$ Meter: M.T. Giken) [16]. After calibration, a PO$_2$ needle-type electrode with a diameter of 10 μm was inserted into the posterior nerve root (Fig. 1d). A differential meter (Model FD-223: WPI, Sarasota, FL, USA) was used to measure the tissue pH in the nerve root [17]. An antimony pH electrode (Product

FIG. 2. **a,b** Change of the intraradicular blood flow volume due to compression. **a** At the proximal side of the clip. **b** At the distal side of the clip. **c,d** Change of PO_2 due to nerve root compression. **c** At the proximal side of the clip. **d** At the distal side of the clip. **e,f** Change of the tissue pH due to nerve root compression. **e** At the proximal side of the clip. **f** At the distal side of the clip

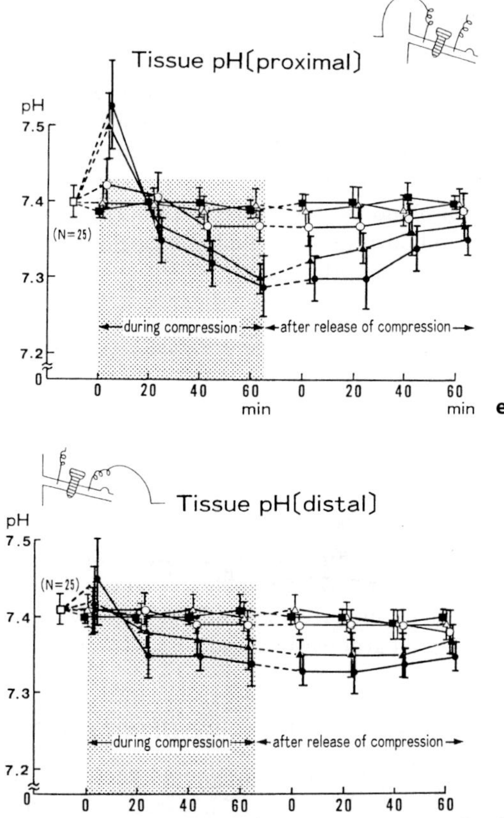

801: Diamond General Ann Arbor, Michigan, USA) with a diameter of 80 μm was inserted into the posterior nerve root, after calibrating the electrode in the standard pH solution before the experiment (Fig. 1e).

Finally, nerve root conduction studies were carried out using an electro-myometer (Dantec Neuromatic 2000c, Skovlunde, Denmark). The sciatic nerve was exposed at the thigh and stimulated with 0.1-ms square-wave voltage pulses at a rate of 2/s using a bipolar electrode. The stimulus intensity was adjusted to 1.5–2 times the motor threshold and 20 responses were summated. The amplitude was recorded directly from the seventh lumbar posterior nerve root at the distal and proximal sides of the clip, and then the sensory nerve conduction velocity was calculated indirectly (Fig. 1f).

Results

The Change of Intraradicular Blood Flow

The intraradicular blood flow at the proximal and distal sides of the clip were 27.1 ± 6.4 and 26.4 ± 5.8 ml/100 g per min (mean ± S.D., $n = 25$), respectively, before clamping the nerve root. The intraradicular blood flow volume at both the proximal and distal sides of the clip decreased during compression. The proximal side of the clip, however, showed a more distinct drop of the flow volume than the distal side on applying compression of 30 and 60 gf. The proximal flow volume decreased by about 40% and 60%, and the distal blood flow volume decreased by about 30% and 25% at 30 and 60 gf, respectively. The proximal and distal flow volume decreased by about 25% on applying compression on 7.5 and 15 gf. When the clamp was released, the proximal blood flow was almost completely restored within 1 h in all groups. The distal blood flow, however, did not recover and persisted at the reduced level after release of compression (Fig. 2a,b).

The Change of PO_2 in the Nerve Root

The PO_2 at the proximal and distal sides of the clip was 36.9 ± 4.2 and 38.0 ± 4.6 mmHg (mean $\pm$ S.D., $n = 25$), respectively, before clamping the nerve root. It was more severely disturbed at the proximal side than the distal side due to compression of 30 and 60 gf. The proximal PO_2 decreased by about 20% and 30% due to 30 and 60 gf compression, respectively, and the distal reduced by about 10% due to both 30 and 60 gf compression. At both sides with compression of 15 and 7.5 gf, the partial oxygen pressure did not show apparent changes during the experiment. When the clamp was released, the proximal and distal PO_2 values were almost completely restored within 1 h in all groups (Fig. 2c,d).

The Change of Tissue pH in the Nerve Root

The tissue pH at the proximal and distal sides of the clip was 7.40 ± 0.03 and 7.41 ± 0.04 (mean $\pm$ S.D., $n = 25$), respectively, before clamping the nerve root. Just after the nerve root was compressed, the proximal and distal sides of the clip showed alkalosis which might have been induced by extravasation of the blood serum [18,19]. This was followed by acidosis at both sides on compression of 30 and 60 gf, probably indicating activation of anaerobic glycolysis [20–22]. The degree of acidosis at the proximal side was greater than at the distal side.

The tissue pH did not show any apparent change during the experiment on nerve root compression of 7.5 and 15 gf. When the compression was released, the tissue pH at both sides did not recover and persisted at the reduced level of 60 and 30 gf (Fig. 2.e,f).

The Change of Nerve Root Action Potential

The proximal amplitude showed a transient augmentation immediately after clipping and the degree of augmentation was maximum on 30 gf compression. This transient augmentation indicated that the blood flow of the ascending radicular artery was intercepted by compression of slow onset, leading to ischemic changes in the nerve root (Fig. 3) [23,24]. The amplitude at the proximal side of compression at 30 and 60 g force decreased by about 30% and 80%, respectively, during 1-h compression. The changes in the amplitude due to compression of 7.5 and 15 gf were minimal (Fig. 4a). This change of amplitude might be attributed to mechanical nerve fiber deformation.

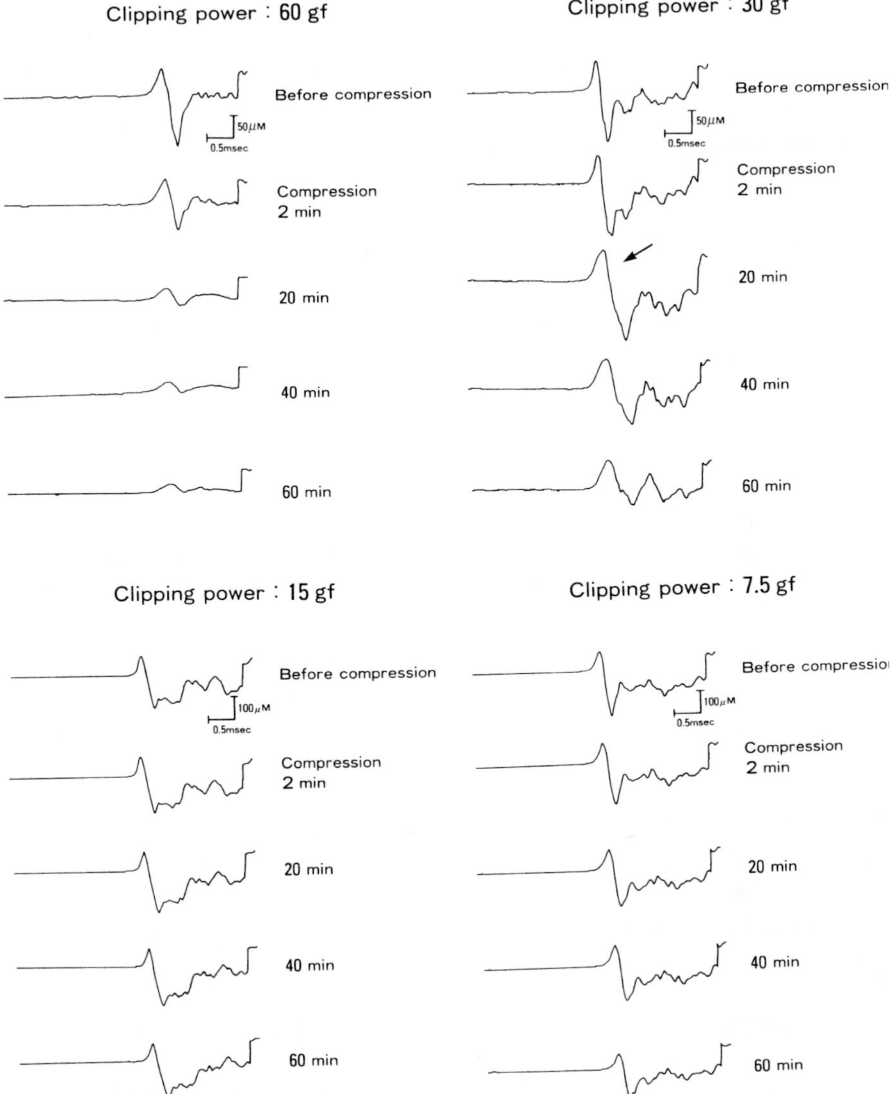

FIG. 3. Amplitude at the proximal side of compression at 60, 30, 15, and 7.5 gf. The proximal amplitude showed a transient augumentation just after clipping, and the degree of augumentation was maximum at 30 gf compression (*arrow*)

At the distal side of the compression, the amplitude did not show any apparent change during the experiment (Fig. 4b).

The nerve root conduction velocity was 91.5 ± 6.4 m/s (mean ± S.D., $n = 23$) before clamping the nerve root. It decreased by about 40% and 50% on applying 30 and 60 gf compression, respectively. When the clamp was released, nerve root conduction velocity did not recover and persisted at the reduced level. It also did not

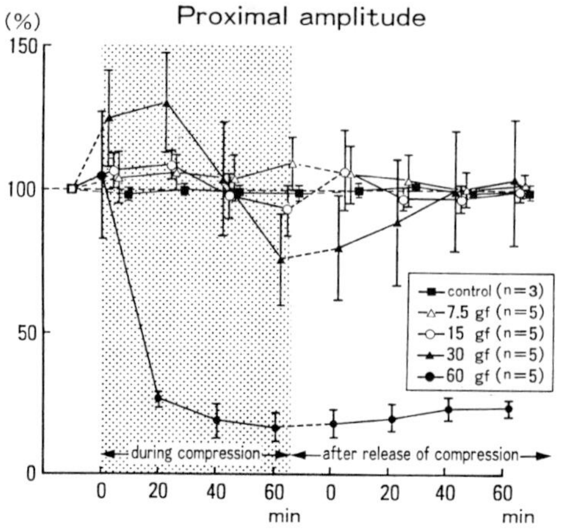

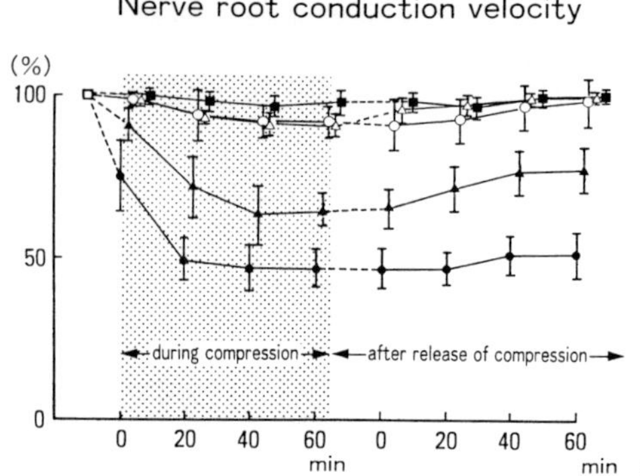

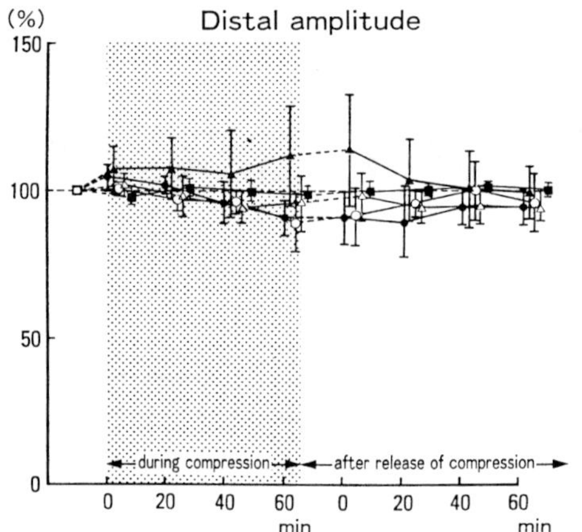

FIG. 4. **a,b** Change of the amplitude due to nerve root compression. **a** At the proximal side of the clip. **b** At the distal side of the clip. The proximal amplitude showed a transient augmentation just after clipping and the degree of augmentation was maximum at 30 gf compression. Then the amplitude at the proximal side of compression at 30 and 60 gf obviously decreased during compression. **c** Change of the conduction velocity due to nerve root compression. The nerve root conduction velocity was more severely disturbed at 60 and 30 gf compression

show any apparent change during the experiment due to 15 and 7.5 gf compression (Fig. 4c).

Discussion

We examined the vasculature of the extradural nerve root in dogs with the aid of high-speed serial photography after injecting India ink into the aorta [25,26]. The radicular artery ascends while the radicular vein descends along the nerve root, at least in the epidural space. Branches of these radicular vessels nourish the nerve roots through the intrinsic vessels on their way. This indicates that the arterial blood supply of the nerve roots in the epidural space comes from the periphery (Fig. 7a).

The nerve root, which is surrounded by cerebrospinal fluid (CSF), has only scanty connective tissue forming the permeable root sheath (Fig. 5a,b). In fact, when horseradish peroxidase (HRP) was injected into the subarachnoid space, HRP was observed in the endoneurial space of the nerve root when examined under the transmission

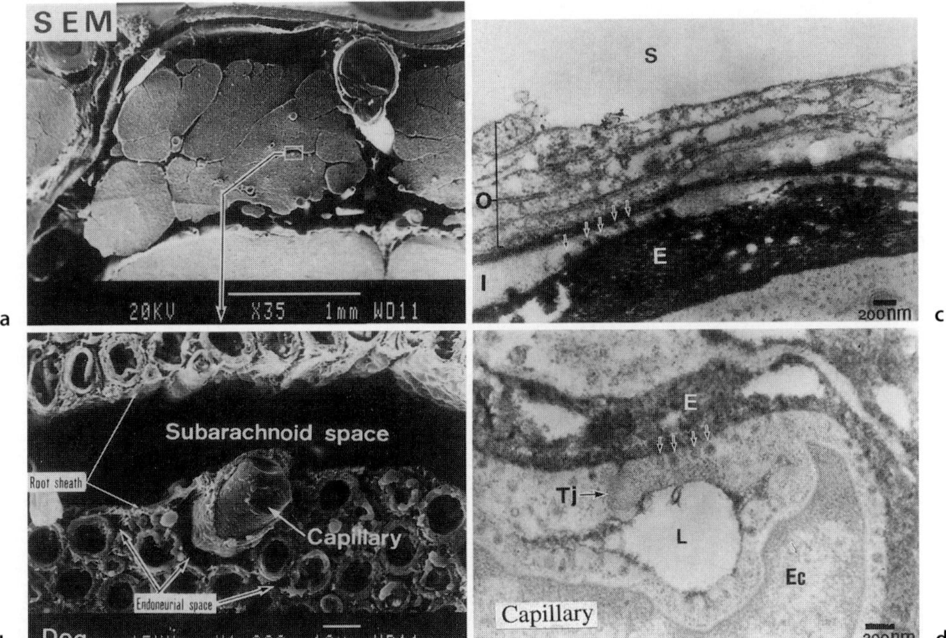

Fig. 5a–f. Electron micrographs of a lumbar nerve root. **a,b** Scanning electron micrographs (*SEM*) of the nerve root obtained after injection of methylmethacrylate into the aorta **c,d** Transverse section of the nerve root seen under a transmmision electron microscope after injecting horseradish peroxidase (HRP) into the subarachnoid space. **c** At 1 h, pinocytotic vesicles (*arrows*) containing the reaction product in the inner layers are thought to move toward the endoneurial space. There is a direct continuity between the endoneurial space of the nerve root and the subarachnoid space. The nerve root sheath does not act as a diffusion barrier like the perineurium of the peripheral nerves. **d** The electron-dense reaction product passed through the nerve root sheath and entered into the capillary lumen in the endoneurial space. In the endothelial cells of the capillaries, pinocytotic vesicles containing the reaction product, about 70 nm in diameter, are throught to move toward the luminal surface by retrograde vesicular transport (*arrows*). However, the tight junctions between the adjacent endothelial cells were never penetrated by HRP. Consequently, cerebrospinal fluid (CSF) invaded the endoneurial flow to the peripheral nerve, and might also have drained into the venous system directly through the endoneurial space. **e,f** Transverse sections of the nerve root segments seen under the electron microscope. HRP was injected intravenously after one-hour compression of 60 gf. **e** The dark reaction product of HRP leaked out of the capillaries under compression. HRP is present in the endoneurial space. The lumen has been cleared of HRP by perfusion fixation. **f** The tight junction between two endothelial cells is broken down and filled with the reaction product of HRP (paracellular transport). Many pinocytotic vesicles appear to carry the reaction product of HRP away from the capillary lumen (*arrows*). HRP is present in the endoneurial space. *E*, endoneurial space; *Ec*, endothelial cell; *I*, inner layer of the nerve root sheath; *L*, capillary lumen; *O*, outer layer of the nerve root sheath; *S*, subarachnoid space; *Tj*, tight junction

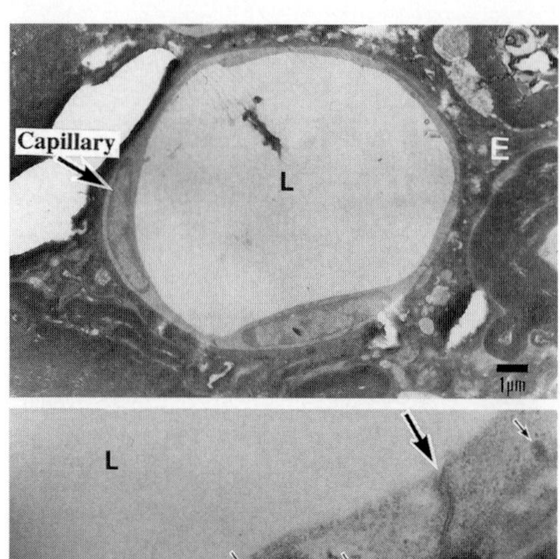

FIG. 5. *Continued*

electron microscope (Fig. 5c) [7]. HRP also appeared in the intraradicular veins through the endothelial transport system in the wall of capillaries (Fig. 5d). This means that it is important for the normal function of the nerve root to be surrounded by a pulsating CSF, and that disturbance of the CSF flow may have an adverse effect on the nerve root.

The capillaries in the nerve root are all of the continuous type. Their endothelial cells are linked with tight junctions, thus constituting a blood–nerve harrier. This barrier in the normal nerve root blocks extravasation of various protein tracers like HRP. To find out what sort of circulatory disturbance will occur in the compressed part of the nerve root, we examined the status of this barrier in the nerve root of dogs directly after 1-h compression, using HRP [7]. A marked extravasation of HRP was induced by 30 and 60 gf compression. After a compression of 15 gf, there was extravasation of HRP only at the peripheral portion of the compressed nerve root (Fig. 6).

With electron microscopy, extravasation of HRP was observed in the endoneurial space between the nerve fibers, especially the perivascular spaces. The tight junctions of the endothelial cells of the capillaries were open, and the dark-stained HRP product extravasated through the junctions into the endothelial space (Fig. 5e,f). This increased paracellular and transcellular transport of the tracer indicated breakdown of the blood–nerve barrier, leading to edema formation in the nerve root.

The blood flow, PO_2, tissue pH, and action potential were more severely affected at the proximal side than at the distal side when the nerve root was compressed at 30 and 60 gf. This may be explained by the vascular system of the nerve root as the degree of ischemic changes at the proximal side was greater than at the distal side. That is, the intrinsic blood circulation in the nerve root at the proximal side was more severely

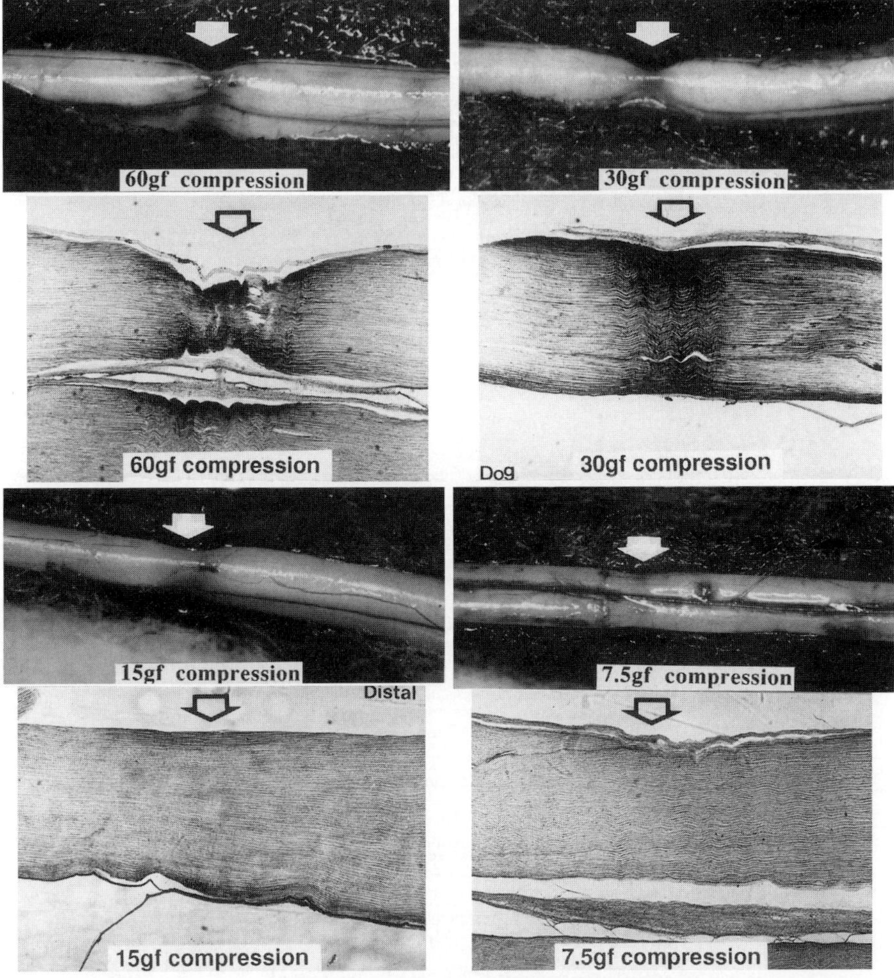

FIG. 6. Just after release of the nerve root compression (*upper*) and longitudinal sections of the nerve root segments after 1-h compression of 60(**a**), 30(**c**), 15(**b**), and 7.5(**d**) gf (*lower*). After intravenous injection of HRP, marked extravasation of HRP in the nerve root was induced after one-hour compression of 60 and 30 gf. After compression of 15 gf, there was extravasation of HRP only at the peripheral portion of the compressed nerve root (*arrows*). There was no extravasation of HRP after compression of 7.5 gf

disturbed while the blood flow at the distal side could be maintained to some degree through the branches when the ascending radicular arteries were clamped together with the nerve root (Fig. 7b).

When the clamp was released, the proximal blood flow of the radicular artery was restored within 1 h in all groups. The distal blood flow and tissue pH at both sides, however, did not recover and persisted at the reduced level after release of the compression at 30 and 60 gf. It is difficult to explain in terms of hemodynamics why these

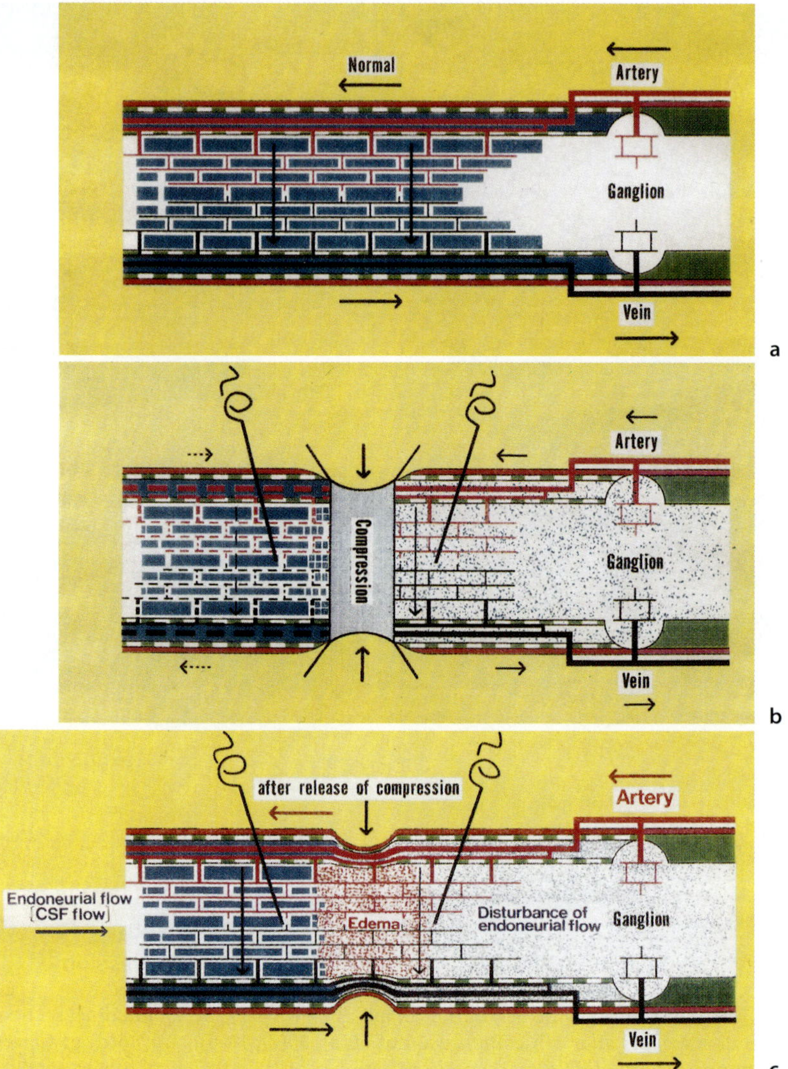

Fig. 7. **a** Normal state of the nerve root. The nerve fibers are soaked in endoneurial fluid (*CSF*). **b** During compression. **c** After release of compression. The distal side of the nerve root is not soaked in CSF although the vascular system has resumed its function. (From [13], with permission)

FIG. 8. The pain mechanism created by the intraradicular acidosis associated with nerve root compression

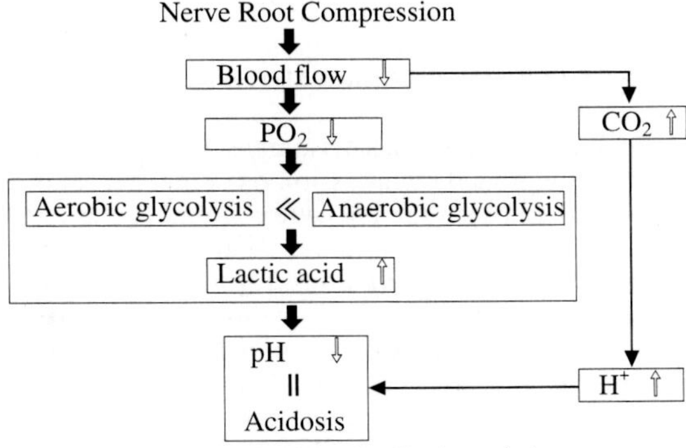

changes did not recover when the clamp was released. We speculated that these phenomena might be due to the effect of intraradicular edema induced by mechanical compression, combined with endoneurial fluid (CSF) flow disturbance and venous congestion (Fig. 7c) [13,27]. This intraradicular edema may lead to acidosis, with subsequent impairment of nerve function. That is, this intraradicular acidosis seems to be a critical factor for development of pain [28–30] associated with nerve root compression (Fig. 8).

References

1. Schmorl G (1926) Uber knorpelknoten an der Hinterflache der Wirbelbandscheiben. Fortschr Geb Rontgenstr 40:629–634
2. Mixter WJ, Barr JS (1934) Rupture of the intervertebral disc with involvement of the spinal canal. N Engl J Med 211:210–215
3. Cornefjord M, Sato K, Olmarker K, Rydevik B, Nordborg C (1997) A model for chronic nerve root compression studies. Presentation of a porcine model for controlled, slow-onset compression with analyses of anatomic aspects, compression onset rate, and morphologic and neurophysiologic effects. Spine 22:946–957
4. Delamarter RB, Bohlman HH, Didge LD, Biro B (1990) Experimental lumbar spine stenosis. Analysis of the cortical evoked potentials, microvasculature, and histopathology. J Bone Joint Surg 72:110–120
5. Gelfan S, Tarlov IM (1956) Physiology of spinal cord, nerve root and peripheral nerve compression. Am J Physiol 185:217–229
6. Iwamoto H, Kuwahara H, Matsuda H, Noriage A, Yamano Y (1995) Production of chronic compression of the cauda equina in rats for use in studies of lumbar spinal canal stenosis. Spine 20:2750–2757
7. Kobayashi S, Yoshizawa H, Hachiya Y, Ukai T, Morita T (1993) Vasogenic edema induced by compression injury to the spinal nerve root. Distribution of intravenously injected protein tracers and gadolinium-enhanced magnetic resonance imaging. Spine 18:1410–1424
8. Naito M, Owen JH, Bridwell K, Oakley DM (1990) Blood flow direction in the lumbar nerve root. Spine 15:966–968
9. Olmarker K, Rydevik B, Hansson T, Holm S (1990) Compression-induced changes of the nutritional supply to the porcine cauda equina. J Spinal Disord 3:25–29

10. Rydevik B, Brown MD, Lundborg G (1984) Pathoanatomy and pathophysiology of nerve root compression. Spine 9:7-15

11. Rydevik B, Holm S, Brown MD (1984) Nutrition of spinal nerve root. Trans Orthop Res Soc 9:276

12. Rydevik B, Pedowicz RA, Hargens AR, Swenson MR, Myers RR, Garfin SR (1991) Effects of acute graded compression on spinal nerve root function and structure: An experimental study on the pig cauda equina. Spine 16:487-493

13. Yoshizawa H, Kobayashi S, Kubota K (1989) Effects of compression on intraradicular blood flow in dogs. Spine 14:1220-1225

14. Yoshizawa H, Kobayashi S, Morita T (1995) Chronic nerve root compression. Pathophysiologic mechanism of nerve root dysfunction. Spine 20:397-407

15. Stossek K, Luebbers DW, Cottin N (1974) Determination of local blood flow (microflow) by electrochemically generated hydrogen: Construction and application of the measuring probe. Pflugers Arch 348:225-238

16. Connelly CM (1957) Methods for measuring tissue oxygen tension; theory and evaluation: the oxygen electrode. Fed Proc 16:681-674

17. Arita H, Ichkawa K, Kuwana S, Kogo N (1989) Possible locations of pH-dependent central chemoreceptors: intramedullary lesions with acidic shift of extracellular fluid pH during hypercapnia. Brain Res 485:285-293

18. Arnold JB, Junck L, Rottenberg DA (1985) In vivo measurement of regional brain and tumor pH using [^{14}C]-dimethyl onazolidinedione and quantitative autoradiography. J Cerebral Blood Flow Metabl 5:369-375

19. Imataka K (1987) Sequential changes of regional brain pH and energy metabolism after cold-induced vasogenic brain edema. Arch Jpn Chir 56:600-612

20. Frei HJ, Wallenfang Th, Poll W, Reulen HJ, Schubert R, Brock M (1973) Regional cerebral blood flow and regional metabolism in cold induced oedema. Acta Neurochir (Wein) 29:15-28

21. Sutton LN, Welsh FA, Bruce DA (1980) Bioenergetics of acute vasogenic edema. J Neurosurg 53:470-476

22. Wagner KR, Tornheim PA, Eichhold MK (1985) Acute changes in regional cerebral metabolite values following experimental blunt head trauma. J Neurosurg 63:88-96

23. Maruhashi J (1967) Effect of oxygen lack on the sinngle isolated mammalian(rat) nerve fiber. J Neurophysiol 30:434-452

24. Seneviratne KN, Peiris OA (1968) The effect of ischemia on the exitability of human sensory nerve. J Neurol Neurosurg Psychiatry 31:338-347

25. Kobayashi S (1990) Experimental study on the blood flow disturbance in the nerve root. Bull Fujita-Gakuen Med Soc 8:107-142

26. Kobayashi S, Yoshizawa H, Kubota K (1990) Circulatory dynamics of lumbosacral spinal nerve root. 18th Ann Meet Int Soc Study Lumbar Spine, Boston, 23 (Abstr)

27. Yoshizawa H, Kobayashi S, Kubota K (1991) Blood supply of nerve roots and dorsal root ganglion. Orthop Clin North Am 22:195-211

28. Lindahl O (1961) Lokale pH-Anderungen das lebenden Gewebes unter Einwirkung Chemischer Reizmittel. Arch Ges Physiol 251:631-644

29. Lindahl O (1961) Experimental skin pain, induced by injection of water-soluble substances in humans. Acta Physiol Scand 51 (suppl):179

30. Lindahl O (1966) Hyperalgesis of the lumbar nerve roots in sciatica. Acta Orthop Scand 37:367-374

Compound Muscle Action Potentials Under Dynamic Stress in Lumbar Spinal Canal Stenosis

YASUNORI FUCHIGAMI, TAKASHI ITOH, SHINYA KAWAI, HIROTSUGU ODA, KAZUO KANEKO, HIROSHI YONEMURA, HIDEAKI FUJIMOTO, and MICHIO SHINOHARA

Summary. Intermittent claudication is one of the characteristic symptoms in lumbar spinal canal stenosis. We recorded compound muscle action potentials (CMAPs) from the extensor digiti brevi (EDB) and the abductor hallucis (AH) before and after dynamic stress elicited by cauda equina electrical stimulation or transcranial magnetic stimulation. In 12 cases of 25 patients, the amplitudes of the CMAPs from the EDB or the AH elicited by cauda equina electrical stimulation decreased transiently, and recovered to the status of the control gradually within 5 min. In four cases of six patients, the amplitudes of the CMAPs elicited by transcranial magnetic stimulation decreased temporarily, and recovered to the status of the control within six minutes. It was suggested that a rapidly reversible physiological block by ischemia on the chronic injured cauda equina was the cause of the neurogenic intermittent claudication.

Key words. Neurogenic claudication, Spinal stenosis, Neural conduction, Compound muscle action potential, Magnetic stimulation

Introduction

Intermittent claudication is one of the characteristic symptoms in lumbar spinal canal stenosis. We have a few reports about the mechanism of the intermittent claudication. To clarify the mechanism of neurogenic intermittent claudication, we tried to record compound muscle action potentials (CMAPs) from the extensor digiti brevi (EDB) and the abductor hallucis (AH) before and after dynamic stress elicited by cauda equina electrical stimulation or transcranial magnetic stimulation.

Materials and Methods

Twenty-five patients (10 men and 15 women), 44 to 77 years old, with symptoms and signs of neurogenic claudication and radiographically narrowed lumbar spinal canal stenosis, were studied.

University of Yamaguchi, School of Medicine, Department of Orthopedic Surgery, 1144 Kogushi, Ube, Yamaguchi,755-8505, Japan

Electrical Stimulation at the Cauda Equina

To stimulate the cauda equina, a catheter electrode was inserted into the epidural space at the level of L1/2. Stimuli consisted of constant current square-wave pulses (0.2 ms duration, stimulus rate 0.5/s to 1/s). The intensity was adjusted from 20 to 40 mA to induce the CMAPs from the EDB and the AH. The patient was seated in a comfortable reclining chair during recording of the potentials. Potentials were recorded with a signal averager (Counterpoint, Dantec Electronics Ltd.). Electrical stimulation was applied once or twice on average. After control CMAPs were recorded by cauda equina electrical stimulation (CEE-CMAPs), the patient stood up and took steps until he could not step any more because typical symptoms, such as sciatic pain, numbness, or weakness developed in the leg to foot. After this dynamic stress the patient was seated again. Then the CEE-CMAPs were recorded every few seconds for 5 min after he had been seated.

Transcranial Magnetic Stimulation

To evaluate the change of muscle potentials after dynamic stress non-invasively, transcranial magnetic stimulation was applied in six patients. The target muscle was the EDB or the AH. During recording of the potentials, the patient was seated in a comfortable reclining chair as for electrical stimulation at the cauda equina, but he needed mild voluntary muscle contraction to facilitate the amplitudes of the CMAPs elicited by transcranial magnetic stimulation (TCM-CMAPs). After dynamic stress the TCM-CMAPs were recorded every minute until 6 min after he had been seated. Magnetic stimulation was applied two or three times in every recording, and these potentials were superimposed.

Results

Electrical Stimulation at the Cauda Equina

CEE-CMAPs Recorded from the EDB

In six cases of 25 patients the CEE-CMAPs could not be evoked because of muscular atrophy which may have been induced by chronic cauda equina compression. In 12 cases the amplitudes of the CEE-CMAPs decreased temporarily, and recovered to the control level gradually within 5 min (Figs. 1, 2). In seven cases the amplitudes of the CEE-CMAPs were not changed. In all patients the latency of the CEE-CMAPs showed no changes after dynamic stress.

CEE-CMAPs Recorded from the AH

In three cases of 25 patients, we could not evoke the CEE-CMAPs because of muscular atrophy. In 12 cases the amplitudes of the CEE-CMAPs decreased temporarily, and recovered to the control level gradually within 5 min (Figs. 3, 4). In 10 cases the amplitudes of the CEE-CMAPs were not changed.

Transcranial Magnetic Stimulation

In four cases of six patients the amplitudes of the TCM-CMAPs decreased transiently, and recovered to the control within 6 min (Figs. 5–7). In one case the amplitudes of

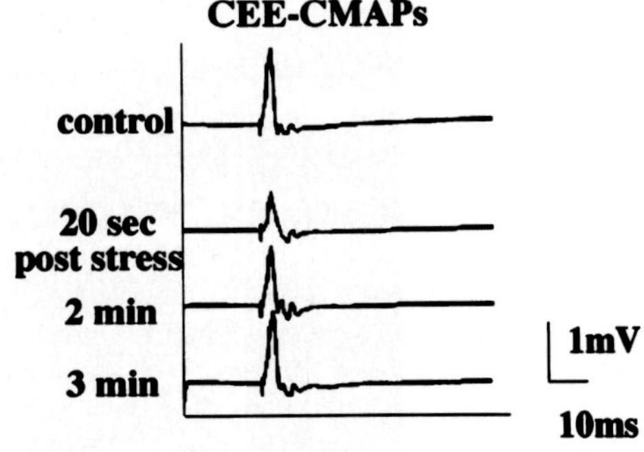

FIG. 1. The amplitude of the cauda equina electrical stimulation–compound muscle action potential (*CEE-CMAPs*) from the extensor digiti brevi (EDB) in a 57-year-old man decreased temporarily at 20 s post-stress

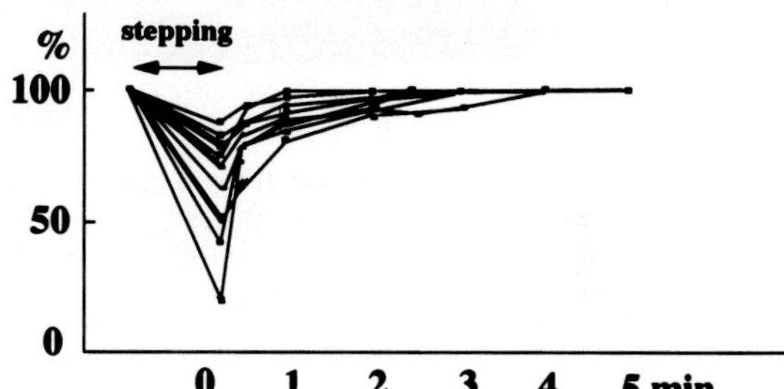

FIG. 2. The amplitude ratio of the CEE-CMAPs from the extensor digiti brevi (EDB) against the control recovered to the control level within 5 min in 12 cases

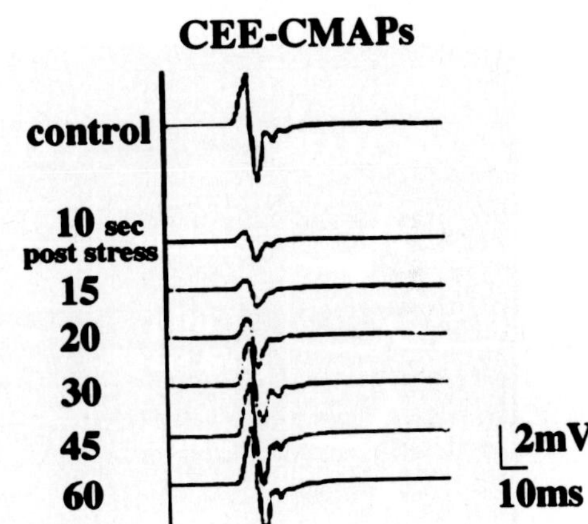

FIG. 3. The amplitude of the CEE-CMAPs from the abductor hallucis (AH) in a 54-year-old woman decreased transiently at 30 s post-stress

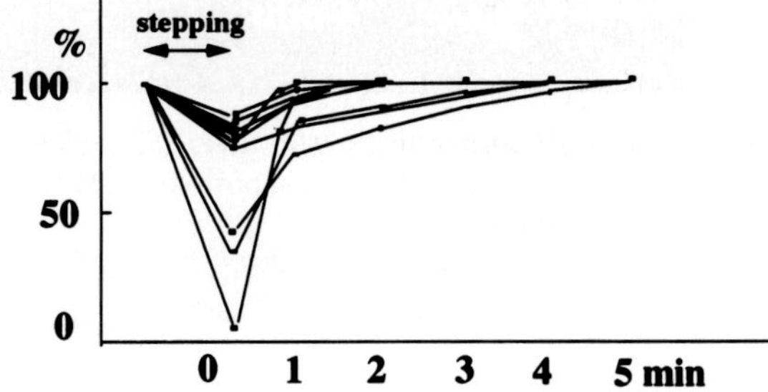

FIG. 4. The amplitude ratio of the CEE-CMAPs from the AH against the control recovered to the control level within 5 min in 12 cases

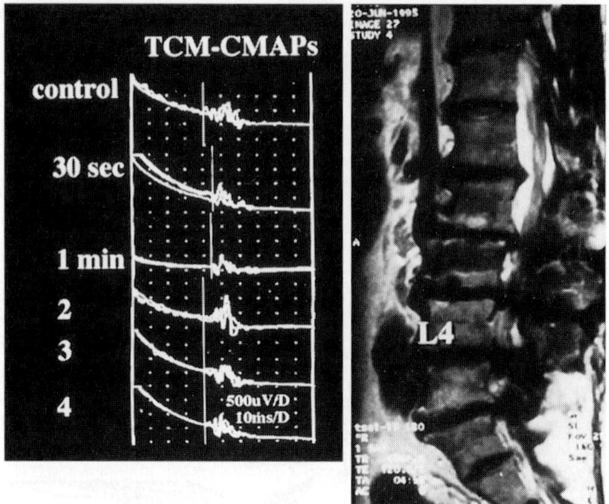

FIG. 5. The amplitudes of the transcranial magnetic stimulation (TCM)-CMAPs from the EDB in a 64-year-old man decreased temporarily within 1 min post-stress. Magnetic resonance imaging (MRI) (*right*) showed multiple-level stenosis of the lumbar spinal canal

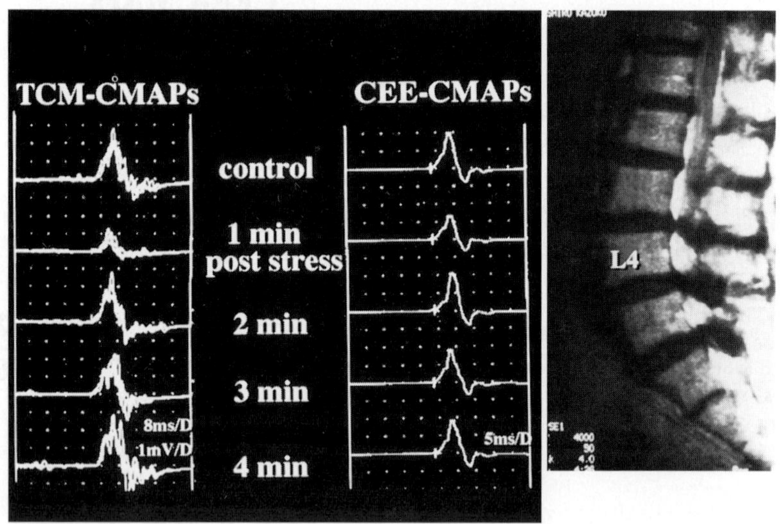

FIG. 6. The amplitudes of the *TCM-CMAPs* and the *CEE-CMAPs* from the AH in a 70-year-old woman decreased transiently at 1 min post-stress. MRI (*right*) showed multiple-level stenosis of the lumbar spinal canal

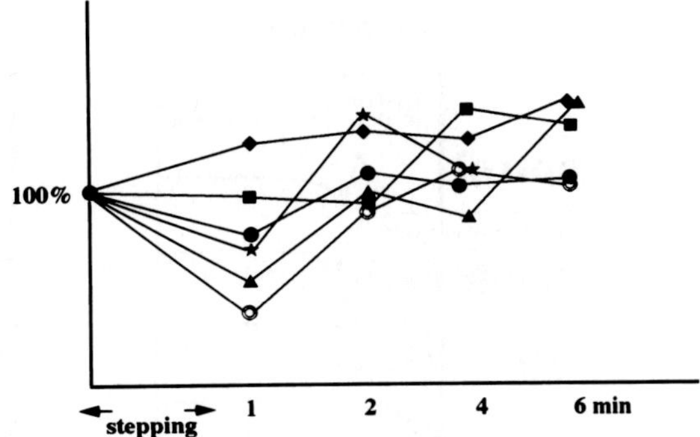

FIG. 7. The amplitude ratio of the TCM-CMAPs against the control recovered to the control level within 6 min in six cases

the TCM-CMAPs were not changed. In another case the amplitudes of the TCM-CMAPs increased.

Discussion

Intermittent claudication in lumbar spinal canal stenosis may be related to direct compression, arterial insufficiency, or impaired venous drainage of the neural elements of the cauda equina. But the actual pathophysiology of neurological claudication is unknown. Symptoms—for example, radicular pain, muscle weakness, or numbness in buttocks—appear when the patient assumes any position which accentuates lumbar lordosis, such as standing and walking. These symptoms were relieved quickly by sitting down or by recumbency. The claudication time varied directly with the oxygen availability, suggesting a relative ischemia of the cauda equina during walking [1]. Dynamic myeloscopic examination showed the blood vessels on the cauda equina were dilated in lumbar spinal canal stenosis with intermittent claudication [2]. These findings suggested that disturbance of microcirculation on the cauda equina might play an important role in the development of neurogenic claudication. There have been some electrophysiological reports on neurogenic claudication under dynamic stress. The amplitudes of the evoked spinal cord potentials recorded from the conus medullaris decreased transiently after walking [3]. The persistence of the F-waves from the EDB or the AH were reduced after walking [4]. These electrophysiologic changes after walking were transient. Recovery from these changes to the control level occurred within several minutes. In our study, the amplitudes of the CEE-CMAPs and the TCM-CMAPs after dynamic stress also decreased transiently and recovered to the control level within 5 or 6 min. These dynamic electrophysiologic changes most likely reflect transient conduction block in the cauda equina.

In an ischemic study using a tourniquet around the upper arm of a human, a rapidly reversible physiological block occurred over 20 min of ischemia in a healthy subject and was reversible within a few minutes [5] (Fig. 8). The electrical conductivity of the nerve fibers was influenced by arterial pressure of oxygen (PaO_2), because the propagating action potentials needed maintaining by the transmembrane potentials which were driven by an energy-dependent sodium-potassium pump. This pump was transporting sodium and potassium continuously, and was consuming adenosine triphos-

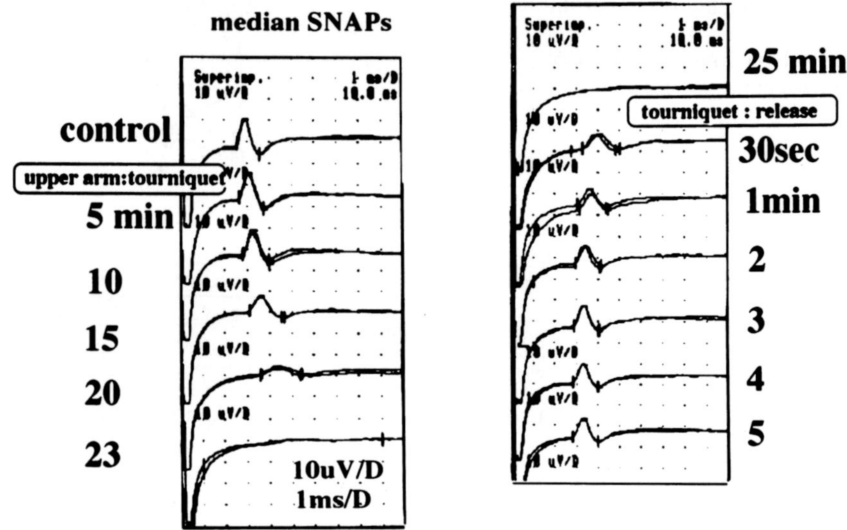

FIG. 8. The amplitudes of the orthodromic median sensory action potentials (*SNAPs*) under ischemic conditions in healthy a 38-year-old man showed progressive reduction after 25 min. When the tourniquet was released, the amplitudes of the SNAPs recovered within seconds

phate (ATP) which required an adequate O_2 supply. This suggested that a possible mechanism of neurogenic claudication was transient ischemia on the cauda equina which had chronic subclinical damage. Recording the CEE-CMAPs and the TCM-CMAPs under dynamic stress in lumbar spinal canal stenosis is useful for detecting the electrophysiological changes in neurogenic intermittent claudication.

Conclusion

To clarify the mechanism of neurogenic intermittent claudication, we recorded the CEE-CMAPs and the TCM-CMAPs from the EDB and the AH before and after dynamic stress. The amplitudes of the CEE-CMAPs and the TCM-CMAPs after dynamic stress decreased transiently and recovered to the control level within 5 or 6 min. We suggest that a rapidly reversible physiological block caused by ischemia on the chronically injured cauda equina is the mechanism of neurogenic intermittent claudication.

References

1. Evans JG (1964) Neurogenic intermittent claudication. Br Med J 2:985–987
2. Ooi Y, Mita F, Satoh Y (1990) Myeloscopic study on lumbar spinal canal stenosis with special reference to intermittent claudication. Spine 15:544–549
3. Tamaki T, Tsuji H, Takano H, Kuwataka K, Noguchi T (1986) Electrophysiological analyses on cauda equina intermittent claudication (in Japanese). Rinsho Seikei Geka 21:513–517

4. London SF, England JD (1991) Dynamic F waves in neurogenic claudication. Muscle Nerve 14:457–461
5. Fullerton PM (1963) The effect of ischaemia on nerve conduction in the carpal tunnel syndrome. J Neurol Neurosurg Psychiatry 26:358–397

Part 5
Human Iliac CFU-F Properties and Potential Uses

Immobilization Osteopenia—Bone Loss After Arthroplastic Surgery

HIROMICHI NORIMATSU, SATOSHI MORI, and JUN KAWANISHI

Summary. Immobilization, physical inactivity, and/or reduced muscle strength, is the cause of osteopenia. We examined 44 patients during the immobilized and remobilized periods after arthroplastic surgery. Bone mineral density (BMD) of the lumbar vertebrae showed no remarkable change, but femoral neck BMD of the contralateral limb decreased temporarily at about 5 months, then gradually returned to the preoperative value about 12 months after surgery. Metabolic bone markers of bone resorption and bone formation increased markedly, on average 3 months after surgery. In conclusion, immobilization alters the mechanical usage of bone in terms of activating bone resorption and depressing bone formation for a short period in the initial phase. Remobilization acts to restore bone mineral in both cortical and trabecular bones.

Key words. Immobilization, Osteopenia, Osteoporosis, Arthroplastic surgery

Introduction

Immobilization by long-term bed rest [1], space flight [2], or simulated weightlessness is known to be a cause of decreased bone mass [3]. Loss of stimulation from muscular inactivity and reduction in weight-bearing might change bone remodelling activity. It has been recognized that immobilization and weight-bearing stimulate the excretion of prostaglandin E2 (PGE2) [4,5], insulin-like growth factor-1 (IGF-1) [6], and nitric oxide (NO) [7] by osteoblasts and osteocytes. Disuse osteopenia has been studied in patients [8], human volunteers [1] and in experimental growing [9] and adult animals [10] by bone histomorphometry, radiographic measurement, quantitative computed tomography of vertebral trabeculae and peripheral bones and single- and dual-energy X-ray absorptiometry. Recovery from immobilization is experienced in humans if the remobilization period and follow-up time are long enough.

We studied the changes in bone mineral density (BMD) of the lumbar vertebrae, femoral neck, and periprosthetic bone and changes in metabolic bone markers during

Department of Orthopedic Surgery, Kagawa Medical University, 1750-1 Ikenobe, Mikichou, Kidagun, Kagawa 761-0793, Japan

TABLE 1. Group A patients[a] ($n = 23$)

Diagnosis	Cases	Men	Women	Age (years)	Procedures	
ANF	7	4	3	23–72	FHR	7
OA	14	2	12	48–77	FHR	8
					THR	6
RA	2	0	2	29, 65	FHR	2

[a] Age, 58 ± 13 years; height, 151 ± 9 cm; weight, 54 ± 11 kg.
ANF, avascular necrosis of the femoral head; OA, osteoarthritis; RA, rheumatoid arthritis; FHR, femoral head replacement; THR, total hip replacement.

immobilization and remobilization periods after arthroplastic surgery of the hip or knee joint in patients.

Materials and Methods

Group A

We examined 23 Japanese patients (17 women, 6 men; age 23–77 years) who had osteoarthritis, rheumatoid arthritis of the hips, and avascular necrosis of the femoral neck (Table 1). They all underwent either total hip replacement (THR, $n = 6$) or femoral head replacement (FHR, $n = 17$). Two weeks postoperatively they began exercising using a three-point gait with no weight-bearing on their operated legs. Weight-bearing exercise was introduced 4–6 weeks after surgery. The BMD of their lumbar vertebrae, contralateral femoral neck, and Gruen's seven zones (Fig. 1) in periprosthetic bone was measured using DXA (Lunar DXA-α Madison) before and after surgery. The follow-up period of measurement was from 9 to 34 months. The study protocol was explained to the patients and their consent was obtained.

Group B

Twenty-one Japanese patients (19 women, 2 men; age 42–84 years) who had osteoarthritis, rheumatoid arthritis of the hip, or avascular necrosis of the femoral head were examined (Table 2). They all underwent osteotomy ($n = 4$), THR ($n = 9$), FHR ($n = 3$), or total knee replacement (TKR $n = 5$). Three-point gait was begun at 2 weeks, and weight-bearing exercise was introduced at 4–6 weeks postoperatively. The following measurements were made before and after surgery (1) BMD of the lumbar vertebrae and contralateral femoral neck by DXA (Lunar Expert), and (b) levels of bone metabolic markers (1CTP, pyridinoline, deoxypyridinoline, osteocalcin, and P1CP). Follow-up time was 4–12 months after surgery.

Results

In group A, BMD of the lumbar vertebrae (L2–4) showed no remarkable recovery to the preoperative value, during the immobilization and remobilization period (Fig. 2, Table 3). Femoral neck BMD of the contralateral limb in half the patients was

Fig. 1. Gruen's seven zones

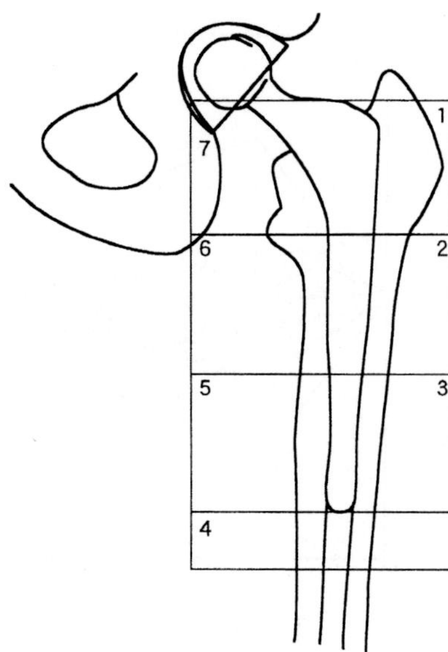

Table 2. Group B patients[a] ($n = 21$)

Diagnosis	Cases	Men	Women	Age (years)	Procedures	
ANF	3	1	2	67–69	FHR	3
OA (hip)	12	2	10	42–84	THR osteotomy	9
						3
OA (knee)	3	1	2	55–77	TKR osteotomy	2
						1
RA	3	0	3	50–80	TKR	3

[a] Age, 63 ± 11 years, height: 148 ± 7 cm, weight, 50 ± 9 kg.
ANF, avascular necrosis of the femoral head; OA, osteoarthritis; RA, rheumatoid arthritis; FHR, femoral head replacement; THR, total hip replacement; TKR, total knee replacement.

Table 3. Changes in bone mineral density in the lumbar spine and femoral neck (Group A)

	Before surgery (g/cm²)	Percent change in BMD, months after surgery				
		6 M	12 M	18 M	24 M	36 M
Lumbar spine (L2–4)	1.01 ± 0.15	-0.3 ± 3.5	$-1.7 \pm 2.3^*$	-1.5 ± 3.0	-2.9 ± 3.5	-2.8 ± 1.8
Femoral neck	0.75 ± 0.18	-0.7 ± 3.5	0.0 ± 3.5	-0.6 ± 2.7	2.1 ± 3.1	5.4 ± 3.7

$^* P < 0.05$.
BMD, bone mineral density.

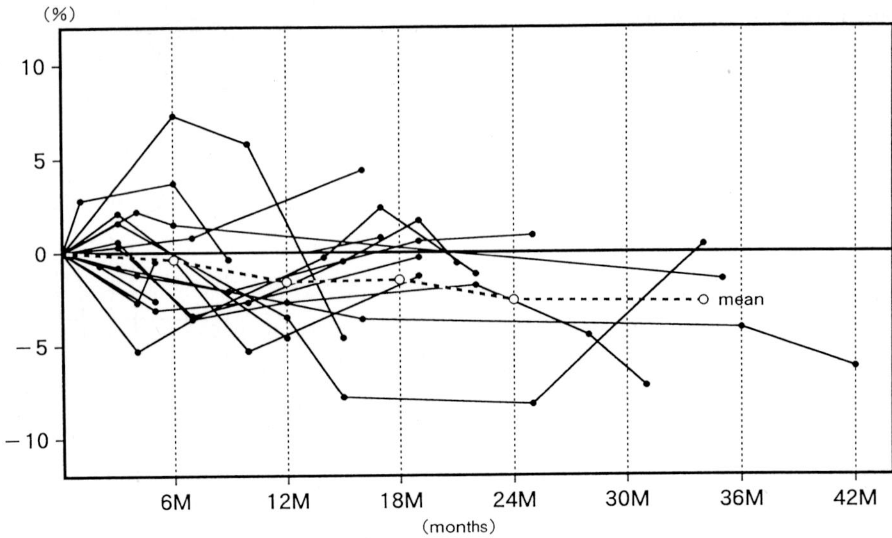

FIG. 2. Percentage of longitudinal deviation in L2–4 bone mineral density (BMD) after surgery. BMD of the lumbar vertebrae showed no marked recovery to the preoperative value during the immobilization and remobilization periods

TABLE 4. Changes in BMD in the lumbar spine and femoral neck (Group B)

	Before surgery (g/cm²)	percent change in BMD, months after surgery	
		6 M	12 M
Lumbar spine (L2–4)	0.98 ± 0.18	−1.2 ± 7.2	−6.3 ± 6.1
Femoral neck	0.70 ± 0.16	−0.5 ± 7.1	−5.1 ± 9.0

decreased temporarily at about 5 months, then it gradually returned to its preoperative level (Fig. 3, Table 3). Patients in Group B showed no marked changes in lumbar and femoral neck BMD during the period immediately after surgery (Table 4). The BMD of all zones other than the first (great trochanter) and seventh (calcar) zones showed a decrease until 24 months, and then recovered gradually. These two proximal zones continued to lose bone mineral, almost 20% to 30% of the preoperative value, until 36 months (Fig. 4, Table 5).

Metabolic markers of bone resorption—pyridinoline and deoxypyridinoline—increased markedly, on average 3 months after surgery (Table 6). Also osteocalcin and P1CP, which are markers of bone formation, increased significantly at 3 or 6 months after surgery (Table 6).

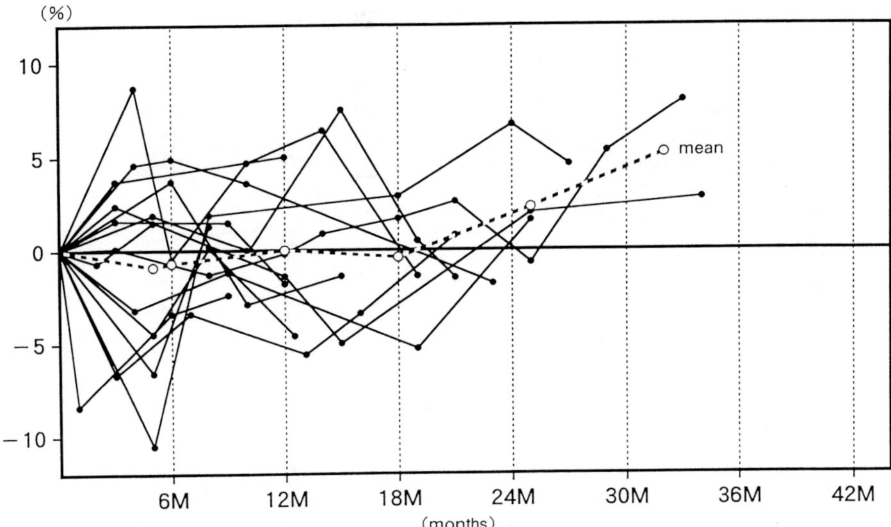

FIG. 3. Percentage of longitudinal deviation in femoral neck BMD after surgery BMD of the femoral neck in half the patients showed a temporary decrease at about 5 months, then gradually recovered to the pre-operative value

Discussion

In the active phase of immobilization, bone resorption increases and bone formation decreases. In animal models of immobilization—tail suspension [11], cast application [12,13], neurectomy, and hind limb bandage to the abdomen [14,15]—osteoclast numbers in trabecular bone increase, and mineral appositional rate and bone formation rate decrease. These observations were mainly on trabecular bone which shows the influence of immobilization faster than does cortical bone.

The calcium endocrine system responds early to skeletal unloading by space flight and bed rest. Plasma parathyroid hormone (PTH) has been reported to decrease during skeletal unloading [16]. Serum $1,25(OH)_2D_3$ was significantly reduced by bed rest on day 5 in 14 patients with spinal cord injury [17]. But some reports have shown no changes in ionized calcium and parathyroid hormone (PTH) with skeletal unloading [18].

Mechanical stress by weight bearing and muscle contraction changes interstitial fluid flow through the canalicular network in the bone. This fluid flow directly acts on osteocytes to enhance the secretion of cytokine, PGE2 and IL-1, for example, which promote osteoblast-like stroma cells and then conduct osteoclast differentiation.

Mechanical usage has an effect on bone growth, modelling, and remodelling. Frost [19] has indicated that bone strains in or above 1500–3000 microstrain cause bone modelling to increase cortical bone mass, while strains below 100–300 microstrains remove existing cortical-endosteal and trabecular bone. The minimum strain that acts to acquire or preserve bone mass is called the minimum effective strain.

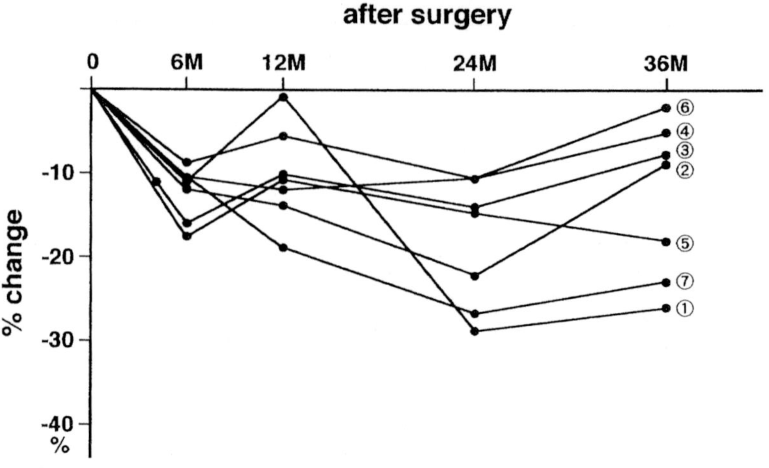

Fig. 4. Percent changes in BMD in the seven zones. All zones other than the 1st and 7th showed a decrease in BMD until 24 months after surgery, then gradually recovered. The 1st (greater trochanter) and 7th zone (calcar) continued to lose BMD, almost 20% to 30% of the preoperative value, until 34 months after surgery

Prolonged immobilization due to poliomyelitis, spinal cord injury [20], cerebrovascular accident [21], muscular dystrophy, and other diseases [22] is known to cause a decrease in skeletal bone mass. Osteoporosis is a disease that includes osteopenia, and the causative factors are intermingled [23]. Bone loss in the initial phase of immobilization has been described as a rapid loss of bone mass within the first 6 months. In this phase osteoclastic bone resorption increases, while osteoblastic bone formation decreases [24]. Remobilization that begins before this irreversible point, activates osteoblast generation and inhibits bone resorption, restoring bone mass to its preimmobilization level.

A change in Bone volume due to immobilization and remobilization has been reported at various skeletal sites. Losses in bone mineral in patients confined to prolonged bed rest have been more marked in the lumbar vertebrae than in the long bones of the extremities, which have relatively higher cortical bone mass [2,25]. In our study, bone mineral density decreased greater more in the lumbar vertebrae than in the femoral neck. Furthermore, bone mineral loss of the femoral neck began to recover at 5 months postsurgery, and reached the preoperative level 12–18 months after surgery. There was a time lag of about 3 months between the beginning of recovery of bone mineral loss and initiation of remobilization. It was suggested that the bone mass level did not return to preimmobilization level after long-term immobilization [10,26].

Dual-energy X-ray absorptiometry has been shown to be an accurate and precise tool for the assessment of periprosthetic BMD. The time-related changes of periprosthetic bone density after total hip arthroplasty mainly reflect bone response to the strain redistribution determined by the insertion of the femoral stem into the

TABLE 5. Changes in BMD in Gruen zones after surgery

	Zone 1	Zone 2	Zone 3	Zone 4	Zone 5	Zone 6	Zone 7
Preoperative value (g/cm^2)	0.76 ± 0.13	1.41 ± 0.27	1.42 ± 0.22	1.40 ± 0.22	1.56 ± 0.23	1.41 ± 0.21	0.91 ± 0.18
Postoperative % change							
at 6 months	−10.6 ± 16.3	−12.0 ± 13.1[#]	−17.8 ± 12.2*	−10.9 ± 7.9*	−15.7 ± 11.2*	−9.3 ± 17.4	−11.7 ± 16.8
12 months	−0.6 ± 26.4	−14.9 ± 10.3**	−11.0 ± 13.8	−12.3 ± 13.0[##]	−10.1 ± 12.0[##]	−5.6 ± 15.0	−19.8 ± 19.5
24 months	−29.1 ± 7.1	−22.9 ± 2.3[##]	−14.2 ± 5.6	−10.8 ± 0.5[##]	−14.5 ± 7.4	−11.1 ± 14.4	−26.8 ± 22.8
36 months	−26.1 ± 12.2	−9.0 ± 15.9	−7.8 ± 3.9	−5.1 ± 4.1	−18.0 ± 1.8**	−2.3 ± 16.8	−23.4 ± 25.0

* $P < 0.001$, ** $P < 0.005$, [#] $P < 0.01$, [##] $P < 0.05$.

TABLE 6. Changes in metabolic markers after surgery

	Before surgery	After surgery	
		3 months	6 months
Bone resorption markers			
ICTP (ng/ml)	6.3 ± 5.2	8.4 ± 3.1	6.9 ± 3.0
pyridinoline (nM/mM creat.)	59.3 ± 15.9	99.5 ± 49.5*	90.5 ± 63.7
deoxypyridinoline (nM/mM creat.)	9.0 ± 2.7	13.1 ± 5.1*	12.8 ± 9.0
Bone formation markers			
osteocalcin (ng/ml)	6.6 ± 4.4	8.7 ± 3.6**	10.5 ± 11.2***
P1CP (ng/ml)	107.5 ± 48.0		147.8 ± 63.3***

* $P < 0.05$; ** $P < 0.02$; *** $P < 0.01$.

medullary canal. Previously published studies reported a widely varing decrease in the periprosthetic regions. The greatest decrease was observed 6 months after surgery in the calcar region (greater than 50% by Trevisan [27], 13.5%–19.2% by Kroger et al. [28,29]) and great trochanter region where stress shielding was greater. There was an increase in the bone density of all of the regions except the calcar region after 3 months [27], but our study showed a decrease until 24 months and then a gradual recovery.

Recently, biochemical assays for monitoring bone turnover have been introduced [30]. The serum levels of skeletal alkaline phophatase and osteocalcin are the most reliable markers of bone formation. Consistently, the most promising markers of bone resorption are urinary levels of collagen degradation products. In this study patients showed increased values of both bone resorption markers (1CTP, pyridinoline, deoxypyridinoline) and bone formation markers (osteocalcin, P1CP) in the acute initial phase after surgery.

In conclusion, immobilization alters the mechanical usage of bone in terms activating bone resorption and depressing bone formation for a short period in the initial phase. Remobilization acts to restore bone mineral density in both cortical and trabecular bones.

References

1. Donaldson CL, Hulley SB, Vogel JM, Hattner RS, Bayers JH, McMillan DE (1970) Effect of prolonged bed rest on bone mineral. Metabolism 19:1071–1084
2. Rambaut PC, Goode AW (1985) Skeletal changes during space flight. Lancet ii:1050–1052
3. Rose GA (1966) Immobilization osteoporosis—A study of the extent, severity, and treatment with bendrofluazide. Br J Surg 53:769–774
4. Binderman I, Zor U, Kaye AM, Shimshoni Z, Harell A, Somjen D (1988) The transduction of mechanical force into biochemical events in bone cells may involve activation of phospholipase A_2. Calcif Tissue Int, 42:261–266
5. Klein-Nulend J, Plas AV, Semeins CM, Ajubi NE, Frangos JA, Nijweide PJ, Burger EH (1995) Sensitivity of osteocytes to biochemical stress in vitro. FASEB J 9:441–445
6. Lean JM, Jagger CJ, Chambers TJ (1995) Increased insulin-like growth factor-1 mRNA expression in osteocytes precedes the increase in bone formation in response to mechanical stimulation. J Bone Min Res, 9 (Suppl 1):S142
7. Klein-Nulend J, Semeins CM, Ajubi NE, Nijweide PJ, Burger EH (1995) Pulsating fluid flow increases nitric oxide (NO) synthesis by osteocytes but not periosteal osteoblasts—correlation with prostaglandin upregulation. Biochem Biophys Res Comm 217:640–648
8. Nishiyama S, Kawahara T, Matsuda I (1986) Decreased bone density in severely handicapped children and adults, with reference to the influence of limited mobility and anticonvulsant medication. Eur J Pediatr, 144:457–463
9. Tuukanenn J, Wallmark B, Jalovaara P, Takara J, Sjogren S, Vaananen K (1991) Changes induced in growing rat bone by immobilization and remobilization. Bone, 12:113–118
10. Mattson S (1972) Reversibility of disuse osteoporosis—Experimental studies in the adult rat. Acta Orthop Scand 144(S):1–135
11. Bourrin S, Palle S, Genty C, Alexandre C (1995) Physical exercise during remobilization restores a normal bone trabecular network after tail suspension-induced osteopenia in young rats. J Bone Min Res 10:820–828
12. Wronski TJ, Morey ER (1983) Inhibition of cortical and trabecular bone formation in the long bones of immobilized monkeys. Clin Orthop 181:269–276
13. Uhthoff HK, Jaworski ZFG (1978) Bone loss in response to long-term immobilization. J Bone Joint Surg 60-B:420–429
14. Norimatsu H, Mori S, Kawanishi J, Kaji Y, Li J (1997) Immobilization as the pathogenesis of osteoporosis: Experimental and clinical studies. Osteoporosis Int, 7 (Suppl. 3):S57–S62
15. Li XJ, Jee WSS, Chow SY, Woodburry DM (1990) Adaptation of cancellous bone to aging and immobilization in the rat: A single photon absorptiometry and histomorphometry study. Anat Rec 227:12–24
16. Arnaud SB, Sherrard DJ, Maloney N, Whalen RT, Fung P (1992) Effects of 1-week head-down tilt bed rest on bone formation and the calcium endocrine system. Aviat Space Environ Med 63:14–20
17. Stewart AF, Adler M, Byers CM, Segre GV, Broadus AE (1982) Calcium homeostasis in immobilization: An example of resorptive hypercalciuria. N Engl J Med 306:1136–1140
18. Halloran BP, Bikle DD, Harris J, Foskett HC, Morey-Holton E (1993) Skeletal unloading decreases production of 1,25-dihydroxyvitamin D. Amer J Physiol, 264:E712–E716
19. Frost HM (1987) Bone "mass" and the "mechanostat": A proposal. Anat Rec 219:1–9
20. Uebelhart D, Demiaux-Domenech B, Roth M, Chantraine A (1995) Bone metabolism in spinal cord injured individuals and in others who have prolonged immobilization—A review. Paraplegia 33:669–673

21. del Puente A, Pappone N, Mandes MG, Mantova D, Scarpa R, Oriente P (1996) Determinants of bone mineral density in immobilization—A study on hemiplegic patients. Osteoporosis Int 6:50–54
22. Yoshikawa T, Uesato T, Nakasone T, Kuniyoshi S, Nakasone S, Ibaraki K, Takara H, Norimatsu H (1990) Influences of immobilization on bone mineral loss after the surgery of the cervical spine or lower extremity. In: Takahashi HE (ed) Bone morphometry. Niigata (Japan) Nishimura, pp 555–558
23. Frost HM (1998) Osteoporosis: a rationale for further definitions? Calcif Tissue Int 62:89–94
24. Haude JP, Shulz LA, Morgan WJ, Breen T, Warhold L, Crane GK, Baran DT (1995) Bone mineral density changes in the forearm after immobilization. Clin Orthop 317:199–205
25. Hansson TH, Roos BO, Nachemson A (1975) Development of osteopenia in the fourth lumbar vertebra during prolonged bed rest after operation of scoliosis. Acta Orthop Scand, 46:621–630
26. Jaworski ZFG, Uhthoff HK (1986) Reversibility of nontraumatic disuse osteoporosis during its active phase. Bone, 7:431–439
27. Trevisan C, Bigoni M, Randelli G, Marinoni EC, Peretti G, Ortolani S (1997) Periprosthetic bone density around fully hydroxyapatite coated femoral stem. Clin Orthop Rel Res 340:109–117
28. Kroger H, Miettinen H, Arnala I, Koski E, Rushton N, Suomalainen O (1996) Evaluation of periprosthetic bone using dual-energy X-ray absorptiometry: precision of the method and effect of operation on bone mineral density. J Bone Miner Res, 11:1526–1530
29. Kroger H, Vanninen E, Overmyer M, Mietinen H, Rushton N, Suomalainen O (1997) Periprosthetic bone loss and regional bone turnover in uncemented total hip arthroplasty: A prospective study using high-resolution single photon emission tomography and dual-energy X-ray absorptiometry. J Bone Miner Res, 12:487–492
30. Eyre DR (1996) Biochemical markers of bone turnover. In: Favus MJ (ed) Primer on the metabolic bone diseases and disorders of mineral metabolism, 3rd ed. Lippincott-Raven New York pp 114–119

Characterization of Osteoblast Progenitor Cells in Human Iliac Bone Marrow

Naoto Endo, Hiroshi Yamagiwa, Saburo Nishida, Kunihiko Tokunaga, Naoki Kinto, Tadashi Hayami, Taizo Horikoshi, Liu Zhang, Tatsuhiko Tanizawa, and Hideaki E. Takahashi

Summary. Osteoblast progenitor cells derive from pluripotent, mesenchymal stem cells in the bone marrow stroma, and play a crucial role in the formation of bone in remodeling and fracture healing. Mechanical stimuli and humoral factors, including systemic and local growth factors, regulate the proliferation and differentiation of bone marrow stroma cells into osteoblasts. When the bone marrow cells are cultured in vitro, osteoblast progenitor cells proliferate to form colonies of cells (colony-forming unit-fibroblastic, or CFU-F), and express alkaline phosphatase (ALP). These CFU-Fs exhibit osteoblastic phenotype, and form calcified nodules in vitro. The number of nucleated cells and ALP-positive CFU-Fs in marrow specimens obtained from human ilia were quantified in order to examine the concentration of osteoprogenitor cells with osteoblastic features. Human bone marrow cells were harvested by aspiration of the anterior iliac crests of 74 female donors whose ages ranged from 2 to 88 years, and who were without systemic or metabolic bone disease. These aspirated human bone marrow cells formed calcified nodules in vitro, and exhibited osteoblastic phenotype such as the expression of ALP, osteopontin (OPN), osteocalcine (OSC), parathyroid hormone-receptor (PTH-R), collagen type III (COL-III), collagen type I (COL-I), core-binding factor-1 (CBFA-1) and bone morphogenetic protein (BMP-2) mRNAs. The 2 ml aspirates of bone marrow yielded an average total number of $81.0 \pm 6.3 \times 10^6$ nucleated cells, and an average of 21.2 ± 2.4 ALP-positive CFU-Fs. There was a decrease in the number of ALP-positive CFU-Fs with age, while there was no significant correlation between the total cell number and age. These results indicate that (a) human bone marrow contains osteoblast progenitor cells, and (b) the total number of cells and the number of ALP-positive CFU-Fs in the iliac bone marrow differ from one another. However, the number of ALP-positive CFU-Fs were negatively correlated with age. These findings suggest that the number of ALP-positive CFU-Fs is one of the indices that reflect bone-forming activity, and bone-forming activity is related to the age-dependent change in the number of osteoprogenitor cells.

Department of Orthopaedic Surgery, Niigata University School of Medicine, 1-757 Asahimachi-dori, Niigata 951-8510, Japan

Key words. Osteoprogenitor cells, Colony-forming unit-fibroblastic (CFU-F), Bone marrow, Osteoblastic differentiation

Introduction

Bone formation during bone remodeling, fracture healing, and bone grafting into a defect is dependent on the proliferation and differentiation of osteoblast progenitor cells into osteoblasts [1–4]. Osteoblasts, the active bone-forming cells, derive from osteoblastic precursors present in the bone marrow stroma [5–10]. The number of osteoblast progenitor cells capable of differentiating into osteoblasts, and/or the functional activity of the differentiated osteoblasts, could regulate bone formation in both pathological conditions and normal conditions such as aging. Numerous osteoblastic cell cultures derived from animal bone have been developed [1,5,7,11–13]. These studies have provided useful information regarding osteoblastic features of progenitor cells. However, these findings may not reflect features of human bone cells because of differences between species and senescence [11,14,15]. A few studies using human osteoblastic progenitor cells in human marrow stroma have been reported [16–20]. This chapter describes the development of human osteoblast progenitor cells harvested by aspiration of iliac bone marrow, and the characteristic phenotype of these osteoprogenitor cells. Furthermore, the total number of nucleated cells and the number of ALP-positive colony forming units-fibroblastic, or CFU-Fs, have been evaluated to determine the concentration of osteoprogenitor cells in human iliac bone marrow.

Human Osteoblast Progenitor Cells from Iliac Bone Marrow Exhibit Osteoblastic Phenotype in Culture

We have developed a procedure for isolating human osteoblast progenitor cells from iliac bone marrow. Human bone marrow cells were harvested during surgery for treatment of acetabular dysplasia or osteoarthritis. Prior informed consent was obtained. The bone marrow cells were harvested by aspiration of the anterior iliac crest with a marrow tapping needle (Komiya's marrow tapping needle, Mizuho Medical, Tokyo, Japan) after the induction of general or spinal anesthesia before the scheduled surgical procedure. Precisely 2 ml of bone marrow fluid was harvested from each tapping with a 5 ml syringe. The bone marrow aspirate harvested from each subject was suspended with α-modified minimal essential medium (α-MEM, Gibco, New York, NY, USA). The bone marrow cells were plated in 6 multi-well plates (Corning, New York, NY, USA) at a density of 4×10^6 nucleated cells. The culture medium was first changed on day 1, and then changed on every third day thereafter. The bone marrow cells in culture form fibroblastic colonies (CFU-Fs) originating from a single cell. These marrow cells express alkaline phosphatase (ALP), and subsequently demonstrate characteristics of the osteoblastic phenotype such as expression of osteopontin (OPN), osteocalcine (OSC), parathyroid hormone-receptor (PTH-R), collagen type III (COL-III), and collagen type I (COL-I) mRNAs in culture. In addition, these cells express mRNAs of core binding factor a-1 (Cbfa-1), an essential transcriptional factor for osteoblast differentiation, and bone morphogenetic protein-2 (BMP-2), a potent factor for osteoblast proliferation and differentiation. These results suggest that Cbfa-1 and BMPs regulate the proliferation and differentiation of osteoblast progenitor cells in the iliac bone marrow. The bone marrow cells from human iliac bone marrow form calcified nodules in the presence of β-glycerophosphate in culture, as detected with von Kossa staining. These findings indicate that osteoblast progenitor cells are present in human iliac bone marrow, and differentiate into mature osteoblasts by expressing osteoblast phenotype [21–24].

Hormone and Growth Factors Affect the Proliferation and Differentiation of Osteoblast Progenitor Cells in Bone Marrow

Bone marrow cells have been shown in animal studies to respond to TGF-β, FGF, BMP, 1,25 (OH)2D3, and PTH [25,27]. In addition to these humoral factors, mechanical loading has been shown to affect bone marrow cells in mice.

In humans, BMP-2, FGF, and TGF-β have been reported to stimulate ALP activity in bone marrow cells in culture [26]. BMP-2 has been shown to be the most potent stimulator of ALP activity, and has profound effects on the proliferation and expression of osteoblastic phenotype [2,12,25–27].

Osteogenic Potential and Bone Formation In Vitro and In Vivo

In vitro studies have shown that bone marrow cells are capable of forming calcified nodules [7]. After we cultured bone marrow cells for 4 weeks in the presence of 10 mM of β-glycerophosphate (Wako Chemical, Osaka, Japan) in α-MEM medium, followed by fixation with 10% neutral buffered formalin in phosphate buffered saline (PBS), and von Kossa staining, the cultures exhibited calcified nodules.

In vivo studies have shown that bone formation occurs when human bone marrow cells are transplanted subcutaneously into immunodeficient mice [21,26].

These in vitro and in vivo studies indicate that human osteoblast progenitor cells obtained from the iliac bone marrow of humans exhibit osteogenic potential with respect to bone formation [8,15,19,20,28].

Aging and Number of ALP-positive CFU-Fs

Bone formation is dependent on the proliferation and differentiation of osteoblast progenitor cells. Age-related bone loss occurs as a result of an imbalance between bone resorption and formation, leading to skeletal disorders such as osteoporosis. This decrease in bone formation may depend on a reduction in the concentration of osteoblast progenitor cells, or on a lower sensitivity to growth factors affecting the differentiation of osteoprogenitor cells in the marrow. In order to study in vivo age-related changes in skeletal tissue, a useful approach is to examine osteoprogenitor cells

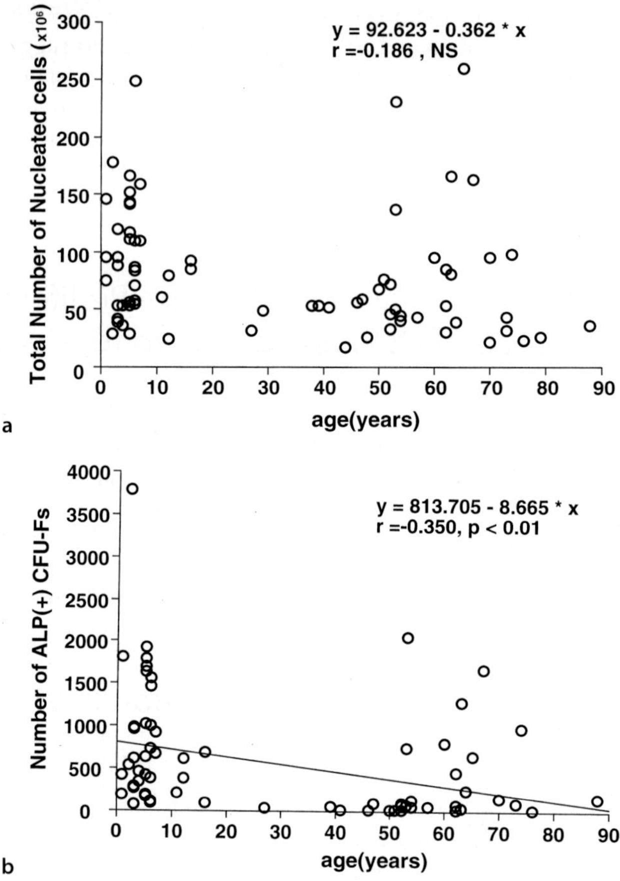

FIG. 1. **a** Relationship between age and the total number of nucleated cells. No correlation was found between age and the total number of nucleated cells. **b** Relationship between age and the number of alkaline phosphatase (*ALP*)-positive colony-forming unit-fibroblastic (*CFU-Fs*) per 2 ml aspirate obtained from human iliac bone marrow. On day 7 in culture, the medium was removed, and the cell layers were fixed with 10% neutral buffered formalin in phosphate buffered saline, and then stained for ALP. The number of ALP-positive colonies consisting of more than 50 cells were counted in each well. The average number of ALP-positive CFU-Fs in 4 wells was computed for each subject. There was a significant negative correlation between age and the number of ALP-positive CFU-Fs. Donor subjects were 74 females, ranging in age from 2 to 88 years.

in the bone marrow. It has been found that the efficiency of CFU-F formation decreases with age in cultures of mice and guinea-pig marrow cells [13,30]. Several studies have been published concerning age-related changes of CFU-Fs in humans [21,22].

Age-dependent changes in the total number of nucleated cells, and in ALP-positive CFU-Fs, on day 7 in culture from aspirates obtained from 74 subjects are shown in Fig. 1a and 1b. The 2 ml aspirates of bone marrow yielded an average total number of

$81.0 \pm 6.3 \times 10^6$ nucleated cells, and an average of 21.2 ± 2.4 ALP-positive CFU-Fs. The number of ALP-positive CFU-Fs declined with age. However, the total number of nucleated cells obtained from the 2 ml aspirates was not related to age. These results indicate that the total number of nucleated cells and the number of ALP-positive CFU-Fs in the iliac bone marrow differ from one another, while the number of ALP-positive CFU-Fs is negatively correlated with age.

With regard to the changes in bone formation with aging, it has been reported that cells in culture from young rats produced three times more bone-like nodules, compared with older rats. The difference in bone-forming activity between the child and adult reflects an age-related decline in the number of marrow osteoblast progenitor cells, or their potential to differentiate into mature osteoblasts [13,29,30].

These findings suggest that (a) the rate of cell proliferation reflects, in part, the change in bone formation, and (b) the number of ALP-positive CFU-Fs is one of the indices that reflect bone-forming activity. Furthermore, the evaluation of the activity of osteoprogenitor cells in iliac bone marrow could be useful for estimating the bone formation activity in individual patients [19,21].

Future Directions

Our results have demonstrated that human bone marrow cells express osteoblastic features such as ALP activity and the formation of calcification nodules. This indicates that osteoblast progenitor cells exist in human bone marrow. Since the rate of bone formation at the tissue level is dependent on the number of osteoblasts, and on the functional activity of each osteoblast, the evaluation of bone marrow cells and the number of ALP-positive CFU-Fs provide an approach for the investigation of the mechanism of bone formation, and the differentiation of osteoblast progenitor cells into osteoblasts. This procedure will eventually be used in the clinic. In addition, osteoblast progenitor cells with osteoblastic properties in the bone marrow could serve as a reservoir for use in bone grafting.

Acknowledgments. We would like to thank Masahumi Homma, MD; Toshiro Iga, MD; and Seiya Hatakeyama, MD, from the Hamagumi Children's Rehabilitation Center Niigata, Niigata City, Japan, for their special assistance in our study. We also acknowledge Ms. Hiroe Kondo for her technical support, and Mr. Shinichi Nishikiori, Mr. Hideki Akazawa, and Mr. Masahumi Saito for their help in the study.

References

1. Aubin JE, Liu F, Malaval L, Gupta AK (1995) Osteoblast and chondroblast differentiation. Bone 17:77S–83S
2. Lian JT, Stein GS (1996) Osteoblast biology. In: Marcus R, Feldman D, Kelsey J (eds) Osteoporosis. Academic, San Diego, pp 23–59
3. Parfitt AM, Villanueva AR, Foldes J, Rao DS (1995) Relations between histologic indices of bone formation: Implication for the pathogenesis of spinal osteoporosis. J Bone Miner Res 10:466–487
4. Rodan GA, Harada S (1997) The missing bone. Cell 89:677–680

5. Caplan AR (1991) Mesenchymal stem cells. J Orthop Res 9:641–650
6. Connolly JF, Guse R, Lippiello L, Dehne R (1989) Development of an osteogenic bone-marrow preparation. J Bone Joint Surg 71-A:684–691
7. Friedenstein AJ (1990) Osteogenic stem cells in the bone marrow In: Heersche JNM, Kanis JA (eds) Bone and mineral research, vol. 7, Elsevier Amsterdam, pp 243–272
8. Kuznetsov SA, Krebsbach PH, Satomura K, Kerr J, Riminucci M, Benayahu D, Robey PG (1997) Single-colony derived strains of human marrow stromal fibroblasts form bone after transplantation in vivo. J Bone Miner Res 12:1335–1347
9. Owen M (1988) Marrow stromal cells. J Cell Sci 10 (Suppl):63–76
10. Prockop DJ (1997) Marrow stromal cells as stem cells for nonhematopoietic tissues. Science 276:71–74
11. Bergman RJ, Grazit D, Kahn AJ, Gruber H, McDougall S, Hahn TJ (1996) Age-related change in osteogenic stem cells in mice. J Bone Miner Res 11:568–577
12. Nishida S, Yamaguchi A, Takahashi HE, Yoshiki S, Suda T (1992) Properties of osteo-progenitor cells in bone marrow of aged and ovariectomized rats. J Bone Miner Res 7 (Supple 1):S113
13. Lian CT, Barnes J, Seedor JG, Quartuccio HA, Bolander M, Jeffrey JJ, Rodan GA (1992) Impaired bone activity in aged rats: Alteration at the cellular and molecular levels. Bone 13:435–441
14. Wergedal JE, Baylink DJ (1984) Characterization of cells isolated and cultured from human bone. Proc Soc Exp Biol Med 176:60–69
15. Yamamoto T, Ecarot B, Glorieux FH (1991) In vivo osteogenic activity of isolated human bone cells. J Bone Miner Res 6:45–51
16. Ashton BA, Adbullah F, Cave J, Williamson M, Sykes BC, Couch M, Poser JW (1985) Characterization of cells with high alkaline phosphatase activity derived from human bone and marrow: Preliminary assessment of their osteogenicity. Bone 6:313–319
17. Auf' Rmklok B, Hauschka PV, Schwartz E (1985) Characterization of human bone cells in culture. Calcif Tissue Int 37:228–235
18. Bab I, Passi-Even L, Gazit D, Sekeles E, Ashton BA, Peylan-Ramu N, Ziv I, Ulmansky M (1988) Osteogenesis in vivo diffusion chamber cultures of human marrow cells. Bone Miner 4:373–386
19. Bruder SP, Jaiswal N, Haynesworth SE (1997) Growth kinetics, self-renewal, and the osteogenic potential of purified human mesenchymal stem cells during extensive sub-cultivation and following cryopreservation. J Cell Biochem 64:278–294
20. Connolly JF, Guse R, Tiedeman J, Dehne R (1991) Autologous marrow injection as a substitute for operative grafting of tibial nonunions. Clin Orthop 266:259–270
21. Majors AK, Boehm CA, Nitto H, Midura RJ, Muschler GF (1997) Characterization of human bone marrow stromal cells with respect to osteoblastic differentiation. J Orthop Res 15:546–557
22. Marie PJ (1994) Human osteogenic cells: A potential tool to assess the etiology of pathologic bone formation. J Bone Miner Res 9:1847–1850
23. Muschler GF, Boehm C, Easley K (1997) Aspiration to obtain osteoblast progenitor cells from human bone marrow: The influence of aspiration volume J Bone Joint Surg 79:1699–1709
24. Robey PG, Termine JD (1985) Human bone cells in vitro. Calcif Tissue Int 37:453–460
25. Fromigue O, Marie PJ, Lomori A (1998) Bone morphogenetic protein-2 and trans-forming growth factor-beta-2 interact to modulate human bone marrow stromal cell proliferation and differentiation. J Cell Biochem 68:411–426
26. Long MW, Robinson JA, Ashcraft EA, Mann KG (1995) Regulation of human bone marrow-derived osteoprogenitor cells by osteogenic growth factors. J Clin Invest 95:881–887
27. Nishida S, Yamaguchi A, Tanizawa T, Endo N, Mashiba T, Uchiyama Y, Suda T, Yoshiki S, Takahashi HE (1994) Increased bone formation by intermittent parathyroid

hormone administration is due to the stimulation of proliferation and differentiation of osteoprogenitor cells in bone marrow. Bone 15:717–723
28. Ashton BA, Allen TD, Howlett CR, Eagleson CC, Hattori A, Owen M (1980) Formation of bone and cartilage by marrow stromal cells in diffusion chambers in vivo. Clin Orthop 151:297–307
29. Inoue K, Ohgushi H, Yoshikawa T, Okumura M, Sempuku T, Tamai S, Dohi Y (1997) The effect of aging on bone formation in porous hydroxyappatite: Biochemical and histological analysis. J Bone Miner Res 12:989–994
30. Quarto R, Thomas D, Liang CT (1995) Bone progenitor cell deficits and age associated decline in bone repair capacity. Calcif Tissue Int 56:123–129

Trabecular Bone Turnover and Bone Marrow Capacity for Bone Cells in Immobilization-Related Bone Loss

AKINORI SAKAI

Summary. Adequate physical exercise promotes bone formation and inhibits bone resorption. Immobilization, in contrast, reduces bone formation and enhances bone resorption. In the present study, it was found that the immobilized tibia of mice after neurectomy of the sciatic nerve showed a decrease in bone formation from 3 to 5 days after the treatment. The bone resorption increased from 7 days, reached a peak level from 14 to 21 days after the start of immobilization, and thereafter gradually decreased. The population of alkaline phosphatase-positive cells among colony-forming units-fibroblastic, which are considered the progenitor cells of osteoblasts, decreased. The formation of colony-forming units for granulocytes and macrophages was not different between the immobilized tibia and the sham-operated tibia; however, the tartrate-resistant acid phosphatase-positive multinucleated cells transiently increased in the immobilized tibial bone marrow under parathyroid hormone stimulation, from 10 to 14 days postsurgery. The terminal process in the osteoclast development was thus thought to be enhanced by immobilization.

Key words. Immobilization, Unloading, Bone marrow, Colony-forming units-fibroblastic (CFU-f); Colony-forming units for granulocytes and macrophages (CFU-GM)

Introduction

Immobilization of bones and joints under conditions such as long-term bed rest, paralysis after spinal cord injury or peripheral nerve injury, and plaster cast fixation leads to systemic or local bone loss. Mechanical stress, such as physical exercise or physical loading, modulates bone metabolism at various levels, from systemic hormonal function to genomic translation. Mechanical stress is essential for bone growth and the activation of bone metabolism [1,2]. The proper amount of physical exercise promotes bone formation and inhibits bone resorption. Immobilization, in contrast, inhibits bone formation and promotes bone resorption, and as a result leads to bone loss known clinically as disuse bone atrophy and disuse osteoporosis.

Department of Orthopaedic Surgery, University of Occupational and Environmental Health, 1-1 Iseigaoka, Yahatanishi-ku, Kitakyushu 807-8555, Japan

Clinical Conditions of Immobilization Osteopenia

Trabecular bone metabolism changes more significantly under the unloaded condition without exercise or bodyweight bearing than under the loaded condition. Urinary and serum calcium levels and bone resorption increase after systemic immobilization such as bed rest [3,4]; bone volume is rapidly lost and the bone strength weakens [5]. Immobilization causes more severe bone loss in infants and the young than in the old [6], and in patients with diseases that promote a bone metabolic condition such as hyperparathyroidism, Paget's disease of the bone, and hypercalcemia due to malignant tumors. The higher the trabecular bone turnover, the larger the bone loss. Thus, the effects of immobilization on bone metabolism depend on the individual basal level of bone turnover.

Continuous bed rest for a few days to a number of weeks causes abnormal bone resorption–formation coupling, reduces bone formation, and enhances bone resorption. Bone loss caused by immobilization for at least 3–4 weeks is detectable by measurement with dual-energy X-ray absorptiometry (DXA). While the rate of bone loss due to postmenopausal osteoporosis is 2%–4% per year, immobilization causes more rapid bone loss. Krolner et al. [7] reported approximately 1% bone loss per week and a 10%–20% loss per every few months in patients confined to bed for the long term.

Mechanism of Immobilization Osteopenia

To investigate the effects of immobilization or non-weight bearing on bone mass, neurectomized animals and tail-suspension animals were used.

The Effects of Immobilization on Bone Formation and Bone Resorption

We treated 6-week-old ddY mice and rats with limb immobilization by sciatic neurectomy and compared histomorphometrically tibial undecalcified samples in the immobilized limbs with those in sham-operated limbs [8–10] (Fig. 1). Bone labeling with an intraperitoneal calceine injection (6 mg/kg bodyweight) was performed twice at 5 and 2 days before the animals were killed.

The bone formation rate decreased significantly from 3 to 5 days and recovered 10 days after start of the immobilization. The trabecular bone volume and trabecular thickness were significantly decreased in the immobilized tibia compared to the sham-operated tibia 14 days after surgery. The percentage of calceine double-labeled trabecular surface was significantly decreased 7 and 12 days in the immobilized tibia after surgery and thereafter returned to the same level observed in the sham-operated tibia. The bone mineral apposition rate was lower in the immobilized tibia than in the sham-operated tibia, but the difference was not significant.

The osteoclast number and osteoclast surface at the trabeculum transiently increased from 7 days, reached the peak level from 14 to 21 days after immobilization and returned to the sham level at 42 days.

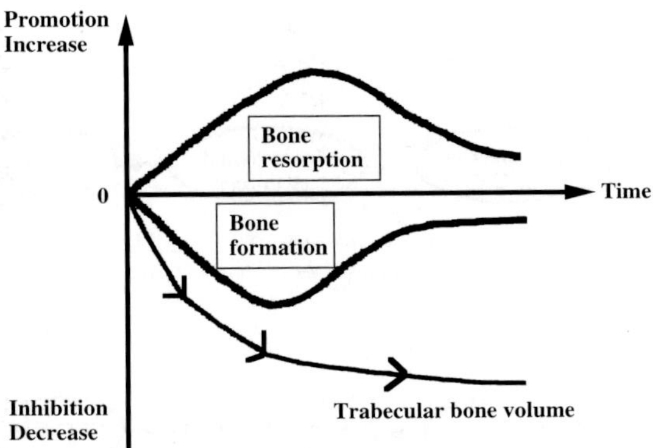

FIG. 1. Time course of trabecular bone dynamics after immobilization

The Effects of Immobilization on Bone Marrow Cells

Bone and cartilage disorders are focused on bone marrow cell differentiation and proliferation, and cytoplasmic or nuclear signal transduction. We studied the effects of immobilization on bone marrow cells by treating 6-week-old ddY male mice with sciatic neurectomy [8]. We compared bone marrow cells obtained from the immobilized tibia with those from the sham-operated tibia in the cell culture system described by Takahashi et al. [11].

We observed that the number of adherent bone marrow stromal cells, i.e., those adhering to the bottom surface of the culture dish, decreased immediately after immobilization and recovered to the same level as that of the sham limbs 12 days after surgery. These adherent cells showed the same level of cell proliferation in the immobilized tibia and the sham tibia, based on the data of [^{3}H]-thymidine incorporation. These results were due to the decrease in the proportion of adherent stromal cells among the total bone marrow cells. The alkaline phosphatase (ALP) activity in the bone marrow cells decreased time-dependently after immobilization. Colony-forming units-fibroblastic (CFU-f) showed a steady-state level throughout the experimental period, with no difference between the immobilized and sham tibiae. The proportion of ALP-positive cells among the fibroblastic cells declined after immobilization (Fig. 2a).

The tartrate-resistant acid phosphatase (TRAP)-positive multinucleated cells formed from the immobilized tibial bone marrow increased transiently from 10 to 14 days after immobilization in the presence of parathyroid hormone (PTH). There was no transient increase in the sham limbs or in the neurectomized limbs in the presence of 1,25(OH)$_2$D$_3$ or prostaglandin E$_2$ (PGE$_2$). The mechanism underlying the enhancement of bone resorption in immobilization was thus thought to be associated with the abnormality in the developmental process of osteoclast differentiation by PTH. Colony-forming units for granulocytes and macrophages (CFU-GM) transiently showed a two-fold increase in both the immobilized tibia and the sham tibia 12 to 14 days after surgery, and then returned to the baseline level. The terminal process in osteoclast development was thus enhanced by immobilization (Fig. 2b).

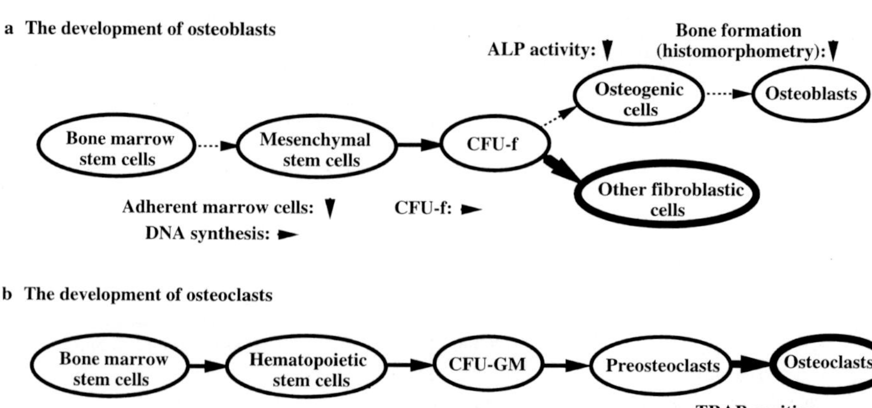

Fig. 2a,b. The effects of immobilization on the development of (a) osteoblasts and (b) osteo-clasts. *CFU-f*, colony-forming units-fibroblastic; *ALP*, alkaline phosphatase; *CFU-GM*, colony-forming units for granulocytes and macrophages; *TRAP*: tartrate-resistant acid phosphatase

The Effects of Unloading on Bone Formation

Conditions such as bed rest present several factors regarding immobilization and unloading which work in combination to affect bone loss. There are some mechanistic differences in the bone loss due to immobilization and that due to unloading. In a rat model, bone formation was shown to stop in the tibia and lumbar body 5 days after the start of tail-suspension, and the bone formation gradually recovered at 15 days with continued tail-suspension [12]. Based on the measurement of serum osteocalcin, the bone formation was estimated to decrease from 2 to 5 days after tail-suspension and recover thereafter [13]. The bone formation rate, which was measured by tetracycline bone labeling, changed in the same manner as serum osteocalcin. However, although the bone formation recovered in the rat model mentioned above, the bone loss during the initial 2 weeks could not be restored [14]. Subsequent loading after a 2-week unloading in this model stimulated bone formation more than usual until the lost bone volume recovered. There were no remarkable changes in bone formation and bone volume in either the humerus or the vertebral body of the cervical spine in tail-suspension rats.

Tail-suspension for 14 days reduced the gain in the bone mineral density (BMD) of the femur at both the metaphysis (rich in trabecular bone) and the diaphysis (rich in cortical bone). Treatment with pamidronate, an inhibitor of bone resorption, could not restore the normal gains in cortical bone mass and strength [15].

Tail-suspension rats had normal serum levels of steroid hormone and PTH. The serum level of $1,25(OH)_2D_3$ decreased significantly in parallel with the level of bone formation. However, even if $1,25(OH)_2D_3$ was administered intravenously until it reached the normal level, bone loss by unloading could not be prevented.

Unloaded bone showed a resistant response to insulin-like growth factor I (IGF-I). IGF-I and IGF-I receptor increased at both the mRNA and protein levels in the tibia of tail-suspension rats. The intravenous administration of IGF-I increased bone volume in the loaded humerus, but did not in the unloaded femur and tibia [16]. Osteoblasts in unloaded bone might show a resistant response to IGF-I at various levels, from cytoplasmic signal transduction to genomic actions.

The Effects of Immobilization on Articular Cartilage

We prepared a knee joint immobilization model by fixing the hind limb of 6-month-old male Japanese white rabbits in a plaster cast [17]. The articular cartilage was degraded 7 days after the immobilization. We found that in a cell culture system, the combination of basic fibroblast growth factor (bFGF) and transforming growth factor-β 1 (TGF-β 1) or that of bFGF and TGF-β 2 synergistically stimulated the DNA synthesis of articular chondrocytes obtained from the articular cartilage of a rabbit immobilized for 7 days. Such a response was not found in the chondrocytes obtained at 4 or 14 days of immobilization. We observed the different responses of cultured articular chondrocytes to growth factors such as bFGF, TGF-β 1 and TGF-β 2 early after immobilization.

The Importance of Parathyroid Hormone

Bone is the site of calcium storage and the supportive organ of the skeleton. In the evolutionary process of animal development from life underwater to life on land, a large calcium storage and a strong structure against gravity were needed. With this evolution, the parathyroid gland developed. Calcium can be utilized effectively through the action of PTH on the parathyroid gland and active vitamin D. Modulation systems of bone metabolism such as bone resorption-formation coupling developed in land animals. The mechanism of immobilization-related bone loss is thought to be related to a bone metabolic modulating system that developed as part of the process of moving from underwater life to land life.

Based on the following findings, the mechanism of immobilization osteopenia appears to involve PTH. The process of osteoclast development from bone marrow cells to TRAP-positive multinucleated cells in the presence of PTH was enhanced in immobilized tibia [8]. Immobilization osteopenia was partially improved by parathyroidectomy [18,19]. WR-2721, an antagonist of PTH, suppressed the number of increased osteoclasts [20]. With a lack of calcium bone resorption was enhanced. This stimulated PTH secretion [21].

Clinical Treatment

In patients with osteopenia due to short-term immobilization without a basic bone metabolic disorder, the clinical symptoms improve. The lost bone volume can recover without specific treatment. For patients with osteopenia due to long-term immobilization, we treat the osteopenia with the standard drugs against postmenopausal or senile osteoporosis and have no specific treatment protocol.

It is thought that PTH antagonist administration is useful to treat or to prevent immobilization osteoporosis. The activity of cyclooxygenase type II (COX-II), prostaglandin synthetase, was recently shown to be up-regulated by PGE_2. Mechanical stress such as loading stimulates the PGE_2 synthesis of osteoblasts, and this stimulative effect is amplified by an increase in COX-II. It is thus possible that immobilization osteopenia could be prevented or treated by the administration of a COX-II selective inhibitor.

Conclusions

The immobilized tibia of mice after neurectomy of the sciatic nerve showed a decrease in bone formation from 3 to 5 days after immobilization surgery. Bone resorption increased from 7 days, reached a peak level from 14 to 21 days after immobilization, and thereafter gradually decreased. The population of ALP-positive cells among the CFU-f colonies (which are considered the progenitor cells of osteoblasts) decreased. There was no difference in CFU-GM formation between the immobilized tibia and the sham tibia, but the TRAP-positive multinucleated cells increased in the immobilized tibial bone marrow under PTH stimulation. The terminal process in osteoclast development was thus enhanced by immobilization.

References

1. Frost HM (1985) The pathomechanics of osteoporosis. Clin Orthop 200:198–225
2. Frost HM (1987) The mechanostat: a proposed pathogenic mechanism of osteoporosis and the bone mass effects of mechanical and non-mechanical agents. Bone Miner 2:73–85
3. Stewart AF, Adler M, Byers CM, Segre GV, Broadus AE (1982) Calcium homeostasis in immobilization: an example of resorptive hypercalciuria. N Engl J Med 306:1136–1140
4. Isales C, Carcangiu ML, Stewart AF (1987) Hypercalcemia in breast cancer. Reassessment of the mechanism. Am J Med 82:1143–1147
5. Jenkins DP, Cochran TH (1969) Osteoporosis: the dramatic effect of disuse of an extremity. Clin Orthop 64:128–134
6. Bergstrom WH (1978) Hypercalciuria and hypercalcemia complicating immobilization. Am J Dis Child 132:553–554
7. Krolner B, Toft B, Pors-Nielsen S, Tondevold E (1983) Physical exercise as prophylaxis against involutional vertebral bone loss: a controlled trial. Clin Sci 64:541–546
8. Sakai A, Nakamura T, Tsurukami H, Okazaki R, Nishida S, Tanaka Y, Norimura T, Suzuki K (1996) Bone marrow capacity for bone cells and trabecular bone turnover in immobilized tibia after sciatic neurectomy in mice. Bone 18:479–486
9. Murakami H, Nakamura T, Tsurukami H, Abe M, Barbier A, Suzuki K (1994) Effects of tiludronate on bone mass, structure, and turnover at the epiphyseal, primary, and secondary spongiosa in the proximal tibia of growing rats after sciatic neurectomy. J Bone Miner Res 9:1355–1364
10. Weinreb M, Rodan GA, Thompson DD (1989) Osteopenia in the immobilized rat hind limb is associated with increased bone resorption and decreased bone formation. Bone 10:187–194
11. Takahashi N, Yamana H, Yoshiki S, Roodman GD, Mundy GR, Jones SJ, Boyde A, Suda T (1988) Osteoclast-like cell formation and its regulation by osteotrophic hormones in mouse bone marrow cultures. Endocrinology 122:1373–1382

12. Globus RK, Bikle DD, Morey-Holton E (1986) The temporal response of bone to unloading. Endocrinology 118:733–742
13. Patterson-Buckendahl P, Globus RK, Bikle DD, Cann CE, Morey-Holton E (1989) Effects of simulated weightlessness on rat osteocalcin and bone calcium. Am J Physiol 257:R1103–R1109
14. Sessions ND, Halloran BP, Bikle DD, Wronski TJ, Cone CM, Morey-Holton E (1989) Bone response to normal weight bearing after a period of skeletal unloading. Am J Physiol 257:E606–E610
15. Kodama Y, Nakayama K, Fuse H, Fukumoto S, Kawahara H, Takahashi H, Kurokawa T, Sekiguchi C, Nakamura T, Matsumoto T (1997) Inhibition of bone resorption by pamidronate cannot restore normal gain in cortical bone mass and strength in tail-suspended rapidly growing rats. J Bone Miner Res 12:1058–1067
16. Bikle DD, Harris J, Halloran BP, Morey-Holton ER (1994) Skeletal unloading induces resistance to insulin-like growth factor I. J Bone Miner Res 9:1789–1796
17. Okazaki R, Sakai A, Nakamura T, Kunigita N, Norimura T, Suzuki K (1996) Effects of transforming growth factor β s and basic fibroblast growth factor on articular chondrocytes obtained from immobilised rabbit knees. Ann Rheum Dis 55:181–186
18. Burkhart JM, Jowsey J (1967) Parathyroid and thyroid hormones in the development of immobilization osteoporosis. Endocrinology 81:1053–1062
19. Lindgren U (1975) The effect of thyroparathyroidectomy on the development of disuse osteoporosis in adult rats. Clin Orthop 118:251–256
20. Shaker JL, Fallon MD, Goldfarb S, Farber J, Attie MF (1989) WR-2721 reduces bone loss after hindlimb tenotomy in rats. J Bone Miner Res 4:885–890
21. Weinreb M, Rodan GA, Thompson DD (1991) Immobilization-related bone loss in the rat is increased by calcium deficiency. Calcif Tissue Int 48:93–100

Cbfa1 Is a Master Gene for Osteoblast Differentiation

Toshihisa Komori

Summary. A transcription factor, Cbfa1, which belongs to the *runt*-domain gene family, is expressed restrictively in fetal development. *Cbfa1* expression was first detected at embryonic day 9.5, which is four days earlier than the beginning of ossification, and was preferentially detected in the osteoblast lineage during osteogenesis. *Cbfa1* deficient mice lacked both intramembranous and endochondral ossification completely. The skeletons of the mutant mice are composed of cartilage and fibrous tissues in calvaria. *Cbfa1* mutant mice expressed alkaline phosphatase and osteonectin, which are the markers for osteoprogenitors, but not osteopontin and osteocalcin, which are the markers for immature osteoblasts and mature osteoblasts respectively. Therefore, the differentiation of osteoblast was blocked in the mutant mice. Further, *Cbfa1* expression in nonosteoblastic cells induced osteoblastic markers in vitro. These data demonstrate that Cbfa1 is an essential transcription factor for osteoblast differentiation. The maturational disturbance of osteoclast and chondrocyte was also observed in the mutant mice, indicating the direct or indirect role of Cbfa1 in the differentiation of osteoclast and chondrocyte. Heterozygously mutated mice in the *Cbfa1* locus showed the similar phenotype with cleidocranial dysplasia, which is an autosomal inherited disease. The mutations of *CBFA1* locus were identified in cleidocranial dysplasia patients.

Key words. Cbfa1, *Runt*-domain gene family, Osteoblast differentiation, Cleidocranial dysplasia, Bone formation

Introduction

Bones are generated by the two mechanisms of intramembranous and endochondral ossification. Both mechanisms require osteoblasts and osteoclasts, and endochondral bone formation involves the proliferation and differentiation of chondrocytes and their replacement by osteoblasts. Osteoclasts originate from hematopoietic precursors of monocytes [1], and osteoblasts and chondrocytes are derived from the common

Third Department of Medicine, Osaka University Medical School, 2-2 Yamada-oka, Suita, Osaka 565-0871, Japan precursors of mesenchymal cells, including osteoblasts, chondrocytes, myoblasts, adipocytes, tendon cells, and dermal fibroblasts [2]. These progenitors acquire specific phenotypes depending on the maturational stage of the particular cell type during the differentiation process. In the case of skeletal muscles, the muscle-specific transcription factors of the MyoD family, which belong to the basic Helix-Loop-Helix family, are necessary for determining the pathway of differentiation into the muscle lineage [3]. In addition, peroxisome proliferator-activated receptor γ_2 (PPARγ_2) plays an important role in determining the pathway of differentiation into the adipocyte lineage [4]. Recently, a specific transcription factor for osteoblast differentiation has been identified [5–7].

The core binding factor (Cbfa1), also called polyoma enhancer binding protein (Pebp2αA), is a transcription factor that belongs to the *runt*-domain gene family. Three *runt*-domain genes (*Cbfa1/Pebp2αA*, *Cbfa2/Pebp2αB*, and *Cbfa3/Pebp2αC*) have been identified [8–10]. They have a DNA-binding domain, *runt*, which is homologous with the Drosophila pair-rule gene *runt* [11] and they form heterodimers with the co-transcription factor Cbfb/Pebp2β, which is expressed ubiquitously, and acquire an enhanced DNA binding capacity in vitro [12,13]. CBF/PEBP2 specifically recognize a consensus sequence, TGPyGGTPy, which was originally identified in the polyoma virus enhancer [14] and murine leukemia virus enhancers [15]. The consensus sequence has also been found in T-cell-specific genes (TCRα, TCRβ, TCRδ, TCRγ, CD3ϵ), enzymes (myeloperoxidase, neutrophil elastase, granzyme B serine protease), and cytokines and their receptors (GM-CSF, IL-3, CSF-1) [5]. In recent studies, cbf/pebp2-related factors were shown to interact with the promoter region of osteocalcin gene [16–18].

CBFA2/PEBP2αB/AML1 and CBFB/PEBP2β are frequently involved in chromosomal translocations in acute leukemia and thought to be related to the luekemogenesis. Knockout mice of *Cbfa2* and *Cbfb* showed similar phenotype and died at the midgestation between embryonic day 10.5 and day 14.5 [19,20]. Both knockout mice exhibited hemorrhage in the central nervous system and lacked fetal liver hematopoiesis. Therefore, it was demonstrated that Cbfa2 is essential for fetal liver hematopoiesis and Cbfb is essential for the function of Cbfa2 in vivo.

Cbfa1 was originally cloned from mouse fibroblasts and *Cbfa1* expression was detected in T-cell lines, NIH3T3 cells, thymus, and testis [21]. Consistent with these observations, there is a Cbf/Pebp2 site (TGPyGGTPy) in the regulatory regions of many T-cell-specific genes, including the T cell receptor α, β, γ, and δ genes, and Cbfa1 binds to T-cell receptor β enhancer and stimulates the enhancer activity in vitro [8]. These observations led to the speculation that Cbfa1 is likely to be involved in T-lymphocyte-specific transcriptional regulation [21]. However, *Cbfa1* knockout mice showed complete lack of bone formation and it was evident that Cbfa1 is an essential transcription factor for bone formation [5,6].

Cbfa1 Gene and its Expression

The *Cbfa1* gene is composed of eight exons, and three N-terminal sequences were reported in mice and humans [7,8,22–24] (Fig. 1). One product starts with a sequence (MRIPVD) encoded by exon 1 (Fig. 1a), and two products contain sequences from

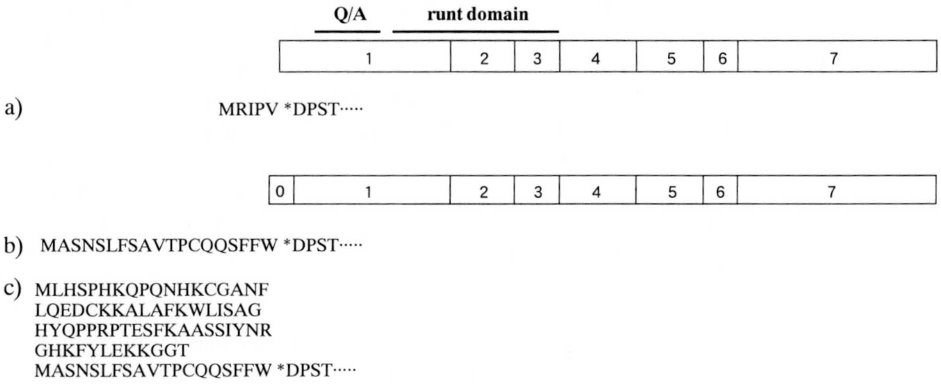

Q/A   **runt domain**

| | 1 | 2 | 3 | 4 | 5 | 6 | 7 |

a)   MRIPV *DPST·····

| 0 | 1 | 2 | 3 | 4 | 5 | 6 | 7 |

b) MASNSLFSAVTPCQQSFFW *DPST·····

c) MLHSPHKQPQNHKCGANF
    LQEDCKKALAFKWLISAG
    HYQPPRPTESFKAASSIYNR
    GHKFYLEKKGGT
    MASNSLFSAVTPCQQSFFW *DPST·····

FIG. 1. Diagrammatic representation of the structure of proteins encoded by mouse *Cbfa1* cDNAs and their *N*-terminal amino acids. Amino acid sequences *a–c* are from references 8, 23, and 7 respectively indicates a glutamine and alanine stretch. *Q/A*

exon 0 spliced to an aspartic acid residue at position 6 of the former sequence (Fig. 1b, 1c). In the latter products, two different translation start sites encoded by exon 0 were used [7,23,24]. Therefore, at least two promoters are regulating *Cbfa1* expression. Further, several variants of *Cbfa1* mRNA by alternative splicing have been reported [23]. However, the functional differences of these products remain to be investigated.

Cbfa1 expression was detected in bones and osteoblasts by Northern blot [7,25], and all skeletons at day 18.5 by in situ hybridization [5]. *Cbfa1* expression was observed strongly in osteoblasts and weakly in chondrocytes. It was also detected in the thymus and tendon, and weakly in the fibroblasts of dermis but not in the tissues including brain, heart, lung, gut, liver, and muscle by in situ hybridization [5]. In embryogenesis, the weak expression of *Cbfa1* was first detected at day 9.5 in the notochord underlying the mid- and hindbrain, at day 10.5 in the mesoderm destined to become shoulder bone, and at day 11.5 in maxillary and mandibular components of the first branchial arch as well as the humerus [6]. At day 12.5, *Cbfa1* expression was observed in the ribs and vertebral bodies of the spinal column, the developing bones of the limbs, the shoulder and pelvic girdles, the jaw, and the skull, and *Cbfa1* expressed strongly in the mesenchymal cells surrounding cartilaginous condensation [6]. Therefore, *Cbfa1* was expressed from osteoblast precursors to mature osteoblasts, but the meaning of the *Cbfa1* expression before the appearance of osteoblast precursors remains to be clarified.

Lack of Bone Formation in Cbfa1 Deficient Mice

Cbfa1 deficient mice died just after birth without breathing [5,6]. The mutant mice exhibited dwarfism uniformly and had short legs. They lacked ossification completely in both endochondral and intramembranous ossification [5,6]. In day-18.5 mutant embryos, the middle part of tibia remained as calcified cartilage without formation of the bone marrow cavity. Neither vascular nor mesenchymal cell invasion was observed in the calcified cartilage. Although alkaline phosphatase (AP)-positive cells appeared in the perichondrial region of the calcified cartilage, no bone was formed [5]. A few tartrate-resistant acid phosphatase (TRAP)-positive cells appeared adjacent to the calcified cartilage, at the perichondrium, but the size of the cells and the number of nuclei were reduced in comparison with those in wild-type embryos [5]. Femurs of mutant embryos were composed of non-calcified cartilage, and neither AP-positive nor TRAP-positive cells appeared at perichondrium of the femurs [5]. Therefore, both the development of osteoblasts and osteoclasts were blocked, and the appearance of AP-positive cells and TRAP-positive cells were correlated with the presence of calcification in the cartilage. Further, the maturation of chondrocytes was also disturbed, because calcification of cartilage was restricted in the tibia, fibula, ulna, and radius, and osteopontin expression was not observed in the hypertrophic chondrocytes in the calcified cartilage. Calvaria of mutant mice were composed of a thin layer of AP-positive cells without ossification and no TRAP-positive cells were observed [5].

Cleidocranial Dysplasia Is Caused by the Heterozygous Mutations in Cbfa1 Locus

Cleidocranial dysplasia (CCD) is an autosomal-dominant disease characterized by hypoplastic clavicle, open fontanelles, supernumerary teeth, short stature, and other changes in skeletal patterning and growth [26]. Heterozygously mutated mice in the *Cbfa1* locus exhibited a similar phenotype with CCD [5,6]. They had hypoplasia of the clavicle, nasal, parietal, interparietal, and supraoccipital bones with open fontanelles and sutures, and multiple Wormian bones. Hypoplastic hyoid bone and xiphoid process with two well-separated ossification centers were also observed. The pubic and ischial bones were widely separated and hypoplastic. However, the development of the primordium of the tooth structure was slightly delayed but structurally normal [6]. These primordia were severely hypoplastic in homozygously mutated mice, although the differentiation into the different layers was recognizable. The lack of supernumerary teeth can be explained by the fact that mice have only one set of teeth, and primary teeth are not affected in humans [24].

A microdeletion in chromosome 6p21 has been shown in one family with CCD [27]. Furthermore, a radiation-induced mutant mouse that carries similarities with CCD (Ccd mouse) has been reported to have the deletion in chromosome 17 distal to the MHC complex in an area that shows homology to human 6p21 [28]. *CBFA1* was mapped to chromosome 6p12–p21 [29–31], and the mutations of the *CBFA1* gene were found in patients with CCD [24,30]. These include the deletion of the *CBFA1* gene, insertion of 16 nucleotides within the polyglutamine stretch which causes a stop codon in the *runt* domain, the deletion of 10 nucleotides within the *runt* domain, a missence mutation in the C-terminal region, an in-frame duplication within the polyalanine stretch leading to 27 alanine residues instead of 17 residues, and missense mutations in the *runt* domain. These patients had typical craniofacial features of CCD except for the patients with the in-frame duplication within the polyalanine stretch. They exhibited minor craniofacial features associated with brachydactyly of hands and feet [24].

Cbfa1 is a Transcription Factor for Osteoblast Differentiation

Cbfa1 mutant mice lacked both endochondral and intramembranous ossification and had maturational arrest of osteoblasts, because they expressed AP and osteonectin, which are the markers for osteoprogenitors, but not osteopontin and osteocalcin, which are the markers for immature osteoblasts and mature osteoblasts respectively [5]. This indicates that the lack of bone formation in *Cbfa1* deficient mice was caused by the maturational arrest of osteoblasts and demonstrates that Cbfa1 is essential for osteoblast differentiation. Does Cbfa1 function as the first transcription factor for the differentiation from pluripotent mesenchymal cells to osteoprogenitor cells? *Cbfa1* expression was detected four days earlier than the beginning of ossification [6]. Further, BSP and osteocalcin were induced by the transfection of a *Cbfa1* expression vector to C3H10T1/2 and skin fibroblasts [7]. Therefore, Cbfa1 seems to function from the early stage of osteoblast differentiation. However, AP was detected in the calvaria and the periphery of calcified cartilage of *Cbfa1* deficient mice [5]. Therefore, Cbfa1 is certainly an essential factor for the maturation of osteoprogenitors, but it remains to be clarified whether Cbfa1 is the earliest factor for the induction of osteoprogenitors from pluripotent mesenchymal cells in vivo.

References

1. Suda T, Udagawa N, Takahashi N (1996) Cells of bone: osteoclast generation. In: Bilezikian JP, Raisz LG, Rodan GA (eds) Principles of bone biology. Academic, London, pp 87–102
2. Aubin JE, Turksen K, Heersche JNM (1993) Osteoblastic lineage. In: Noda M (ed) Cellular and molecular biology of bone. Academic, London, pp 1–45
3. Weintraub H (1993) The MyoD family and myogenesis: redundancy, networks, and thresholds. Cell 75:1241–1244
4. Tontonoz P, Hu E, Spiegelman BM (1994) Stimulation of adipogenesis in fibroblasts by PPARγ₂, a lipid-activated transcription factor. Cell 79:1147–1156
5. Komori T, Yagi H, Nomura S, Yamaguchi A, Sasaki K, Deguchi K, Shimizu Y, Bronson RT, Gao YH, Inada M, Sato M, Okamoto R, Kitamura Y, Yoshiki S, Kishimoto T (1997) Targeted disruption of Cbfa1 results in a complete lack of bone formation owing to maturational arrest of osteoblasts. Cell 89:755–764
6. Otto F, Thornell AP, Crompton T, Denzel A, Gilmour KC, Rosewell IR, Stamp GWH, Beddington RSP, Mundlos S, Olsen BR, Selby PB, Owen MJ (1997) Cbfa1, a candidate gene for cleidocranial dysplasia syndrome, is essential for osteoblast differentiation and bone development. Cell 89:765–771
7. Ducy P, Zhang R, Geoffroy V, Ridall AL, Karsenty G (1997) Osf2/Cbfa1: a transcriptional activator of osteoblast differentiation. Cell 89:747–754
8. Ogawa E, Maruyama M, Kagoshima H, Inuzuka M, Lu J, Satake M, Shigesada K, Ito Y (1993) PEBP₂/PEA₂ represents a new family of transcription factor homologous to the products of the Drosophila *runt* and the human *AML1* gene. Proc Natl Acad Sci USA 90:6859–6863
9. Bae SC, Yamaguchi-Iwai Y, Ogawa E, Maruyama M, Inuzuka M, Kagoshima H, Shigesada K, Satake M, Ito Y (1993) Isolation of PEBP2αB cDNA representing the mouse homolog of human acute myeloid leukemia gene, *AML1*. Oncogene 8:809–814
10. Bae SC, Takahashi E, Zhang YW, Ogawa E, Shigesada K, Namba Y, Satake M, Ito Y (1995) Cloning, mapping and expression of PEBP2αC, a third gene encoding the mammalian Runt domain. Gene 159:245–248

11. Kania MA, Bonner AS, Duffy JB, Gergen JP (1990) The Drosophila segmentation gene *runt* encodes a novel nuclear regulatory protein that is also expressed in the developing nervous system. Genes Dev 4:1701–1713

12. Ogawa E, Inuzaka M, Maruyama M, Satake M, Naito-Fujimoto M, Ito Y, Shigesada K (1993) Molecular cloning and characterization of PEBP2β, the heterodimeric partner of a novel Dorosophila runt-related DNA binding protein PEBP2α. Virology 194:314–331

13. Wang S, Wang Q, Crute BE, Melnikova IN, Keller SR, Speck NA (1993) Cloning and characterization of subunits of the T-cell receptor and murine leukemia virus enhancer core-binding factor. Mol Cell Biol 13:3324–3339

14. Kamachi Y, Ogawa E, Asano M, Ishida S, Murakami Y, Satake M, Ito Y, Shigesada K (1990) Purification of a mouse nuclear factor that binds to both the A and B cores of the polyomavirus enhancer. J Virol 64:4808–4819

15. Wang S, Speck NA (1992) Purification of core-binding factor, a protein that binds the conserved core site in murine leukemia virus enhancers. Mol Cell Biol 12:89–102

16. Geoffroy V, Ducy P, Karsenty G (1995) A PEBP2α/AML-1-related factor increases osteocalcin promoter activity through its binding to an osteoblast-specific cis-acting element. J Biol Chem 270:30973–30979

17. Merriman HL, van Wijnen AJ, Hiebert S, Bidwell JP, Fey E, Lian J, Stein J, Stein GS (1995) The tissue-specific nuclear matrix protein, NMP-2, is a member of the AML/CBF/PEBP2/*Runt domain* transcription factor family: interaction with the osteocalcin gene promoter. Biochemistry 34:13125–13132

18. Banerjee C, Hiebert SW, Stein JL, Lian JB, Stein GS (1996) An AML-1 consensus sequence binds an osteoblast-specific complex and transcriptionally activates the osteocalcin gene. Proc Natl Acad Sci USA 93:4968–4973

19. Sasaki K, Yagi H, Bronson RT, Tominaga K, Matsunashi T, Deguchi K, Tani Y, Kishimoto T, Komori T (1996) Absence of fetal liver hematopoiesis in mice deficient in transcriptional coactivator core binding factor β. Proc Natl Acad Sci USA 93:12359–12363

20. Wang Q, Stacy T, Miller JD, Lewis AF, Gu TL, Huang X, Bushweller JH, Bories JC, Alt FW, Ryan G, Liu PP, Wynshaw-Boris A, Binder M, Marín-Padilla M, Sharp AH, Speck NA (1996) The CBFβ subunit is essential for CBFα2 (AML1) function in vivo. Cell 87:697–708

21. Satake M, Nomura S, Yamaguchi-Iwai Y, Takahama Y, Hashimoto Y, Niki M, Kitamura Y, Ito Y (1995) Expression of the runt domain-encoding PEBP2α genes in T cells during thymic development. Mol Cell Biol 15:1662–1670

22. Ahn MY, Bae SC, Maruyama M, Ito Y (1996) Comparison of the human genomic structure of the Runt domain-encoding *PEBP2/CBFα* gene family. Gene 168:279–280

23. Stewart M, Terry A, Hu M, O'hara M, Blyth K, Baxter E, Cameron E, Onions DE, Neil JC (1997) Proviral insertions induce the expression of bone-specific isoforms of PEBP2αA (CBFA1): evidence for a new *myc* collaborating oncogene. Proc Natl Acad Sci USA 94:8646–8651

24. Mundlos S, Otto F, Mundlos C, Mulliken JB, Aylsworth AS, Albright S, Lindhout D, Cole WG, Henn W, Knoll JH M, Owen MJ, Mertelsmann R, Zabel BU, Olsen BR (1997) Mutations involving the transcription factor CBFA1 cause cleidocranial dysplasia. Cell 89:773–779

25. Banerjee C, McCabe LR, Choi J, Hiebert SW, Stein JL, Stein GS, Lian JB (1997) Runt homology domain proteins in osteoblast differentiation: AML3/CBFA1 is a major component of a bone-specific complex. J Cell Biochem 66:1–8

26. Jarvis JL, Keats TE (1974) Cleidocranial dysostosis, a review of 40 new cases. Am J Radiol 121:5–16

27. Mundlos S, Mulliken JB, Abramson DL, Warman ML, Knoll JH M, Olsen BR (1995) Genetic mapping of cleidocranial dysplasia and evidence of a microdeletion in one family. Hum Mol Genet 4:71–75

28. Mundlos S, Huang LF, Selby P, Olsen BR (1996) Cleidocranial dysplasia in mice. Ann NY Acad Sci 785:301–302
29. Levanon D, Negreanu V, Bernstein Y, Bar-Am I, Avivi L, Groner, Y (1994) AML1, AML2, and AML3, the human members of the *runt* domain gene-family: cDNA structure, expression, and chromosomal localization. Genomics 23:425–432
30. Lee B, Thirunavukkarasu K, Zhou L, Pastore L, Baldini A, Hecht J, Geoffroy V, Ducy P, Karsenty G (1997) Missense mutations abolishing DNA binding of the osteoblast-specific transcription factor *OSF2/CBFA1* in cleidocranial dysplasia. Nature Genet 16:307–310
31. Zhang Y, Bae S, Takahashi E, Ito Y (1997) The cDNA cloning of the transcripts of human *PEBP2αA/CBFA1* mapped to 6p12.3–p21.1, the locus for cleidocranial dysplasia. Oncogene 15:367–371

Which Activates Mechanotransduction in Bone—Extracellular Fluid Flow or Mechanical Strain?

Ichiro Owan[1], Kunio Ibaraki[1], Randall L. Duncan[2],
Charles H. Turner[2], and David B. Burr[2]

Summary. We have defined mechanocoupling as the transduction of applied mechanical forces into a local mechanical signal which bone cells can perceive. Two candidates for this localized phenomenon are substrate strain or fluid flow within the bone matrix. Studies using the rat tibial 4-point bending model show that dynamic loads but not static loads increase bone formation, suggesting fluid flow as the machanical determinant of bone adaptation. To study the effects of these candidates on the osteoblast, MC3T3-E1 cells were grown on type I collagen-coated plastic plates and subjected to 4-point bending. Varying levels of substrate strain and fluid effects can be created independently in this system. Osteopontin (OPN) mRNA expression was used to assess the anabolic response of MC3T3-E1 cells. When fluid flow was low, neither strain magnitude nor strain rate was correlated with OPN expression. However, a higher magnitude of fluid flow significantly increased OPN mRNA expression independent of the strain magnitude or rate. We conclude that extracellular fluid flow might be more important than deformation of cell substrate in bone formation in response to mechanical loading.

Key words. Mechanical strain, Fluid flow, Mechanotransduction, Osteoblasts, Osteopontin

Introduction

Bone cell function is modulated by mechanical forces. Removal of mechanical stimulation, as in extended periods of immobilization or weightlessness, is characterized by reduced matrix protein production [1,2], mineral content [3], and bone formation [4,5] as well as an increase in bone resorption [6–8] resulting in a rapid loss of total body calcium [7,9]. Conversely, increased skeletal loading can increase bone formation and decrease bone resorption [10,11].

[1] Department of Orthopedic Surgery, Faculty of Medicine, University of the Ryukyus 207 Uehara, Nishihara, Okinawa 903-0125, Japan
[2] Department of Orthopedic Surgery and The Biomechanics and Biomaterials Research Center Indiana University Medical Center, Indianapolis, IN 46202, USA

The types of mechanical signals the bone cells perceive in vivo remain unclear. One school of thought suggests that the osteoblasts and osteocytes detect small deformations in the bone tissue brought on by external forces. Osteoblasts respond to strain in vitro. But, the magnitude of the strain used in most in vitro experiments was greater than 10000 µstrain [12–14] while typical strains incurred in bone tissue in humans during vigorous exercise are less than 2000 µstrain [15].

An alternative proposal is that the extracellular fluid flow mediates the response of bone to mechanical loading. Fluid is driven through the bone tissue by stress gradients resulting from external loads [16]. Cyclic mechanical forces, such as those produced by 4-point bending, cause fluid flow through the canaliculi as well as deformations in the extracellular matrix. It has also been reported that continuous fluid shear rapidly increases nitric oxide, cAMP, inositol triphosphate and prostaglandin (PGE_2) levels in osteoblast cultures [17–19]. Therefore, we hypothesized that stress-induced fluid flow rather than mechanical deformation plays a key role in mechanotransduction.

Rat Tibial 4-Point Bending

When external loads produced by a 4-point bending device are applied to the tibiae of rats, the bone tissue responds with increased bone formation after a threshold of 1050 µstrain is surpassed [20]. It has also been observed that the bone formation rate is dependent upon the applied strain rate [21]. When bending loads were applied to rat tibiae that created equivalent peak strains in the tissue but with varied rates of strain, bone formation was significantly increased in the two experimental groups with the highest strain rates compared to the groups with lower strain rates. The amount of new bone formation was directly proportional to the rate of strain in the bone tissue (Fig. 1a,b). Thus, the rate of change of deformation appears to be a more important stimulus for bone formation than the deformation itself. Likewise, applied loading at frequencies less than 0.5 Hz has no effect on bone formation in rats [22]. These results are strong evidence that bone cells are sensitive to dynamic loading and the corresponding extracellular fluid forces.

Cell Loading System

We developed an in vitro cell loading system using 4-point bending, in which mechanical deformation and fluid effects can be varied independently. MC3T3-E1 cells on the plates cultured in α-MEM with 10% serum were subjected to compressive strain with the Vitrodyne 1000 Universal Material Tester (Liveco, Burlington, VT, USA). The magnitude of strain on the plates was calculated as:

$$\varepsilon = td/a(L - 1.33a)$$

where ε is strain, t is plate thickness, d is displacement, and a and L are lengths shown in Fig. 2. Thicker plates or larger displacements result in larger strains. The magnitude of the fluid effects on bone cells is proportional to the displacement rate, that is, speed of the actuator ram movement. Thus, varying levels of substrate strain and fluid effects can be created by varying the plate thickness, displacement, and displacement rate. The calculated strain distribution on the plate was verified by measuring actual

Fig. 1. **a** Loading waveforms applied to the rat tibia. The peak magnitude of the applied load was 54 N for all groups, but the magnitude of the cyclic fraction of the load was varied from 0 N (Group 1) to 54 N (Group 4). Cyclic loading was applied at 36 cycles/day for 2 weeks. **b** Relative bone formation rate (*BFR/BS* of right tibia–BFR/BS of left tibia) expressed as means ± SEM. Bone formation rate was proportional to the magnitude of the cyclic fraction of the load waveform, which varied from 0 N for Group 1 to 54 N for Group 4. * Significant difference from Group 1; ** significant difference from Group 2. (Adapted from [21])

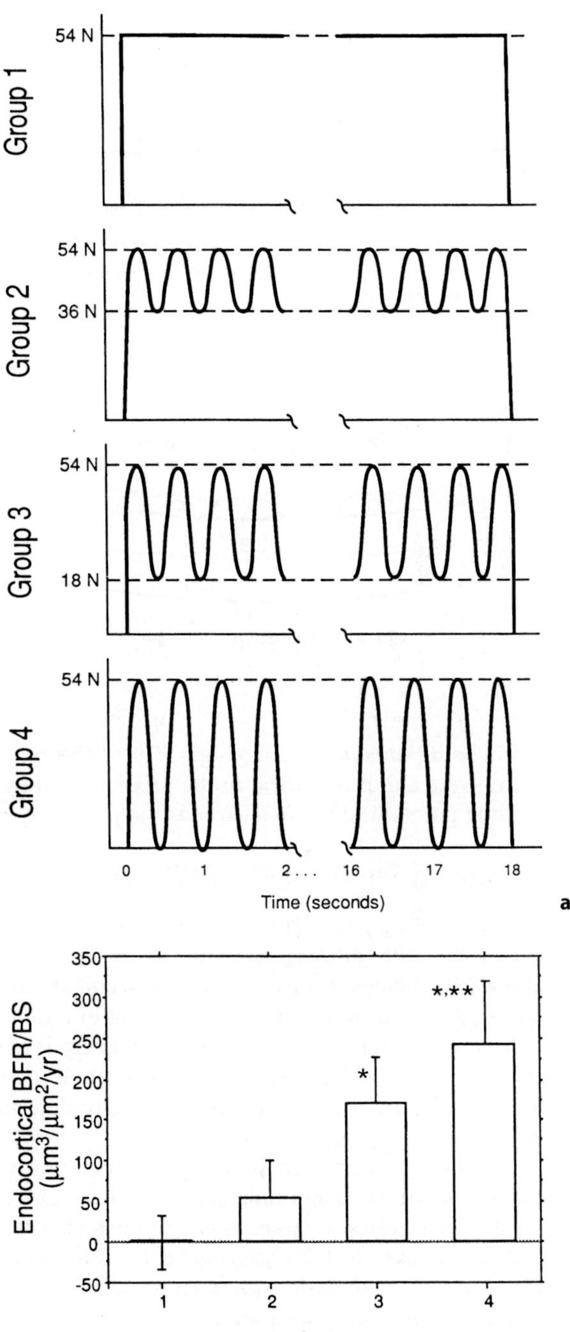

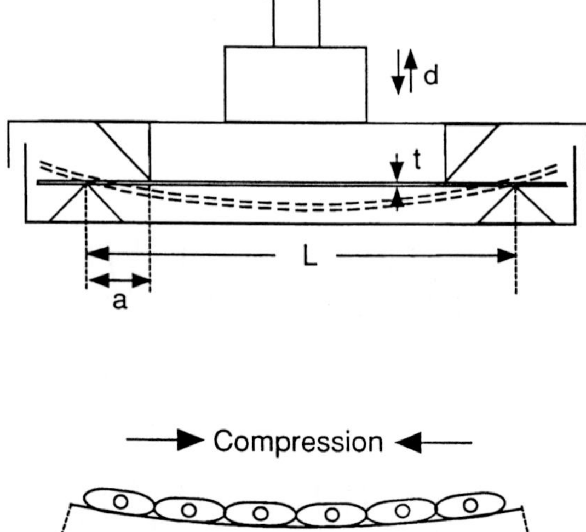

FIG. 2. Diagram of cell loading system. Cells are grown on type I collagen-coated plates. The plates are bent by applying 4-point loading, causing compressive strains on the cells. The strain on the cells is proportional to the product of plate thickness (t) and displacement (d). As the plate is pushed through the culture medium, fluid shear forces and pressures are imposed on the cells. These fluid effects are proportional to the displacement rate of the plate. Adapted from Owan et al., (1997)

strain using uniaxial strain gauges. The measured mechanical strains on the culture plates were almost identical to the predicted values in the region between the upper loading points, and no area exceeds the predicted value.

Substrate Strain or Fluid Effects

The anabolic response of MC3T3-E1 cells to mechanical stimuli was assessed by measuring the OPN mRNA expression after mechanical loading. Bending strains were applied at 4200 μstrain with a displacement rate of 3 mm/s for 24 h. Cells were harvested at 24, 48, 72 and 96 h following initiation of mechanical loading, and total RNA was extracted for Northern blot analysis. Time-course experiments demonstrated that MC3T3-E1 cells expressed a 4-fold increase at 72 h following the onset of loading (Fig. 3). This time point was used to determine maximal stimulation of OPN expression.

The strain magnitude and displacement rate were varied independently. Three ranges of strain magnitude, low, medium and high, as well as three different displacement rates ($\dot{d}$) were applied to osteoblasts for 24 h at 0.5 Hz (Table 1). There was no increase in OPN expression $\dot{d} = 2$ mm/s at regardless of strain magnitude. However, OPN expression was significantly increased at $\dot{d} = 3$ and 4 mm/s compared to each control, and compared to $\dot{d} = 2$ mm/s (Fig. 4). These studies demonstrated that strain magnitude had no effect on OPN expression, but application of larger displacement rates, that is, greater fluid forces, significantly increased OPN expression [23].

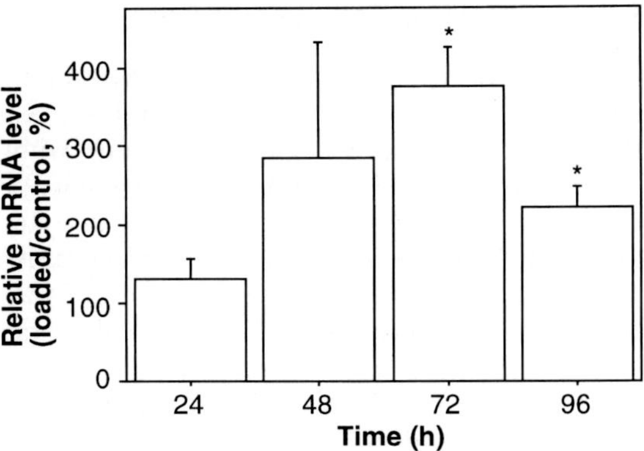

FIG. 3. Time course of osteopontin (OPN) mRNA expression in response to mechanical loading. Densitometric measurements of OPN expression from Northern blots (normalized by GAPDH expression; means ± SEM of three individual experiments). *Asterisks* indicate a significant difference compared to control ($P < 0.01$, using the Student's t-test; there was no change in OPN expression in the control samples with time, $P = 0.83$ by ANOVA). (Adapted from [23])

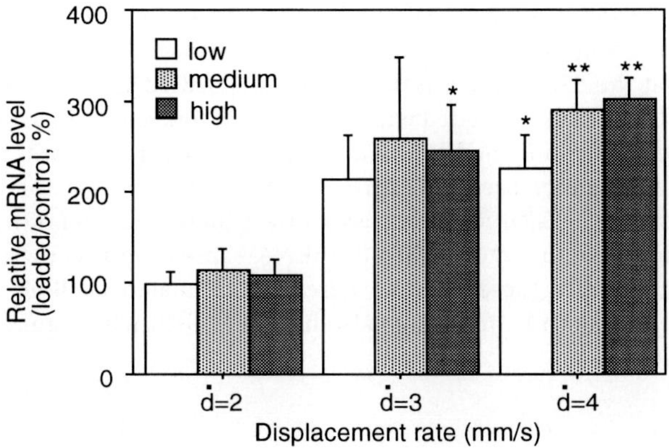

FIG. 4. Effects of different strain magnitudes and displacements on OPN mRNA expression. Fluid forces on the cells were approximately proportional to the displacement rate. Data were generated from densitometric measurements of OPN expression from Northern blots (normalized by GAPDH expression; means ± SEM of three individual experiments). *Asterisks* indicate significant differences compared to control (*$P < 0.05$, **$P < 0.005$, using the Student's t-test). Displacement rates of 3 mm/s and 4 mm/s significantly increased OPN expression compared to a displacement rate of 2 mm/s ($P < 0.01$, using Fisher's PLSD test). There was no effect of strain magnitude on OPN expression ($P = 0.46$, using two-way ANOVA). (Adapted from [23])

TABLE 1. Maximum displacement (d, mm), displacement rate ($\dot{d}$, mm/s), plate thickness (t, μm), and resultant peak strain magnitude ($\mu strain$) used in this experiment[a]

d (mm)	$\dot{d}$ (mm/s)	Strain magnitude (μstrain)		
		low	medium	high
2	2	1890 (t = 510)	2820 (t = 760)	4710 (t = 1270)
3	3	1390 (t = 250)	2840 (t = 510)	4230 (t = 760)
4	4	1850 (t = 250)	3780 (t = 510)	5640 (t = 760)

[a] Adapted from [23].

Shear Stress or Streaming Potentials

In our culture system, OPN expression was induced by fluid pressures or shear stresses applied to cells. Others have shown that bone cells are more sensitive to fluid shear stress than to fluid pressure [24]. Fluid flow within bone causes fluid shear stresses on the osteocytes and their cell processes, but it also creates electrical potentials called streaming potentials. From the results of this study, we cannot distinguish whether osteoblast function is modulated by shear stresses or streaming potentials. Reich et al. [17] found that increased viscosity of the fluid media caused an increased osteoblastic response even though the flow rate was held constant. This result indicated that the osteoblastic response was attributable to fluid shear stresses, which are dependent upon viscosity, rather than streaming potentials, which are viscosity-independent.

The exact mechanism through which mechanical stimuli affect gene expression is unknown. However, Resnick et al. [25,26] have identified a shear stress response element (SSRE) in the promoter region of several genes responsive to fluid shear in endothelial cells. Computer analysis of the OPN promoter regions of several species has revealed that the SSRE core binding sequence (GAGACC) or its complementary sequence (GGTCTC) is also encoded within the mouse, rat, and human OPN promoter. Whether OPN expression is mediated via this promoter region is still unclear.

Mechanical loading increased the expression of several other factors in addition to OPN. Both c-*fos* and COX-2 mRNA expression were increased after 30 min of loading, and transforming growth factor (TGF)-β_1 mRNA expression was increased after 6 h of loading. Additionally, these mRNAs were also regulated by fluid effects. These factors, such as TGF-β_1 and c-*fos*, which also have the SSRE, may regulate OPN mRNA expression.

Conclusion

In summary, using a 4-point bending device which enables us to independently vary the magnitudes of strain and fluid effects, we found that fluid flow, and not strain, alters OPN expression in cultured osteoblast-like cells. These data indicate that fluid shear is an important mediator of the osteogenic response to mechanical loading.

References

1. Simmons DJ, Russell JE, Winter F, Tran Van P, Vignery A, Baron R, Rosenberg GD, Walker WV (1983) Effect of spaceflight on the non-weight-bearing bones of rat skeleton. Am J Physiol 244:R319–R326
2. Patterson-Buckendahl PE, Grindeland RE, Martin RB, Cann CE, Arnaud SB (1985) Osteocalcin as an indicator of bone metabolism during spaceflight. Physiologist 28:S227–S228
3. Uhthoff HK, Jaworski ZFG (1978) Bone loss in response to long term immobilization. J Bone Joint Surg 60B:420–429
4. Morey ER, Baylink DJ (1978) Inhibition of bone formation during spaceflight. Science 201:1138–1141
5. Wronski TJ, Morey ER (1983) Inhibition of cortical and trabecular bone formation in the long bones of immobilized monkeys. Clin Orthop Rel Res 181:269–276

6. Cann CE, Adachi RR (1983) Bone resorption and mineral excretion in rats during spaceflight. Am J Physiol 244:R327–R331

7. Weinreb M, Rodan GA, Thompson DD (1991) Immobilization-related bone loss in rat is increased by calcium deficiency. Calcif Tissue Int 48:93–100

8. Vico L, Chappard D, Alexandre C, Palle S, Minaire P, Riffat G, Murukov B, Rakhmanov S (1987) Effects of a 120-day period of bed rest on bone mass and bone cell activities in man: attempts at countermeasure. Bone Miner 2:383–394

9. Rambaut PC, Johnston RS (1979) Prolonged weightlessness and calcium loss in man. Acta Astronaut 6:1113–1122

10. Rubin CT, Lanyon LE (1984) Regulation of bone formation by applied dynamic loads. J Bone Joint Surg 66A:397–402

11. Sessions ND, Halloran BP, Binkle DD, Wronski TJ, Cone CM, Morey-Holton ER (1989) Bone response to normal weight bearing after a period of skeletal unloading. Am J Physiol 257:E606–E610

12. Somjen D, Binderman I, Burger EH, Harell A (1980) Bone remodeling induced by physical stress is prostaglandin E_2 mediated. Biochim Biophys Acta 627:91–100

13. Binderman I, Shimshoni Z, Somjen D (1984) Biochemical pathways involved in the translation of physical stimulus into biological message. Calcif Tissue Int 36 (Suppl):582–585

14. Sandy JR, Meghji S, Farndale RW, Meikle MC (1989) Dual evaluation of cyclic AMP and inositol phosphates in response to mechanical deformation of murine osteoblasts. Biochim Biophys Acta 1010:265–269

15. Burr DB, Milgrom C, Fyhrie D, Forwood M, Nyska M, Finestone A, Hoshaw S, Saiag E, Simkin S (1996) In vivo measurement of human tibial strains during vigorous activity. Bone 18:405–410

16. Otter MW, Palmieri VR, Wu DD, Seiz KG, MacGinitie LA, Cochran GVB (1992) A comparative analysis of streaming potentials in vivo and in vitro. J Orthop Res 10:710–719

17. Reich KM, Gay CV, Frangos JA (1990) Fluid shear stress as a mediator of osteoblast cyclic adenosine monophosphate production. J Cell Physiol 143:100–104

18. Reich KM, Frangos JA (1993) Protein kinase C mediates flow-induced prostaglandin E_2 production in osteoblasts. Calcif Tissue Int 52:62–66

19. Johnson DL, McAllister TN, Frangos JA (1996) Fluid flow stimulates rapid and continuous release of nitric oxide in osteoblasts. Am J Physiol 271:E205–E208

20. Turner CH, Forwood MR, Yoshikawa T (1994) Mechanical loading thresholds for lamellar and woven bone formation. J Bone Min Res 9:87–97

21. Turner CH, Owan I, Takano Y (1995) Mechanotransduction in bone: role of strain rate. Am J Physiol 269:E438–E442

22. Turner CH, Forwood MR, Otter MW (1994) Mechanotransduction in bone: do bone cells act as sensors of fluid flow? FASEB J 8:875–878

23. Owan I, Burr DB, Turner CH, Qui J, Tu Y, Onyia JE, Duncan RL (1997) Mechanotransduction in bone: osteoblasts are more responsive to fluid forces than mechanical strain. Am J Physiol 273:C810–C815

24. Klein-Nulend J, Van Der Plas A, Semeins CM, Ajubi NE, Frangos JA, Nijweide PJ, Burger EH (1995) Sensitivity of osteocytes to biomechanical stress in vitro. FASEB J 9:441–445

25. Resnick N, Collins T, Atkinson W, Bonthron RT, Dewey CF Jr, Gimbron MA Jr (1993) Platelet-derived growth factor B chain promoter contains a cis-acting fluid shear-stress-responsive element. Proc Natl Acad Sci USA 90:7908–7910

26. Resnick N, Gimbrone MA Jr (1995) Hemodynamic forces are complex regulators of endothelial gene expression. FASEB J 9:874–882

Bone Resorption Is Inhibited by an Osteocyte-Derived Protein

AKIKO IKEDA[1], MARI AOKI[1], KATSUKI TSURITANI[1], KAYO KAMIOKA[2], KENJI HIURA[3], TOSHIO MIYOSHI[1], HIROSHI HARA[1], and MASAYOSHI KUMEGAWA[2]

Summary. In the process of bone resorption, osteoclasts encounter a large number of osteocytes excavated from the bone tissue. For instance, osteocytes released from the collagen matrix have been shown to be engulfed into osteoclasts by phagocytosis. After the osteoclast–osteocyte encounter or incorporation of osteocytes into osteoclasts, it is possible that osteocytes transmit some signals to osteoclasts.

To investigate roles of osteocytes in bone resorption, we examined the homogenate and conditioned medium from purified chick calvarial osteocytes in a pit-formation assay. The osteocyte homogenate markedly inhibited pit formation by unfractionated bone cells, whereas the conditioned medium of the cells had no effect. A novel bone-resorption-inhibitory protein was purified from collagenase-digested chick calvarial fragments enriched in osteocytes. The inhibitory protein, of molecular mass 18.5 kDa, showed significant inhibition of pit formation by purified osteoclasts as well as by unfractionated bone cells. Microinjection of the protein into osteoclasts caused disruption of podosomes in the cells. Thus osteocytes may be involved in the regulation of bone resorption by osteoclasts.

Key words. Osteocyte, Osteoclast, Bone resorption, Pit formation

Introduction

More than 90% of bone cells are osteocytes [1]. The cells, which originate from osteoblasts, are enclosed within a calcified bone matrix, and contact each other or surface bone cells such as osteoclasts and osteoblasts through a large number of cytoplasmic processes via gap junctions [2–4]. This cell-to-cell communication is thought to play an important role in bone metabolism. It has been suggested that osteocytes, which are the most abundant cells in the bone cell networks, are involved in the regulation of bone remodeling.

[1] Medicinal Research Laboratories, Taisho Pharmaceutical Co., Ltd., 1-403 Yoshino-cho, Ohmiya, Saitama 330-8530, Japan
[2] Department of Oral Anatomy, Meikai University School of Dentistry, Sakado, Saitama, Japan
[3] Department of Orthodontics, School of Dentistry, The University of Tokushima, Tokushima, Tokushima, Japan

Osteocytes are thought to control the differentiation of osteoblasts to osteocytes by cell-to-cell contact through cytoplasmic processes [5–7]. The cells are also reported to express the mRNA of the bone-formation-stimulatory proteins, insulin-like growth factor-1 [8], and bone morphogenetic proteins BMP-6 and -7 [9]. Furthermore, osteocytes are thought to respond to mechanical stress and exert a biological stimulation on osteoblasts [3,8,10–12]. These findings suggest that osteocytes are involved in the modulation of osteoblast generation and bone formation. However, little is known about the role of osteocytes in osteoclastic bone resorption.

Contact of Osteocytes with Osteoclasts

In the resorption phase of bone remodeling, mature osteoclasts degrade bone constituents by secreting H^+ and cysteine proteases into the osteoclast-bone interspace, and finally osteoclasts stop their function and leave the bone surface [13]. Several possible mechanisms by which osteoclasts finish bone resorption have been proposed. For example, estrogen and glucocorticoids are reported to trigger apoptotic cell death of osteoclasts, resulting in inhibition of osteoclastic bone resorption [14,15]. However, the precise mechanism is still unclear.

In the process of bone resorption, osteoclasts are thought to excavate a large number of osteocytes from the bone collagen matrix. Some of excavated osteocytes and residual collagen fibril fragments containing osteocytes are incorporated into osteoclasts by phagocytosis [13,16–19]. In electron microscopic studies, osteocytes are shown to be engulfed and destroyed by osteoclasts during bone degradation [18,19]. Therefore, it is speculated that osteocytes may transmit some signals to osteoclasts after the osteoclast–osteocyte encounter or after their incorporation into osteoclasts.

Inhibition of Bone Resorption by Osteocytes

Previously, we investigated the possible roles of osteocytes in osteoclastic bone resorption [20]. As it was found that osteoclastic bone resorption was inhibited by co-cultivation of osteoclasts with osteocytes, we examined the homogenate and conditioned medium from purified chick calvarial osteocytes in a pit-formation assay using unfractionated bone cells from mice. A marked inhibitory activity toward osteoclastic bone resorption was found in the chick osteocyte homogenate, but not in the conditioned medium from chick osteocytes.

These results suggest that a bone-resorption-inhibitory protein is present in osteocytes, and that the inhibitory protein is not secreted to extracellular environment under normal culture conditions. Our data also suggest that the inhibitory activity emerges after osteoblasts have differentiated into osteocytes, because the homogenates of osteoblastic cell lines such as MC3T3-E1 and ROS17/2.8 had no effect on osteoclastic bone resorption.

An osteocyte-derived inhibitory protein was prepared from chick calvarial fragments from which non-osteocytic cells on the bone surface had been removed by collagenase digestion. The purified protein showed a single form, of 18.5 kDa,

TABLE 1. Effect of the 18.5 kDa protein on pit formation

Addition	Pit formation (% of control)
Unfractionated bone cells	
None	100.0 ± 17.0
18.5 kDa protein	47.4 ± 11.5*
Purified osteclasts	
None	100.0 ± 13.3
18.5 kDa protein	47.9 ± 25.6*

* Significance is indicated in comparison with the corresponding untreated control value (* $p < 0.05$).
Unfractionated bone cells (4×10^5/well) or purified osteoclasts (200/well) from rabbits were injected into dentine slices and incubated for 24 h in the absence or presence of the 18.5 kDa protein (1.65 µg/ml of medium).
Values are the means $\pm$ S.D., $n = 3$.
From [20], with permission.

on sodium dodecyl sulfate/polyacrylamide gel electrophoresis (SDS/PAGE) with silver staining. The purified 18.5 kDa protein significantly inhibited pit formation by unfractionated bone cells from mice and rabbits, as well as that by human giant tumor cells. IC_{50} values were 24–56 nM in cell populations.

To investigate whether this inhibitory protein acts directly on osteoclasts or through other effector cells, the protein was examined in a pit-formation assay using purified rabbit osteoclasts. The 18.5 kDa protein showed inhibitory effect on pit formation by purified osteoclasts (Table 1). The inhibitory activity toward purified osteoclasts corresponded with that toward unfractionated bone cells, suggesting that the 18.5 kDa protein acts directly on osteoclasts and not via other effector cells.

To examine whether the 18.5 kDa protein can act on osteoclasts within the cells, the protein was microinjected into rabbit osteoclasts and the podosomes in the cells were examined (Fig. 1). FITC-labeled α-actinin pre-microinjected into osteoclasts was incorporated into podosomes which lined the periphery of the cells. Although the podosomes were still observed after the injection of buffer (Fig. 1a), microinjection of the 18.5 kDa protein caused disruption of the podosomes within 30 min of the injection (Fig. 1b).

The N-terminal amino acid sequence of the 18.5 kDa protein was 68% identical to a partial sequence of chick and bovine Rho-GTP-dissociation inhibitor (Rho-GDI). Rho, belonging to the Ras-related small G-protein superfamily, is known to be involved in cytoskeletal control via the actomyosin system. It has been shown that inactivation of Rho in osteoclasts caused disappearance of the F-actin-containing podosomes, resulting in functional inactivation of the cells [21]. Rho-GDI is a GDP/GTP-exchange-inhibitory protein for the Rho family members. The microinjection of Rho-GDI into Swiss 3T3 cells was shown to make the cells become round by causing the disappearance of stress fibers [22]. Microinjection of the 18.5 kDa protein also led to disappearance of the podosomes from osteoclasts, suggesting that the protein may be taken up by the cells and modulate the function of Rho by a mechanism similar to that of Rho-GDI.

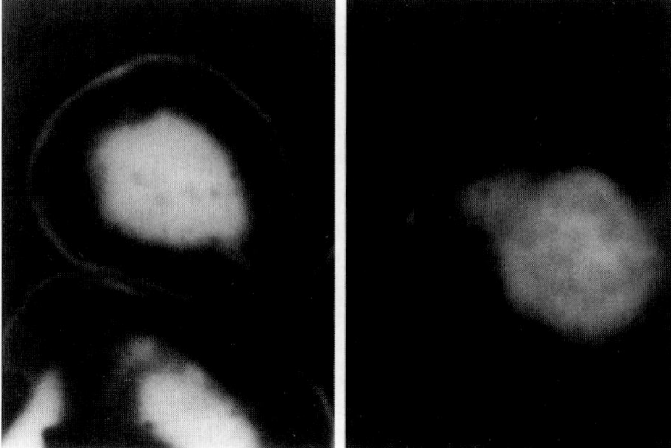

FIG. 1. Microinjection of the 18.5 kDa protein into rabbit osteoclasts. Rabbit osteoclasts were microinjected with buffer **a** or the 18.5 kDa protein (22 µg/ml) **b** 30 min after preinjection of FITC-labeled α-actinin, and incubated for 30 min. (From [20], with permission) ×400

Conclusion

We found that an osteoclastic bone-resorption-inhibitory protein is present in chick calvarial osteocytes. This inhibitory protein appears to affect osteoclasts directly, resulting in inhibition of their function. Although the mechanism by which the protein inhibits bone-resorbing activity of osteoclasts remains unclear, our findings suggest that osteocytes may participate in the regulation of osteoclastic bone resorption.

References

1. Parfitt AM (1977) The cellular basis of bone turnover and bone loss. Clin Orthop Relat Res 127:236–247
2. Palumbo C, Palazzini S, Zaff D, Marotti G (1990) Osteocyte differentiation in the tibia of newborn rabbit: an ultrastructural study of the formation of cytoplasmic processes. Acta Anat 137:350–358
3. Aarden EM, Buerger EH, Nijweide PJ (1994) Function of osteocytes in bone. J Cell Biochem 55:287–299
4. Jones SJ, Gray C, Sakamaki H, Arora M, Boyde A, Gourdie R, Green C (1993) The incidence and size of gap junctions between the bone cells in rat calvaria. Anat Embryol 187:343–352
5. Nefussi JR, Sautier JM, Nicolas V, Forest N (1991) How osteoblasts become osteocytes: a decreasing matrix forming process. J Biol Buccale 19:75–82
6. Palumbo C, Palazzani S, Marotti G (1990) Morphological study of intercellular junctions during osteocyte differentiation. Bone 11:401–406
7. Marotti G, Ferretti M, Muglia MA, Palumbo C, Palazzini S (1992) A quantitative evaluation of osteoblast-osteocyte relationships on growing endosteal surface of rabbit tibiae. Bone 13:363–368
8. Lean JM, Jagger CJ, Chambers TJ, Chow JWM (1994) Increased insulin-like growth factor-1 mRNA expression in osteocytes precedes the increase in bone formation in response to mechanical stimulation. J Bone Miner Res 9 (Suppl 1):S142
9. Price JS, Suswillo RFL, Houston B, Zaman G, Nijweide PJ, Lanyon LE (1995) The expression of bone morphogenetic proteins 6 and 7 in osteocytes: The effects of mechanical strain. J Bone Miner Res 10 (Suppl 1):S307

10. Mikuni-Takagaki Y, Suzuki Y, Kawase T, Saito S (1996) Distinct responses of different populations of bone cells to mechanical stress. Endocrinology 137(5):2028–2035
11. Lozupone E, Palumbo C, Favia A, Ferretti M, Palazzini S, Cantatore FP (1996) Intermittent compressive load stimulates osteogenesis and improves osteocyte viability in bones cultured "in vitro". Clin Rheumatol 15(6):563–572
12. Mullender MG, Huiskes R (1997) Osteocytes and bone lining cells: which are the best candidates for mechano-sensors in cancellous bone? Bone 20(6):527–532
13. Bonucci E (1981) New knowledge on the origin, function and fate of osteoclasts. Clin Orthop Relat Res 158:252–269
14. Kameda T, Mano H, Yuasa T, Mori Y, Miyazawa K, Shiokawa M, Nakamaru Y, Hiroi E, Hiura K, Kameda A, Yang NN, Hakeda Y, Kumegawa M (1997) Estrogen inhibits bone resorption by directly inducing apoptosis of the bone-resorbing osteoclasts. J Exp Med 186(4):489–495
15. Dempster DW, Moonga BS, Stein LS, Horbert WR, Antakly T (1997) Glucocorticoids inhibit bone resorption by isolated rat osteoclasts by enhancing apoptosis. J Endocrinol 154(3):397–406
16. Marks SC (1983) The origin of osteoclasts. J Pathol 12:226–256
17. Takahashi T, So S, Wang D, Takahashi K, Kurihara N, Kumegawa M (1986) Phagocytosis of different matrix components by different cell types at bone-forming sites in cultured mouse calvariae. Cell Tissue Res 245:9–17
18. Tonna EA (1972) An electron microscopic study of osteocyte release during osteoclasis in mice of different ages. Clin Orthop Relat Res 87:311–317
19. Elmardi AS, Katchburian MV, Katchburian E (1990) Electron microscopy of developing calvaria reveals images that suggest that osteoclasts engulf and destroy osteocytes during bone resorption. Calcif Tissue Int 46:239–245
20. Maejima-Ikeda A, Aoki M, Tsuritani K, Kamioka K, Hiura K, Miyoshi T, Hara H, Takano-Yamamoto T, Kumegawa M (1997) Chick osteocyte-derived protein inhibits osteoclastic bone resorption. Biochem J 322:245–250
21. Zhang D, Murakami H, Udagawa N, Nakamura I, Saito S, Shibasaki Y, Mori N, Narumiya S, Takahashi N, Suda T (1994) The small GTP-binding protein Rho is involved in osteoclastic bone resorption by regulating podosome formation. J Bone Miner Res 9 (Suppl 1):S131
22. Miura Y, Kikuchi A, Musha T, Kuroda S, Yaku H, Sasaki T, Takai Y (1993) Regulation of morphology by rho p21, its inhibitory GDP/GTP exchange protein (rho GDI) in Swiss 3T3 cells. J Biol Chem 268:510–515

Subject Index

LIFE UNIVERSITY
1269 BARCLAY CIRCLE
MARIETTA, GA 30060
(770) 426-2688

LIFE UNIVERSITY
1269 BARCLAY CIRCLE
MARIETTA, GA 30060
(770) 426-2688